Modern Monitoring
in Anesthesiology
and Perioperative Care

Modern Monitoring in Anesthesiology and Perioperative Care

Edited by

Andrew B. Leibowitz, MD
Icahn School of Medicine at Mount Sinai

Suzan Uysal, PhD
Icahn School of Medicine at Mount Sinai

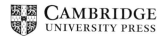

CAMBRIDGE
UNIVERSITY PRESS

University Printing House, Cambridge CB2 8BS, United Kingdom

One Liberty Plaza, 20th Floor, New York, NY 10006, USA

477 Williamstown Road, Port Melbourne, VIC 3207, Australia

314–321, 3rd Floor, Plot 3, Splendor Forum, Jasola District Centre,
New Delhi – 110025, India

79 Anson Road, #06–04/06, Singapore 079906

Cambridge University Press is part of the University of Cambridge.

It furthers the University's mission by disseminating knowledge in the pursuit of
education, learning, and research at the highest international levels of excellence.

www.cambridge.org
Information on this title: www.cambridge.org/9781108444910
DOI: 10.1017/9781108610650

© Cambridge University Press 2020

First published 2020

Printed in the United Kingdom by TJ International Ltd, Padstow Cornwall

A catalogue record for this publication is available from the British Library.

Library of Congress Cataloging-in-Publication Data
Names: Leibowitz, Andrew B., editor.
Title: Modern monitoring in anesthesiology and perioperative care / edited by Andrew B. Leibowitz.
Description: Cambridge ; New York, NY : Cambridge University Press, 2020. | Includes bibliographical
references and index.
Identifiers: LCCN 2019042016 | ISBN 9781108444910 (paperback)
Subjects: LCSH: Anesthesia. | Intraoperative monitoring. | Point-of-care testing. | Anesthesiology – Apparatus
and instruments. | Surgical technology.
Classification: LCC RD82 .M62 2020 | DDC 617.9/6–dc23
LC record available at https://lccn.loc.gov/2019042016

ISBN 978-1-108-44491-0 Paperback

....

Contents

The colour plate section can be found between pp. 110 and 111.

Contributors

Elvera Baron, MD, PhD
Assistant Professor
Department of Anesthesiology, Perioperative
and Pain Medicine
Department of Medical Education
The Icahn School of Medicine at Mount Sinai
New York, NY

Karsten Bartels, MD, PhD
Associate Professor
Department of Anesthesiology
University of Colorado
Aurora, CO

Adel Bassily-Marcus, MD
Associate Professor of Surgery
Icahn School of Medicine at Mount Sinai
New York, NY

David S. Beebe, MD
Professor
Department of Anesthesiology
University of Minnesota Medical School
Minneapolis, MN

Lester A. H. Critchley, MD
Retired Professor and Consultant Anesthetist
The Chinese University of Hong Kong

Neha S. Dangayach, MD, MSCR
Assistant Professor of Neurology and Neurosurgery
The Icahn School of Medicine at Mount Sinai
New York, NY

Liza Enriquez, MD
Montefiore Medical Center
Bronx, NY

Erica Fagleman, MD
Department of Anesthesiology, Perioperative and
Pain Medicine
Icahn School of Medicine at Mount Sinai
New York, NY

Myro Figura, MD
Clinical Instructor
Department of Anesthesiology and Perioperative
Medicine

David Geffen School of Medicine
University of California
Los Angeles, CA

Samuel Gilliland, MD
Assistant Professor
Department of Anesthesiology
University of Colorado
Aurora, CO

Ira S. Hofer, MD
Assistant Professor
Director, Division of Bioinformatics and Analytics
Department of Anesthesiology and Perioperative
Medicine
David Geffen School of Medicine
University of California, Los Angeles

Daniel W. Johnson, MD, FCCM
Division Chief & Fellowship Director,
Critical Care
Medical Director, Cardiovascular ICU
Associate Medical Director, Nebraska
Biocontainment Unit
Associate Professor
Department of Anesthesiology
University of Nebraska Medical Center
Omaha, NE

Ronald A. Kahn, MD
Professor of Anesthesiology, Perioperative & Pain
Medicine, and Surgery
Icahn School of Medicine at Mount Sinai
New York, NY
Professor of Anesthesiology, Pain,
and Critical Care
The Tel Aviv Medical Center
Tel Aviv

Daniel Katz, MD
Vice Chair of Education
Associate Professor of Anesthesiology, Perioperative
and Pain Medicine
Icahn School of Medicine at Mount Sinai
New York, NY

Subhash Krishnamoorthy, MD
Department of Anesthesiology

College of Physicians & Surgeons of Columbia
University
New York, NY

Zachary Kuschner, MD
Department of Emergency Medicine
Long Island Jewish Medical Center, Northwell Health
New Hyde Park, NY
Department of Internal Medicine, Division of Critical
Care
Mather Hospital, Northwell Health
Port Jefferson, NY

Andrew B. Leibowitz, MD
Chair of Anesthesiology, Perioperative & Pain
Medicine
Mount Sinai Health System
Professor of Anesthesiology, Perioperative & Pain
Medicine, and Surgery
Icahn School of Medicine at Mount Sinai
New York, NY

Torsten Loop, MD
Professor and Vice Chair
Department of Anesthesiology and Critical Care
University of Freiburg Medical Center
Freiburg, Germany

John M. Oropello, MD, FACP, FCCP, FCCM
Professor of Surgery and Medicine
Program Director, Critical Care Medicine
Icahn School of Medicine at Mount Sinai
Director, Transplant Intensive Care Unit
Mount Sinai Health System
New York, NY

Oliver Panzer, MD
Assistant Professor of Anesthesiology
College of Physicians & Surgeons of Columbia
University
New York, NY

Peter J. Papadakos, MD, FCCM, FAARC
Director of Critical Care Medicine
Tenured Professor of Anesthesiology and
Perioperative Medicine, Surgery, Neurology and
Neurosurgery
University of Rochester
Rochester, NY

Jacob Raphael, MD
Carl Lynch III Professor of Anesthesiology

Department of Anesthesiology and Perioperative
Medicine
University of Virginia Health System
Charlottesville, VA

Lindsay Regali, MD
Anesthesiology Consultants of Virginia, Inc.
Roanoke, VA

Kyle James Riley, MD
Department of Anesthesia, Critical Care and Pain
Medicine
Massachusetts General Hospital
Boston, MA

Benjamin Salter, DO
Assistant Professor of Anesthesiology
Department of Anesthesiology, Perioperative and
Pain Medicine
The Icahn School of Medicine at Mount Sinai
New York, NY

Linda Shore-Lesserson, MD, FAHA, FASE
Past-President, Society of Cardiovascular
Anesthesiologists
Professor of Anesthesiology
Zucker School of Medicine at Hofstra Northwell
Vice Chair for Academic Affairs
Director, Cardiovascular Anesthesiology
Long Island, NY

Julia Sobol, MD, MPH
Assistant Professor of Anesthesiology
College of Physicians & Surgeons of Columbia
University
New York, NY

Robert H. Thiele, MD
Associate Professor
Department of Anesthesiology
University of Virginia
Charlottesville, VA

Shaun L. Thompson, MD
Assistant Professor
Associate Program Director of the Critical Care
Medicine Fellowship
Medical Director of ECLS Services at UNMC
Department of Anesthesiology, Division of Critical
Care
University of Nebraska Medical Center
Omaha, NE

David B. Wax, MD
Professor of Anesthesiology, Perioperative & Pain Medicine
Icahn School of Medicine at Mount Sinai
New York, NY

Albert Yu MD
Assistant Professor of Anesthesiology and Perioperative Medicine

University of Rochester
Rochester, NY

Samson Zarbiv, MD, MPH
Department of Critical Care Medicine
Cooper University Health Care
Cape Regional Health System
Cape May Court House, NJ

Preface

Our current practice environment is daunting. Providing safe quality care using technology and receiving feedback that didn't even exist 15 years ago should be easy, but it isn't. The plethora of information and the number and variety of monitors available for use has increased in an almost exponential fashion. On October 27, 2019, a PubMed search of "noninvasive monitoring of cardiac output" yielded 809 references, a Google search for "anesthesiology guidelines" 25,700 references, and there are at least 9 different technologies for monitoring of cardiac output incorporated into commercially available products.

This book aims to be different than other monitoring books and focuses on the "practical." Chapters on statistics and electronic distraction are unique and provide a framework for evaluation of all monitors, and reveal the risk that too much information poses to the care that we provide. Other chapters focus on the "why" monitoring a certain variable may be advantageous, the basics of "how" the monitor works, and "what" is the evidence of the impact on patient outcome.

A basic theme of the chapters is that just because we can do something does not mean we should, and sometimes less may be more, but a working knowledge of the whys, hows, and whats of modern monitoring in anesthesiology and perioperative care will allow every provider to optimize their patient's safety and the quality of care they provide.

Andrew B. Leibowitz, MD

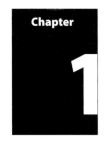

Statistics Used to Assess Monitors and Monitoring Applications

Lester A. H. Critchley

Introduction

An evidence-based approach now prevails when recommending medical treatments. This applies as much to the latest therapies as to appropriate methods to monitor patients and their response to treatment. For an evidence-based approach to be successful, however, it must be based on good-quality clinical data from well-conducted research. The quality of clinical studies and their data is now graded according to the level of evidence they provide,[1] and guidelines exist on how to properly conduct clinical research. Cochrane reviews have set standards for best evidence. Working groups such as the National Institute for Clinical Excellence (NICE) and Resuscitation Council (UK) demonstrate how such an approach can be transformed into up-to-date guidelines and courses. When assessing the value of emerging clinical monitoring technologies for perioperative, emergency room, and critical care use, researchers should be aware that clinical validation studies must be of a sufficient standard to be of use in evidence-based reviews. This perspective drives the approach of this chapter, with a focus on cardiac output (CO) monitoring, since most of the literature on these statistical methods has arisen from analysis of this variable.

Cardiac Output Measurement

Cardiac output is the sum of stroke volumes expelled from the heart over one minute; it can be measured from either the pulmonary or the systemic circulations. As the arterial system leaving the heart branches, it is not possible to measure total CO at a distal point such as the arm or descending aorta, and corrections are needed (e.g., arterial pulse contour analysis and esophageal Doppler).[2,3] Measurement of CO at its source, the heart, is also difficult to achieve in the clinical setting because of restricted access, unless one is performing open-heart surgery.

Instead, at-a-distance (e.g., transthoracic Doppler) or surrogate (e.g., bioimpedance) methods are utilized, which result in lack of precision.[4,5] Compared to measuring other more accessible hemodynamic variables such as blood pressure or heart rate, lack of accuracy and precision has hampered the development of routine CO monitoring in the clinical setting.[5]

Cardiac output can be measured accurately using techniques such as the Fick method and radionuclide imaging studies. These methods, however, have several limitations. They are only applicable in settings such as the physiology laboratory or radiology department; they are inapplicable at the point of care and therefore cannot be used in operating room, emergency medicine, or critical care settings. Furthermore, Fick and radionuclide studies only provide single readings, and there is need for technologies that measure CO on a frequent or continuous basis. The clinical significance of being able to assess changes or trends in CO is only now being recognized, and this is highlighted by the designs of recently marketed CO devices and the statistical approaches to their validation.

All validation studies require a reliable reference method against which comparisons are made. For CO monitoring, the accepted reference method has been and remains single bolus thermodilution using a pulmonary artery Swan–Ganz catheter. The pulmonary artery catheter, however, is now seldom used in clinical practice, and its use is associated with significant risk to patients.[6,7] Clinical validation studies incorporating pulmonary artery catheter measurements are mostly restricted to cardiac surgery and liver transplant. Some recent research studies have used the less invasive transpulmonary thermodilution method, which is employed in the PiCCO (Pulsion, Munich, Germany) and VolumeView (Edwards Lifesciences, Irvine, CA, USA) systems. Errors arise in thermodilution measurement because of injectate and dead space issues,[8] and the degree of inaccuracy varies between clinical settings and different manufactured devices.[9] The precision of the thermodilution method is generally accepted to be ± 20%,[10,11] and this margin of error has played a significant role in the ongoing development of validation statistics.

Cardiac output is not a static variable; its value constantly changes. Achieving a steady state in which simultaneous comparative readings can be taken often proves difficult, and this hampers the collection of good-quality validation data.

Protocol Design and Data Collection

The need for ethical approval and patient consent is an obvious prerequisite for publication. Poorly planned data collection and inadequate sample size will limit the usefulness of collected data and thus the ability to publish the study findings. Common mistakes are (i) failure to blind investigators to comparative readings, (ii) failure to achieve simultaneous readings during steady-state hemodynamics, (iii) failure to have sufficient range of readings, (iv) failure to collect sufficient data resulting in inconclusive results, (v) inconsistent number and timing of repeated measurements from individuals (i.e., irregular data collection), and (vi) failure to collect serial data pairs that show adequate changes and hence fail to facilitate trend analysis. A well-designed study has clearly defined times of data collection, which are of sufficient number to allow comprehensive analysis.[12]

Sample size is difficult to calculate in this type of research, even if a pilot study is performed, because of the range of different variables and outcomes involved. A more pragmatic approach may be based on reviewing the sample sizes used in previous studies that were successful in detecting effects. Comparative studies with cohorts of over 30 patients and 6 or more serial data pairs are recommended.[12]

Background to Validation

Thirty years ago scatter plots and regression and correlation analyses were the principal analytical methods used to show how reliably a new measurement method compared to a reference standard.[13] Regression and correlation, however, only evaluate the degree of association between two measurement methods; they do not quantify accuracy. Quoting correlation coefficients and p values confirms little.

The whole approach to validation statistics changed in the 1980s when J. M. Bland and D. G. Altman introduced a new method of comparing measurements based on bias, the difference between pairs of comparative readings.[14] Bias was plotted against the average of each pair, and the standard deviation of the bias provided a statistic called *limits of agreement* (i.e., 95% confidence intervals for the bias). Bland and Altman, however, never provided guidance as to how the limits of agreement should be used to confirm clinical utility, leaving this to the discretion of the user. This was particularly unsatisfactory when Bland–Altman analysis was applied to CO studies where the reference method, usually thermodilution, was imprecise. Limits of agreement of less than 1 liter/min were considered to be acceptable,[15,16] but no provision for (i) variations in baseline CO or (ii) imprecision of the reference method was made.

To enable outcomes from Bland–Altman style CO studies to be compared in 1999, Critchley proposed the use of percentage error (PE), a statistic calculated from the limits of agreement (i.e., 95% confidence interval of the bias) divided by the baseline CO for the study.[10] A benchmark for acceptance of a new technique of less than 28.4% was set, which was rounded up to less than 30%. This benchmark was based on a reference method's precision of 20% and acceptance of the test method also being set at 20%. Although PE has been criticized over the years for being too strict,[11,17,18] its simplicity and robustness as an analytical tool have withstood the test of time.

In more recent decades, following advances in clinical medicine and monitoring technology, it has become increasingly important to have bedside monitors that accurately follow the vital signs of hospitalized patients. Unfortunately, Bland–Altman analysis does not assess the ability of devices to detect changes; it is limited to assessing accuracy of readings and agreement between methods.[19,20] Thus, new statistical approaches were developed, referred to as *trend analysis.*[21] Many researchers new to clinical monitoring, however, fail to recognize the need to show trending and restrict data collection to that suitable for Bland–Altman analysis.

How to effectively address the issue of trending capability has not been fully resolved in the literature. In a recent review of CO studies, Critchley and colleagues reported that only 20% of the studies performed some form of trend analysis; the analytical methods employed were (i) Bland–Altman analysis of tables and histograms, (ii) regression analysis of scatter plots, and (iii) analysis of direction of change.[21]

When analyzing CO data from hospital patients, commonly used trend analysis methods are (i) concordance on a four-quadrant plot and (ii) polar plot analysis.[22,23] Both these analyses rely on comparing serial data from reference and test methods, calculating the serial change in consecutive readings (ΔCO), and excluding data where the change is small (i.e., < 10–15% change). The polar method involves transforming the data from a simple (x, y) Cartesian format to a radial format (radius, angle). Polar plots provide greater information about the agreement between two methods that is lost when just direction of change is used. Criteria for acceptable trending have been proposed for CO monitoring.[21,23] A more detailed description of these methods follows.

Bland–Altman Analysis

Practically all CO validation studies published today use Bland–Altman analysis and provide a Bland–Altman plot (Figure 1.1). The plot shows bias collected from the whole or subgroups of the study.

Each plot should display horizontal lines indicating mean bias and the 95% confidence intervals or limits of agreement. Inspection of the plot allows one to assess (i) the distribution or spread of data, (ii) the degree of agreement between methods (i.e., size of the limits of agreement), and (iii) any systematic changes in bias as CO increases (i.e., offsets in calibration). One common problem with presenting Bland–Altman plots is using inappropriate scales, especially when more than one plot is shown. Rather than choosing scales that fill the page with data points, the axis of each plot should have similar scales and ranges. Otherwise visual comparisons between plots are difficult to perform. Very often the Bland–Altman plot is accompanied by an (x, y) scatter plot that shows the raw data (Figure 1.1), but regression lines and correlation coefficients are often omitted.

Bland–Altman analysis requires each data pair to be independent of all other pairs and ideally from separate subjects.[14] If data pairs are related (i.e., they come from the same subject), the size of 95% confidence intervals and limits of agreement for the analysis will be reduced. Use of repeated measures (i.e., data pairs from the same subject) is common in CO studies; thus, the data analysis should correct for

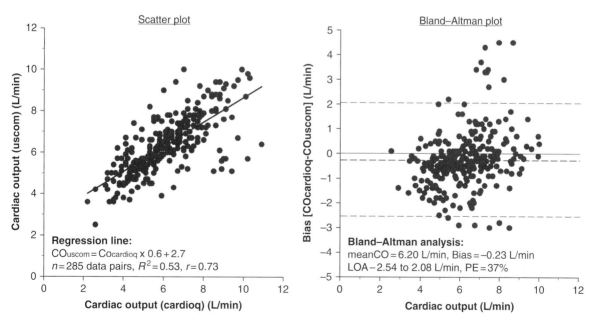

Figure 1.1 Scatter plot with regression line and accompanying Bland–Altman plot. Statistical analysis data are added to each plot. The Bland–Altman plot also displays the mean bias and limits of agreement of the analysis (dashed horizontal lines). Data are from a study that compared two Doppler CO measurement methods, transthoracic (USCOM) and esophageal (CardioQ).

Source: Huang L, Critchley LA. An assessment of two Doppler-based monitors to track cardiac output changes in anaesthetized patients undergoing major surgery. *Anaesth Intens Care* 2014;42:631–9. LOA: limits of agreement, PE: percentage error.

repeated measures by either (i) Bland and Altman or (ii) Myles and Cui methods, which differ slightly in complexity.[24,25] Statistical software programs that perform Bland–Altman analysis should also adjust for repeated measures; journal editors and reviewers expect that authors will employ such corrections and describe them in their manuscripts.

Percentage error is a key outcome statistic arising from CO studies that perform a Bland–Altman analysis.[10] It is used to compare findings of CO studies with findings of other published studies. It also allows criteria to be set for acceptance of a new CO monitor prior to starting a study. Most authors will use the less than 30% benchmark, from Critchley's 1999 paper that based the criteria on a 20% precision for thermodilution CO measurement and the need for less than 20% measurement error (i.e., 95% confidence intervals or precision).[11] A 20% error represented up to a 1 liter/min variation in CO if the mean CO was 5 liter/min.

Cecconi and colleagues have questioned the logic of assuming a 20% error in the reference method.[26] They recommended measuring its precision and using the error to set new acceptance criteria a priori. Their rational was that (i) the error in thermodilution or other reference method is very variable and 20% is just an approximation, and (ii) any significant variation from 20% would result in lesser or greater errors in the test method to be accepted, if the acceptance criteria are set at the standard 30%. Their approach to measuring the reference method's precision was to perform serial steady-state measurements from which the coefficient of variation was calculated and precision derived.[26]

Trend Analysis

Trending capability, the ability to follow changes in CO, can be assessed either by (i) multiple paired comparisons in a small number of subjects (i.e., $n = 6$–10 laboratory animals) or (ii) as part of a larger scale clinical trial with up to 8–10 comparative measurements in 20 or more patients. Statistical approaches are different for the two settings. Small cohort studies are dealt with later in the section Time Plots and Regression Analysis.

Concordance Analysis

For larger cohort clinical trials the current approach is concordance analysis using direction of change.[21,22] This analysis is based on serial data, and ΔCO is the study variable calculated from the difference between consecutive readings. Direction of change in CO can either be increased (i.e., positive direction change) or decreased (i.e., negative direction change); the magnitude of change is not included in the analysis. In the trial a test method is compared to a reference method, which provides pairs of directions of change of readings that can either agree (i.e., concord) or disagree. Concordance is measured as the proportion of readings that agree.

To make concordance analysis easier to visualize, a four-quadrant plot is drawn of ΔCO reference against ΔCO test (Figure 1.2). Data where directions of change agree fall into the right upper and left lower quadrants. The ratio of the number of data pairs where directions of change agree over the total number of data pairs for the study provides the concordance presented as a percentage.

Data pairs where the serial change in CO is small, however, can often have directions of change that disagree due to random errors in measurement; this is referred to as *statistical noise*. To eliminate statistical noise from the concordance analysis an exclusion zone is used that removes data where the change in CO is less than 10–15% of the mean CO for the study. The setting of limits for the exclusion zones is based on a receiver operator characteristic (ROC) curve analysis.[22]

Current advice for acceptable trending ability in CO studies is greater than 92%.[21] Ideally, confidence limits should be calculated for the concordance, which is based on sample size. The ΔCO data is treated as a binomial (i.e., direction of change either agrees or disagrees), and the standard deviation of the concordance ratio (p) is $\sqrt{[np(1-p)]}$, where n is the number of data points. A good example of how this statistic is generated and used is found in Axiak-Flammer and colleagues.[27]

Polar Plots

The introduction of polar plots (Figure 1.2) was to address the problems that (i) the four-quadrant plot method did not include magnitude of change and (ii) all data pairs were treated equally despite size.[14,21,23] By converting the data to (i) a radial distance that represented the size of the combined changes in CO from the two paired readings (i.e., average absolute change in ΔCO) and (ii) an angle that represented the degree of agreement (i.e., the greater the degree of disagreement the larger the angle), more information about the comparison between the two measurement

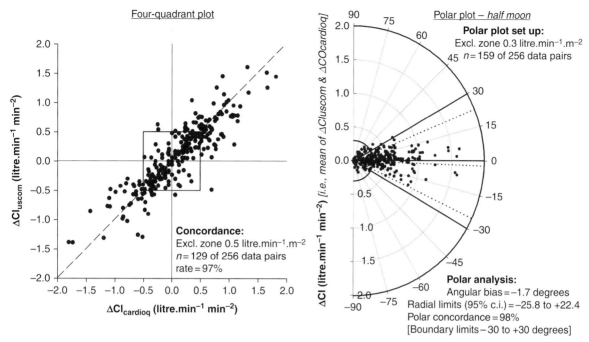

Figure 1.2 Four-quadrant and polar plots showing changes (ΔCO). Four-quadrant plot has zero axes crossing at its center, creating four zones. A central exclusion zone (square) is shown: Data lying within this zone are excluded because they contain a high level of random variation compared to changes in CO (i.e., statistical noise). The line of identity $y = x$ (dashed line) also is shown. Ideally, all data points should lie along this line. Data that lie within the upper right and lower left quadrants agree (i.e., direction of change agrees). Results of concordance analysis are printed in the plot. Polar plot is of a semicircle, or half-moon, design in which both positive and negative changes in CO are shown together. A central exclusion zone also is shown (half circle). Zero- and 30-degree axes are highlighted (solid lines). Mean polar angle and 95% radial limits of agreement for the polar analysis also are shown (dotted lines). Polar concordance rate is based on the proportion of data points that lie within 30 degrees of the polar axis (zero degrees). Results of the polar analysis are shown.

Source: Huang L, Critchley LA. An assessment of two Doppler-based monitors to track cardiac output changes in anaesthetized patients undergoing major surgery. *Anaesth Intens Care* 2014;42:631–9.

methods was retained. The concept of excluding data pairs where changes in CO were small and statistical noise may corrupt the analysis was also applied. However, the exclusion zone was reduced from 15% to 10% of the mean CO for the study because the combined change in ΔCO on the polar diagram (i.e., radial length) was derived from the average of the two ΔCO values, whereas in the four-quadrant plot the combined change was derived from the hypotenuse of a triangle produced by test and reference values and was √2 (or 1.42) times larger in size. The mean angle for all the data pairs provided a measure of misalignment in calibration or offset between methods. Empirically, a limit of ± 5% was set as the criterion for an acceptable offset. The radial limits of agreement were set at ± 30% and were based on a 2:1 ratio in size between ΔCO readings. These limits, however, were not based on sound statistical theory. To make the polar plot more visually friendly, one can rotate

negative change data through 180 degrees to become a positive change, thus producing a half-moon rather than full-moon plot. Generating polar data from Cartesian (x, y) ΔCO data and drawing polar plots can be technically challenging. Some of the newer statistical programs now provide polar plot drawing and analysis software. Guidance can also be found in the original paper describing polar plots.[23] The polar method is probably best reserved for research groups performing high-quality validation studies. Mastering the technique of polar plots provides a greater appreciation of the data and trending ability.

Time Plots and Regression Analysis

Understanding the structure of one's data is the key to knowing which statistical methods are most appropriate. Data arising from validation studies can be considered as a two-dimensional matrix of paired readings representing subjects in one plane and serial measurements from individual subjects in the other plane. Bland–Altman analysis is most appropriate when there are many subjects and few, if any, serial measurements, because the primary attribute being tested is the accuracy of a measurement technique as it is applied to a study sample. In studies where trending capability is being analyzed, multiple serial measurement pairs ($n = 10$ or more) are needed. For this type of study design, data can be analyzed on an individual subject basis (i.e., within subject) using regression analysis. Huang and colleagues performed a number of clinical studies comparing Doppler CO with bioimpedance CO methods during anesthesia for major surgery.[3,28] Their surgical model provided a range of ever-changing CO values. They plotted within subject serial changes in CO over time, for each monitoring modality and for each patient ($n = 7$ to 27 data points). They were able to visually identify divergences in the trend lines for CO between the different monitoring modalities and relate them to interventions during the surgery (Figure 1.3). They also used regression analysis as a method of quantifying the degree trending between the monitoring modalities for each subject. For CO studies using Doppler methods as the reference, they were able to set criteria

when trending capability of the test bioimpedance method was considered acceptable. However, when regression analysis was applied to group data, the systematic differences in calibration between subjects introduced a second source of variation, and trending capability could no longer be easily evaluated using the correlation coefficients.

Reporting Validation Study Data

Since 1999 there have been concerns in the literature regarding how validation study data have been reported, especially for studies using Bland–Altman analysis.[29–32] As recently as 2016, Abu-Arafeh and colleagues published a review of 111 papers from a two-year period, which concluded that Bland–Altman study data were poorly reported and of limited usefulness to evidence-based reviews.[33] Additionally, they proposed a list of 13 key issues to be included in reports and called for journals to provide more guidance on how Bland–Altman studies should be conducted and reported. In 2010, Critchley and colleagues reported similar findings in relation to reporting trend analysis data.[21] Based on the present author's experience as a researcher and journal

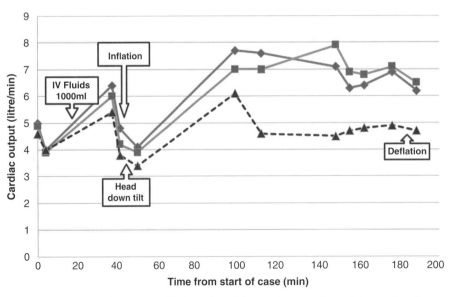

Figure 1.3 Time plot of comparative CO data collected during a laparoscopic surgical procedure. The two uppermost trend lines represent reference Doppler readings (diamond-USCOM and square-CardioQ). The lower dashed line represents a new bioimpedance device (triangles). Note how after 100 minutes there was a definite downward divergence of bioimpedance readings relative to the Doppler readings. Major interventions such as inflation and deflation of the pneumoperitoneum are shown. The precise cause of the downward divergence was unclear yet present in a number of other cases. Detection of this type of change in monitor readings is very important to developers yet does not show up in more classical group statistics using Bland–Altman and concordance analyses.

reviewer in the field of validation studies, the following recommendations are provided:

1. Provide a clear and thorough description of the study design, including (i) recruitment, (ii) number of subjects, (iii) how readings were taken, including blinding of investigators and steady-state synchronous readings, and (iv) timing of data collection points. Remember to mention ethical approval and consent.

2. Provide a well-described plan for analyzing the data in the methods section. Ideally, one should measure the precision of the reference method and use it when setting a priori criteria for acceptance of the test method.[26] A typical sequence for a simple test versus reference comparison study would be (i) results of any pilot studies such as reference method precision and power calculation (i.e., study size), (ii) inspection of study data using scatter plots, (iii) Bland–Altman analysis with details, and (iv) trend analysis using concordance and possibly polar plots. Acceptance criteria with references should be added to the relevant subsections.

3. The results section should start with the general demographics of the study population, including number of subjects and how many subjects were excluded and why. The power calculations justifying the size of the study, if performed, could be included at this point (see previous comments on study size).

4. Draw a scatter plot (optional) that shows the distribution of raw data (Figure 1.1). Multiple plots may be needed if subgroups of subjects have been included in the study design. Addition of a regression line and correlation coefficients is optional, as Bland–Altman recommended their exclusion.[14] Plots should contain, within the diagram or legend, essential information such as number of data points and relevant statistical outcomes, for example regression line equation and correlation coefficient (i.e., r or R^2).

5. Draw the Bland–Altman plot(s) (Figure 1.1). Make sure axes are appropriately scaled with sensible data ranges. If more than one plot is presented, the scales and ranges should be similar to facilitate visual comparison. Add horizontal lines for the mean bias and limits of agreement (i.e., 95% confidence intervals of the bias). Make sure the limits have been corrected for repeated measures, citing which methodology was

used.[24,25] Some authorities are now asking for confidence intervals of the limits of agreement to also be included.[34] It is best to stick to simple numerical measurement units (i.e., CO in liter/min) rather than percentage changes; however, indexing variables to body surface area (BSA) (i.e., cardiac index = CO/BSA) is acceptable. Diagrams and legends should display essential numerical information about the plot(s).

6. Sufficient data to calculate the PE should be provided, including (i) the standard deviation of the bias or 95% confidence interval and (ii) mean CO for all the study data. Ideally, the PE should also be presented. The PE facilitates comparison of data with previous studies; one may wish to make such comparisons in the discussion section. In the methods section the criterion threshold should be set a priori that defines a PE that supports acceptance of the new technique. This requires some consideration regarding the precision of the reference method. Cecconi and colleagues recommend estimating the precision from coefficient of variation measurements for the reference method.[26] The current benchmark for PE is less than 30%, but this criterion should be set in the context of the precision of the reference method as a 20% error is presumed (see Axiak-Flammer et al. for guidance if an alternative reference method has been used[27]).

7. Depending on the study design and data structure, if a trend analysis is performed, then a four-quadrant plot should be drawn (Figure 1.2). Concordance analysis should be performed for studies with grouped data of sufficient numbers (e.g., $n > 20$ subjects) and serial data pairs (e.g., $n > 3$). An exclusion zone should be employed (i.e., 15% of mean CO for the study) to remove data where changes are small and data points lie close to zero. For CO studies the zone is set at 15% of the mean CO value. Remember that concordance is based on the variable ΔCO, *not* CO. Criteria for accepting a CO monitor as having good trending ability have been set at greater than 92%, where the reference method was single bolus thermodilution.[21] For studies with a small number of data pairs, the confidence intervals for the concordance also need to be calculated.[27]

8. A polar plot analysis may also be employed (Figure 1.2), following advice on generating the data from paired readings, creating the plots, and

interpreting the results.[11,21,23] Exclude central zone data that are less than 10% of the mean CO for the study. Key outcome data are the mean angle and 95% radial limits of agreement. They should be added to the polar plot as radial lines. The 30-degree radial axes should also be highlighted. Negative direction data points can be rotated through half a turn (i.e., 180 degrees), but not reflected, to provide a half-moon plot. Ideally, the main data outcomes, including number of data points, exclusion zone size, mean angle, and radial limits of agreement, should be added to the diagram or legend. Polar plots demonstrate (i) offsets in calibration between methods (i.e., mean angle of greater than 5 degrees) and (ii) the level of agreement between the methods (i.e., tightness of alignment of radial data points to the zero-degree axis or mean angle line). The 30-degree lines act as guides to good trending when 95% of data points fall within their boundaries.

9. For less commonly used methods of assessing trending, one should refer to the papers that describe them.

Noncardiac Output Studies

The application of validation statistics is not limited to just CO monitoring data. They can also be applied to blood pressure, oxygen saturation, and hemoglobin level monitoring. The main difference is the criteria used to determine acceptance thresholds and exclusion zones, because of their reliance on the precision of the reference method.

References

1. Oxford Centre for Evidence-based Medicine – Levels of Evidence (March 2009). www.cebm.net/oxford-centre-evidence-based-medicine-levels-evidence-march-2009/ (Accessed November 2017).

2. Sun JX, Reisner AT, Saeed M, Heldt T, Mark RG. The cardiac output from blood pressure algorithms trial. *Crit Care Med* 2009;**37**:72–80.

3. Huang L, Critchley LA. An assessment of two Doppler-based monitors to track cardiac output changes in anaesthetised patients undergoing major surgery. *Anaesth Intens Care* 2014;**42**:631–9.

4. Chong SW, Peyton PJ. A meta-analysis of the accuracy and precision of the ultrasonic cardiac output monitor (USCOM). *Anaesthesia* 2012;**67**:1266–71.

5. Wang DJ, Gottlieb SS. Impedance cardiography: more questions than answers. *Curr Cardiol Rep* 2006;**8**:180–6.

6. Koo KK, Sun JC, Zhou Q, et al. Pulmonary artery catheters: evolving rates and reasons for use. *Crit Care Med* 2011;**39**:1613–8.

7. Harvey S, Harrison DA, Singer M, et al. Assessment of the clinical effectiveness of pulmonary artery catheters in management of patients in intensive care (PAC-Man): a randomized controlled trial. *Lancet* 2005;**366**:472–7.

8. Reuter DA, Huang C, Edrich T, Shernan SK, Eltzschig HK. Cardiac output monitoring using indicator dilution techniques: basics, limits, and perspectives. *Anesth Analg* 2010;**110**:799–811.

9. Yang XX, Critchley LA, Rowlands DK, Fang Z, Huang L. Systematic error of cardiac output measured by bolus thermodilution with a pulmonary artery catheter compared with that measured by an aortic flow probe in a pig model. *J Cardiothorac Vasc Anesth* 2013;**27**:1133–9.

10. Critchley LA, Critchley JA. A meta-analysis of studies using bias and precision statistics to compare cardiac output measurement techniques. *J Clin Monit Comput* 1999;**15**:85–91.

11. Critchley LA. Bias and precision statistics: should we still adhere to the 30% benchmark for cardiac output monitor validation studies? *Anesthesiology* 2011;**114**:1245.

12. Biancofiore G, Critchley LA, Lee A, et al. Evaluation of an uncalibrated arterial pulse contour cardiac output monitoring system in cirrhotic patients undergoing liver surgery. *Brit J Anaesth* 2009;**102**:47–54.

13. Fuller HD. The validity of cardiac output measurement by thoracic impedance: a meta-analysis. *Clin Invest Med* 1992;**15**:103–12.

14. Bland JM, Altman DG. Statistical methods for assessing agreement between two methods of clinical measurement. *Lancet* 1986;**1**:307–10.

15. LaMantia KR, O'Connor T, Barash PG. Comparing methods of measurement: an alternative approach. *Anesthesiology* 1990;**72**:781–3.

16. Wong DH, Tremper KK, Stemmer EA, et al. Noninvasive cardiac output: simultaneous comparison of two different methods with thermodilution. *Anesthesiology* 1990;**72**:784–92.

17. Michard F. Thinking outside the (cardiac output) box. *Crit Care Med* 2012;**40**:1361–2.

18. Peyton PJ, Chong SW. Minimally invasive measurement of cardiac output during surgery and critical care: a metaanalysis of accuracy and precision. *Anesthesiology* 2010;**113**:1220–35.

19. Critchley LA. Validation of the MostCare pulse contour cardiac output monitor: beyond the Bland and Altman plot. *Anesth Analg* 2011;**113**:1292–4.

20. Critchley LA. Meta-analyses of Bland-Altman-style cardiac output validation studies: good, but do they provide answers to all our questions? *Brit J Anaesth* 2017;**118**:296–7.

21. Critchley LA, Lee A, Ho AM. A critical review of the ability of continuous cardiac output monitors to measure trends in cardiac output. *Anesth Analg* 2010;**111**:1180–92.

22. Perrino AC, O'Connor T, Luther M. Transtracheal Doppler cardiac output monitoring: comparison to thermodilution during noncardiac surgery. *Anesth Analg* 1994;**78**:1060–6.

23. Critchley LA, Yang XX, Lee A. Assessment of trending ability of cardiac output monitors by polar plot methodology. *J Cardiothorac Vasc Anesth* 2011;**25**:536–46.

24. Bland JM, Altman DG. Agreement between methods of measurement with multiple observations per individual. *J Biopharm Stat* 2007;**17**:571–82.

25. Myles PS, Cui J. Using the Bland-Altman method to measure agreement with repeated measures. *Br J Anaesth* 2007;**99**:309–11.

26. Cecconi M, Rhodes A, Poloniecki J, Della Rocca G, Grounds RM. Bench-to-bedside review: the importance of the precision of the reference technique in method comparison studies – with specific reference to the measurement of cardiac output. *Crit Care* 2009;**13**:201.

27. Axiak-Flammer SM, Critchley LA, Weber A, et al. Reliability of lithium dilution cardiac output in anaesthetized sheep. *Brit J Anaesth* 2013;**111**:833–9.

28. Huang L, Critchley LA, Zhang J. Major upper abdominal surgery alters the calibration of BioReactance cardiac output readings, the NICOM, when comparisons are made against suprasternal and esophageal Doppler intraoperatively. *Anesth Analg* 2015;**121**:936–45.

29. Mantha S, Roizen MF, Fleisher LA, Thisted R, Foss J. Comparing methods of clinical measurement: reporting standards for Bland and Altman analysis. *Anesth Analg* 2000;**90**:593–602.

30. Dewitte K, Fierens C, Stöckl D, Thienpont LM. Application of the Bland-Altman plot for interpretation of method comparison studies: a critical investigation of its practice. *Clin Chem* 2002;**48**:799–801.

31. Berthelsen PG, Nilsson LB. Researcher bias and generalization of results in bias and limits of agreement analyses: a commentary based on the review of 50 Acta Anaesthesiologica Scandinavica papers using the Altman Bland approach. *Acta Anaesthesiol Scand* 2006;**50**:1111–3.

32. Bein B, Renner J, Scholz J, Tonner PH. Comparing different methods of cardiac output determination: a call for consensus. *Eur J Anaesthesiol* 2006;**23**:710.

33. Abu-Arafeh A, Jordan H, Drummond G. Reporting of method comparison studies: a review of advice, an assessment of current practice, and specific suggestions for future reports. *Br J Anaesth* 2016;**117**:569–75.

34. Drummond GB. Limits of agreement with confidence intervals are necessary to assess comparability of measurement devices. *Anesth Analg* 2017;**125**:1075.

Multimodal Neurological Monitoring

Samson Zarbiv, Erica Fagleman, and Neha S. Dangayach

Introduction

Patients with acute neurological injuries are susceptible to injury progression and clinical deterioration. The goal of neurological monitoring in these patients is to rapidly treat the primary neurological injury, prevent progression to secondary neurological injury, and ultimately improve outcome.

The current monitoring paradigm for patients with acute neurological injuries includes frequent neurological examination, neuroimaging, and multimodal monitoring, depending upon the severity of the primary neurological injury and likelihood of deterioration. Clinical examination, including assessment of mental status and level of consciousness, may be confounded by comorbidities (e.g., facial trauma confounding eye-opening response, tracheostomy precluding verbal response) and use of sedatives or analgesics. Furthermore, clinical examination and neuroimaging assessment are limited because they are performed intermittently and may miss crucial changes that occur between examinations, and because they are to some extent subjective. By contrast, continuous multimodal monitoring provides objective real-time measurement and trending of critical parameters such as intracranial pressure (ICP), cerebral blood flow (CBF), cerebral oxygenation, cerebral metabolism, and systemic hemodynamics. This chapter presents an overview of the principles of multimodal neuromonitoring that may be used in perioperative and intensive care unit (ICU) settings.

Brain Physiological Principles

There are two fundamental aspects of brain physiology that provide the framework for understanding neuromonitoring and management of brain injury: (1) the Monroe–Kellie doctrine and (2) cerebral autoregulation.

The Monroe–Kellie Doctrine

Intracranial pressure is determined by the volume of intracranial contents (i.e., brain parenchyma, cerebrospinal fluid [CSF], and blood) in patients with an intact cranial vault. Under normal circumstances ICP ranges from 5 to 15 mmHg, with brain parenchyma accounting for 80% of the intracranial volume and CSF and blood each accounting for 10%. The Monroe–Kellie doctrine stipulates that the total volume of these three intracranial components remains constant. An increase in the volume of any one of these three components must be accompanied by either a reduction in the volume of the other components or a shift of volume to outside of the cranial vault.

In a compensated state, ICP will remain normal when there is an increase in volume of any of the three intracranial contents, primarily through reducing venous blood volume by displacement out of the intracranial space, reducing intracranial CSF volume by diversion into the spinal subarachnoid space, or a combination of the two.[1] When these compensatory mechanisms fail, ICP will increase rapidly and brain parenchyma will herniate from areas of high pressure to areas of low pressure.[1,2] Intracranial pressure monitoring can guide therapy to reduce the intracranial volume (e.g., hyperventilation, hyperosmolar therapy, CSF diversion, targeted temperature management) and prevent or treat increases in ICP.[3,4]

Cerebral Autoregulation

The second physiological principle in the management of ICP is cerebral autoregulation. Cerebral autoregulation maintains CBF despite variation in mean arterial pressure (MAP). The cerebral perfusion pressure (CPP), which is the pressure gradient driving CBF, is simply the difference between the MAP and the ICP. Under normal circumstances (i.e., with MAPs in the range of 50–150 mmHg) autoregulation is accomplished by vasoconstriction or vasodilation of the cerebral vasculature to maintain a constant CBF. With MAPs outside the 50–150 mmHg range, autoregulation is impaired. Cerebral blood flow will vary with MAP, and may be inadequate and cause secondary ischemic insult.[5]

Intracranial Pressure Monitoring

Intracranial pressure monitoring is the oldest and most commonly used physiologic neurologic monitor. There are several methods of ICP monitoring that are invasive or noninvasive, and continuous or intermittent. Intracranial pressure monitoring is always used in conjunction with other forms of systemic hemodynamic and neuromonitoring. Regardless of the method of ICP monitoring, the objective always is to detect changes in ICP before irreversible injury occurs. A transient and/or minor increase in ICP may not be harmful, but a sustained and/or significant increase in ICP may cause a critical decrease in CPP and CBF, herniation, and death. Intracranial pressure monitoring provides an early "danger" warning that cannot be detected by neurological exam in patients who already have a depressed level of consciousness or are pharmacologically sedated.

Invasive Intracranial Pressure Monitoring

Invasive ICP monitoring should be considered in all patients with clinical and/or radiographic findings indicative of increased ICP, as often accompanies severe traumatic brain injury (TBI), subarachnoid hemorrhage (SAH), intracerebral hemorrhage (ICH), bacterial meningitis, and fulminant hepatic failure. Invasive ICP monitoring devices directly measure ICP via probes that are placed in the intraventricular, intraparenchymal, subarachnoid, subdural, or epidural compartments. Two methods of invasive ICP monitoring that are commonly employed in clinical practice are external ventricular drains (EVDs) and implantable microtransducer systems such as strain gauge devices and fiber optic sensors.

External ventricular drains are considered the gold standard of ICP monitoring. In addition to measuring ICP, they can be used therapeutically to drain CSF (i.e., CSF diversion) to treat increased ICP. Microtransducer devices measure localized ICP, and their measurements correlate well with those of EVDs.[2] They lack therapeutic potential but compared to EVDs they have lower rates of complications such

as intracranial hemorrhage, seizures, and catheter-associated infections.

The Brain Trauma Foundation guidelines recommend invasive ICP monitoring with an EVD to guide management of patients with severe TBI, defined as Glasgow Coma Scale (GCS) score of less than 8 *after* initial resuscitation, or an abnormal head computed tomography (CT) scan (class II evidence).[6,7] The guidelines offer a weaker recommendation for ICP monitoring in patients with a normal head CT scan and two of the three following criteria: systolic blood pressure less than 90 mmHg, age greater than 40 years, or early unilateral or bilateral motor posturing (class III evidence).[7] A study conducted in severe TBI patients found that therapy guided by ICP monitoring was independently associated with a reduction in two-week mortality by 64%, compared to patients in whom neurological examination and routine imaging alone were used to guide clinical care.[3]

In patients with poor-grade aneurysmal SAH, EVD placement is recommended for ICP monitoring and CSF diversion.[8] In spontaneous ICH, EVD placement should be considered in patients with a GCS less than 9, clinical signs of transtentorial herniation, significant intraventricular hemorrhage (IVH), or hydrocephalus.[9]

The ICP waveform may be used to evaluate intracranial compliance. Under normal physiologic conditions the morphology of the ICP waveform has three components: P1 (percussion wave) represents arterial pulsation, P2 (tidal wave) represents the overall intracranial compliance, and P3 (dicrotic wave) represents the venous pulsations. When intracranial compliance diminishes, the P2 wave will increase in amplitude and may exceed the P1 wave's amplitude. Pathological waveforms, known as Lundberg A and B waves, occur during sustained intracranial hypertension and represent a state of reduced compliance. Lundberg A waves last several minutes and represent sustained ICP elevation to greater than 50 mmHg and concomitant reduction in CPP; they indicate evolving brain injury. Lundberg B waves last only 1–3 minutes and represent an elevation of ICP that is less than the 50 mmHg range. They may indicate a compromise in the intracranial compliance and may precede the development of A waves. Lundberg A waveforms are always pathological, but B waveforms vary in their clinical significance.

Noninvasive Intracranial Pressure Monitoring

There are two noninvasive indirect measures of ICP that can be performed at the bedside, transcranial Doppler ultrasound and transocular ultrasound.

Transcranial Doppler (TCD) is the primary modality for noninvasive measurement of ICP. It emits ultrasound waves that travel through various layers of tissue until they encounter red blood cells (RBCs) in blood vessels. After contacting the RBCs, the ultrasound waves are reflected back and the frequency of the returning ultrasound waves indicates the direction and velocity of blood flow in the large arteries of the brain, most commonly the middle cerebral artery (MCA). Transcranial Doppler can be used to calculate the pulsatile index (PI), which is the difference between systolic and diastolic blood flow velocities divided by the mean blood flow velocity. The PI correlates with invasively measured ICP.[10] Pulsatile index values greater than 1.4 are indicative of elevated ICP and are associated with worse clinical outcomes (sensitivity 88%, specificity 97%).[11] Transcranial Doppler does not have the risks of invasive methods, but its main disadvantage is that it also does not provide continuous data.

Transocular ultrasound of the optic nerve sheath diameter is another noninvasive ICP monitoring modality. Increased optic nerve sheath diameter correlates with increased ICP, because in between the optic nerve sheath and the nerve itself, there is subarachnoid space that is in communication with the subarachnoid space of the brain. Optic nerve sheath diameter greater than 5 mm is pathological.[12–14] This noninvasive method of ICP monitoring is easily performed at the bedside, but its accuracy is inferior to invasive ICP measurement and it does not provide continuous data.

Cerebral Blood Flow Monitoring

As reviewed above, CBF is normally maintained within a wide range of MAPs (50–150 mmHg) by adjusting blood vessel diameter, so that CPP is maintained between 50 and 70 mmHg. Impaired autoregulation, increased ICP, or decreased MAP may reduce CBF and result in brain injury. Cerebral blood flow monitoring may detect changes before they lead to injury and be used to guide preventive measures.

Invasive Cerebral Blood Flow Monitoring

Thermal diffusion flowmetry (TDF) is an invasive technique that provides quantitative assessments of regional CBF (rCBF). The TDF catheter utilizes a distal thermistor heated to a few degrees above the regional tissue temperature, and a second, more proximal temperature probe.[15] The difference in temperature between the two probes reflects the absolute blood flow between them and is expressed in mL/100g/min. Thermal diffusion flowmetry can provide continuous CBF data and has been shown to correlate with rCBF data obtained from simultaneous xenon-enhanced CT imaging. Normal rCBF values range between 40 and 70 mL/100g/min; values less than 20 mL/100g/min will result in cerebral ischemia without a concomitant reduction in metabolic demand (e.g., hypothermia, drug-induced coma). Thermal diffusion flowmetry catheters are usually placed in white matter regions that are deemed to be at greatest risk of ischemia. In conjunction with other monitoring devices, they may also assist detection of cerebral vasospasm in SAH patients.[16]

Cerebral blood flow monitoring with TDF can also be used to estimate brain water content (BWC). In a study of 36 comatose brain-injured patients, brain regions that appeared edematous on CT imaging showed higher TDF-calculated BWC than normal-appearing brain regions.[17] These same patients had a calculated decrease in BWC after administration of hyperosmolar therapy, as would be expected. These findings suggest that BWC monitoring utilizing TDF is feasible.

Unfortunately, TDF may only be possible in 30–40% of cases due to high rates of monitor failure and loss of data during recalibration.[5] Given the high rates of failure, TDF is usually used in conjunction with other brain monitoring.

Noninvasive Cerebral Blood Flow Monitoring

In addition to noninvasive measurement of ICP, TCD can also be used to noninvasively measure CBF (ml/gm/min). A blood flow velocity (BFV) in the MCA greater than 120 cm/sec is considered pathological and correlates with cerebral vasospasm (sensitivity 73%, specificity 80%).[8,15]

Patients with SAH should have periodic TCD assessments for early diagnosis of cerebral vasospasm. Prompt management of vasospasm may prevent delayed cerebral ischemia (DCI), a frequent and critical complication of SAH that occurs in up to 70% of cases.[8] The severity of vasospasm can be graded using the Lindegaard ratio (LR), which is the ratio of the MCA BFV to the extracranial internal carotid artery (ICA) BFV. An LR less than 3 is considered normal, whereas LR 3–6 is associated with mild to moderate vasospasm and LR greater than 6 with severe vasospasm.[18]

There are two main limitations to this application. Although cerebral vasospasm is the most common cause of elevated CBF, it is not the only pathologic cause. Common conditions such as fever and increased cardiac output due to any cause (e.g., peripheral shunting, hyperthyroidism, catecholamine administration) will increase BFV.[15] Therefore, BFV should be interpreted in the context of the patient's condition. Another limitation is that TCD is not a continuous monitoring technique, and there is risk of missing significant CBF changes between exams.

Brain Oxygen Monitoring

Critically ill patients recovering from neurologic injury are vulnerable to decreased brain oxygenation. As with increased ICP, transient decreased brain oxygenation may not have any consequence, but sustained cerebral hypoxia can be devastating. There are several invasive and noninvasive methods of monitoring brain oxygenation used to guide therapy.

Invasive Brain Oxygen Monitoring

Jugular Venous Oxygen Saturation

Jugular venous oxygen saturation ($SvjO_2$) can be measured intermittently by sampling blood from the jugular venous bulb from a catheter placed in a retrograde direction, or continuously using a fiber optic catheter similarly placed. It is used to assess oxygen demand–supply mismatch. An increase in the demand-to-supply ratio will result in a decrease in the oxygen saturation of blood draining from the brain. The normal range of $SvjO_2$ is 55–75%, and lower values correlate with poorer outcomes.[19] Current guidelines recommend maintaining $SvjO_2$ greater than 50%.[7] Any condition resulting in arteriovenous shunting or decreased brain metabolism (e.g., hypothermia, drug-induced coma, and brain death) will result in a higher $SvjO_2$; fever, shivering, and seizures will reduce the $SvjO_2$.[20] The main risks of

this monitoring technique are vascular injury of the internal jugular vein, inadvertent cannulation of the carotid artery, and thrombosis of these vessels.

Intraparenchymal Catheters

The partial pressure of oxygen in brain parenchyma ($PbtO_2$) can be directly measured using catheters that are usually inserted into the subcortical white matter. These catheters employ the Clark cell method, utilizing a semipermeable membrane that allows dissolved oxygen to pass through it and generate an electrical current proportional to the $PbtO_2$.[21] Most clinical data regarding $PbtO_2$ monitoring are from studies in severe TBI and, to a lesser extent, SAH patients.[22] When placed in normal parenchyma, $PbtO_2$ values represent global cerebral oxygenation; placement in injured areas will result in regional oxygenation assessment.

In general, $PbtO_2$ monitors are placed when the GCS is ≤ 8 (i.e., similar to indications for ICP monitoring). There is no consensus where in the brain these devices should be placed, but in TBI the right frontal lobe is usually chosen, and in a focal injury the side of maximal pathology is chosen. In SAH, the $PbtO_2$ monitor should be placed in the brain region most likely impacted by the expected vasospastic response.[23] Once placed and confirmed with CT imaging, an "oxygen challenge" should be conducted by increasing FiO_2 from baseline to 1.0 for approximately five minutes; a functional probe will reveal an increase in the $PbtO_2$. The increase is less robust when the probe is in a hypoperfused region (e.g., CBF is less than 20 ml/100 g/min).[24]

The $PbtO_2$ is a more complex variable to interpret than $SvjO_2$ because it may vary significantly by site of placement and might be more sensitive to small changes. It is influenced by global determinants of oxygen delivery (i.e., cardiac output and blood oxygen content), ICP, CPP, autoregulation, and specifically cerebral oxygen tissue gradients (i.e., nonhomogenous cerebral oxygenation), which are more prominent in the injured brain.

Normal $PbtO_2$ values range from 25 to 35 mmHg. Values less than 20 mmHg are suggestive of cerebral ischemia, and those less than 15 mmHg predict poor outcome in severe TBI and SAH patients.[25] Monitoring of $PbtO_2$ should be used when secondary brain injury is likely, and it is best used in an integrated fashion with other monitors, clinical evaluation, and imaging studies.[26] In TBI and SAH, $PbtO_2$ monitoring should always be used in conjunction with ICP monitoring because cerebral hypoxia may occur even when ICP and CPP are normal and would otherwise go undetected and be potentially injurious.[25,27]

Noninvasive Brain Oxygen Monitoring

Near-infrared spectroscopy (NIRS) is the primary noninvasive method of measuring cerebral oxygenation. This technique determines the concentration of oxygenated hemoglobin in the brain (rSO_2) using sensors placed on the forehead that determine the absorption of light in the near-infrared wavelength by brain tissue and hemoglobin.[28] Changes in cerebral oxyhemoglobin concentration help detect impaired regional brain oxygenation that may be due to reduced blood oxygen content or blood flow. Values for cerebral oxyhemoglobin less than 60% are considered pathologic and are associated with cerebral hypoxia. Unfortunately, incorporating NIRS monitoring with other invasive strategies has not been shown to improve outcome (see Chapter 3).[29]

Cerebral Autoregulation Monitoring

Current Brain Trauma Foundation guidelines recommend maintaining CPP between 60 and 70 mmHg in patients with TBI; this goal is often extrapolated to other conditions.[7]

Preservation of normal cerebral autoregulation is the most important factor for determining the lowest target CPP.[30] Aggressive attempts to increase CPP above 70 mmHg by administering fluids and/or vasoactive agents are not recommended due to the associated risk of acute lung injury.[7]

Cerebral perfusion pressure is a crude target used in the absence of more sophisticated monitoring. Intracranial pressure, cerebral oximetry, and TCD measurements, however, may be used to assess cerebral autoregulation and have been studied primarily in the setting of TBI.[31]

Intracranial pressure data can be used to compute the pressure reactivity index (PRx), which reflects the degree of cerebral autoregulation. The PRx is the Pearson correlation coefficient of the MAP and ICP derived from 30 consecutive, 10-second averaged values over a 5-minute period. Correlation coefficients range from +1.0 to −1.0; PRx values near 0 indicate that there is no correlation between the ICP and MAP and that autoregulation is intact. Values closer to +1.0 indicate a positive linear correlation and that autoregulation is impaired. In patients with TBI such values predict greater morbidity and mortality. A plot of CPP on the x-axis and PRx on the y-axis results in a U-shaped curve, and the nadir point represents the optimal CPP. This point is patient-specific and differs based on underlying injury and degree of autoregulation preservation.[32]

The oxygen reactivity index (ORx) is the Pearson correlation coefficient of the CPP and $PbtO_2$.[30] Understanding the relationship between CBF and oxygen/metabolic demand and delivery can help guide management in real time.[33]

Monitoring of PRx and ORx requires continuous data processing, which may be expensive and time-consuming, limiting their use as a bedside modality. An observational study of low-frequency, minute-by-minute assessment of MAP and ICP data found that real-time measurement of optimal CPP was possible and that continuous processing may not be required.[26] Despite encouraging results from small clinical trials supporting the hypothesis that individualized CPP monitoring yields improved outcomes in TBI patients, there is insufficient evidence to support widespread adoption.

Brain Metabolism Monitoring: Cerebral Microdialysis

Cerebral microdialysis (MD) is a technique that allows for direct assessment of the brain's extracellular biochemical milieu by a fine-tipped double-lumen probe with a semipermeable membrane inserted into the subcortical white matter. The fundamental principle of MD is the same as that of hemodialysis; substances will cross a semipermeable membrane along their concentration gradient. The final concentration of substances in the dialysate depends on the difference between their baseline concentration in the probe and their uptake from the brain's extracellular fluid (ECF). Perfusate, a fluid isotonic to the ECF, is introduced into the catheter, and molecules at high concentration in the ECF equilibrate through the semipermeable membrane. The resulting microdialysate can then be analyzed. Several substances, including glucose, lactate, pyruvate, glutamate (an excitatory neurotransmitter associated with the inflammatory cascade), and glycerol (a marker of neuronal cell breakdown associated with irreversible cell injury), can be measured at the bedside.[33]

Glucose serves as the brain's primary energy source, and its metabolism to adenosine triphosphate (ATP) provides the fuel for brain function. During glycolysis the production of pyruvate enters the citric acid cycle to produce energy at the cellular level. During ischemia, seizures, and other situations in which oxygen demand exceeds supply, pyruvate is shunted to the anaerobic metabolic pathway and is converted to lactate.[33] The lactate-to-pyruvate ratio (LPR) is considered to be the most reliable marker of cerebral metabolic derangement due to impaired oxidative metabolism. Elevated LPR may be the result of ischemic injury and is associated with neuronal cell death.[34]

Microdialysis can be used to detect early signs of secondary neurological insult and may be clinically useful as part of multimodality monitoring paradigm in patients with acute brain injury. Microdialysis studies, conducted primarily in patients with severe TBI and poor-grade SAH,[22] reveal significant and predictable patterns of metabolic derangement, including elevated levels of lactate, pyruvate, LPR, glutamate, and glycerol, as well as low levels of glucose after periods of sustained cerebral ischemia.[35]

Values of LPR greater than 40 represent cerebral "metabolic distress," whereas the combination of LPR greater than 40 and brain glucose levels less than 0.7 mmol/L represents brain "metabolic crisis."[35–37] These abnormalities have been associated with poor outcomes in TBI patients.[33,38] Detected metabolic changes can predict vasospasm in patients with high-grade SAH and may be used to guide timely treatment to help prevent DCI and neurologic deterioration.[39–41]

Electrophysiology

Electroencephalography

Continuous electroencephalography (cEEG) monitoring with video patient recording and remote monitoring capability is now fairly routine in neurological ICUs. In addition to its value in diagnosing non-convulsive seizures, cEEG is integral to guide careful titration of sedatives and antiepileptics in status epilepticus, minimizing deleterious side effects while suppressing seizure activity.[42] It is recommended in patients with an unexplained persistently altered mental status or whose mental status does not recover following a clinical seizure.[43,44] In comatose patients, it is estimated that 30% have a cEEG-detected seizure after 24 hours of monitoring that would have gone undiagnosed in the absence of monitoring.[43] As with other neuromonitoring modalities, the goal of cEEG in the ICU setting is early detection so that potential secondary neurologic injury may be avoided by early administration of antiepileptics. Prompt recognition and treatment of seizures prevents resistance to antiepileptic therapy.[45,46]

Continuous EEG also has been used to detect vasospasm and increased ICP as a component of multimodal prognostication in cardiac arrest.[43]

Evoked Potentials

Somatosensory evoked potentials (SSEPs) are electrical signals emitted from the cerebral cortex in response to a sensory stimulus delivered at the periphery. These are often used in combination with motor evoked potentials (MEPs), electrical signals emitted from muscles in response to stimulation of the motor cortex via scalp electrodes. Evoked potential monitoring helps to evaluate the integrity of the ascending somatosensory and descending motor pathways, and is an important component of intra-operative monitoring for surgical complications during spine and brain surgery.[47] Somatosensory evoked potential signals are much smaller in amplitude than typical EEG signals, and therefore the SSEP waveform represents an average of many signals in response to multiple stimuli recorded over a brief period of time.[48] Somatosensory evoked potentials serve as an important noninvasive method of assessing subcortical structures, and unlike many other neuromonitoring modalities, they are not subject to interference by intravenous hypnotics or sedatives.[43,48] Evoked potential monitoring, however, requires specialized equipment and onsite interpretation by a technician who is dedicated to a single patient and in communication with a neurologist. The equipment and expertise required make the timely application of this monitoring challenging.

"Big Data" in Critical Care

The goal of multimodal neuromonitoring is continuous assessment of ICP, CBF, PbtO$_2$, brain metabolism, and neurophysiological function in order to establish baseline status, identify early signs of deterioration that are treatable, and prevent secondary neurologic injury. Multimodal neuromonitoring data may also be used to refine prediction of morbidity and mortality, and help to allocate expensive and scarce resources such as ICU beds.

Intensive care units are data-rich environments. The complexity of critical care and the enormous amount of data generated present an exciting opportunity. Display and trending of information and data from clinical examination, devices, laboratories, and imaging should be able to drive evidence-based decision support and improve outcomes.[49] Despite the promise, most research has focused on using this information to validate patient outcome scoring systems, and has not utilized it in decision support to a significant degree.[50] Commercially available programs that integrate data from various monitors and electronic health records (EHRs) for display and decision support have not been widely adapted. Electronic health records alone could potentially evolve into artificial intelligence systems and move beyond their current feature "best practice alerts" into continuous evidence-based practice drivers.[51,52]

There are several promising databases that are designed for integrating data from general critical care patients.[53,54] The Multiparameter Intelligent Monitoring in Intensive Care (MIMIC) database is a large open-access database that contains demographic, physiological, medication, and outcome data recorded from thousands of ICU patients admitted to Beth Israel Deaconess Medical Center (Boston, Massachusetts, USA).[55] These types of databases can be important resources for patient monitoring research and will support efforts in medical data mining and knowledge discovery.[56]

The International Initiative for Traumatic Brain Injury Research has developed the Federal Interagency TBI Research Informatics System platform to collect patients' phenotypic, genomic, and imaging information. As part of this initiative, the Center-TBI database collects detailed information from thousands of ICU patients in Europe.[57] These databases have been shown to help better understand patient outcomes.[57]

Some programs developed for research purposes have also shown promising results to understand time-synchronized relationships between different neuromonitoring parameters. The *ICM+*, developed at Cambridge University, integrates ICP waveform data with MAP data to monitor autoregulation. Another recent addition is the Moberg Research© multimodal neuromonitoring platform that includes measures of cerebrovascular autoregulation, brain tissue oxygenation, microdialysis, and cEEG to enhance decision support.[58]

In sum, neurocritical care depends on complex bedside monitoring, even though the specifics of what should be monitored and how remain unanswered. The exact impact and costs of the various strategies discussed herein are largely unknown. Successfully integrating monitoring with all the other data available into the clinical workflow while avoiding injury and data misinterpretation is difficult. Achieving improved patient outcomes as a result of these efforts, however, is clearly within reach.

References

1. Jones RF, Dorsch NW, Silverberg GD, Torda TA. Pathophysiology and management of raised intracranial pressure. *Anaesth Intensive Care* 1981;**9**:336–51.

2. Kirkman MA, Smith M. Intracranial pressure monitoring, cerebral perfusion pressure estimation, and ICP/CPP-guided therapy: a standard of care or optional extra after brain injury? *Br J Anaesth* 2014;**112**:35–46.

3. Treggiari MM, Schutz N, Yanez ND, Romand, JA. Role of intracranial pressure values and patterns in predicting outcome in traumatic brain injury: a systematic review. *Neurocrit Care* 2007;**6**:104–12.

4. Muizelaar JP, Wei EP, Kontos HA, Becker DP. Mannitol causes compensatory cerebral vasoconstriction and vasodilation in response to blood viscosity changes. *J Neurosurg* 1983;**59**:822–8.

5. Akbik OS, Carlson AP, Krasberg M, Yonas H. The utility of cerebral blood flow assessment in TBI. *Curr Neurol Neurosci Rep* 2016;**16**:72.

6. Brain Trauma Foundation. Guidelines for the management of severe traumatic brain injury. VI. Indications for intracranial pressure monitoring. *J Neurotrauma* 2007;**24 Suppl 1**: S37–44.

7. Carney N, et al. Guidelines for the management of severe traumatic brain injury, Fourth Edition. *Neurosurgery* 2017;**80**:6–15.

8. Bederson JB, et al. Guidelines for the management of aneurysmal subarachnoid hemorrhage: a statement for healthcare professionals from a special writing group of the stroke council, American Heart Association. *Stroke* 2009;**40**:994–1025.

9. Steiner T, Al-Shahi Salman R, Christensen H, et al. European Stroke Organisation (ESO) guidelines for the management of spontaneous intracerebral hemorrhage. *Int J Stroke* 2014;**9**:840–55.

10. Bathala L, Mehndiratta MM, Sharma VK. Transcranial Doppler: technique and common findings (part 1). *Ann Indian Acad Neurol* 2013;**16**:174–9.

11. Cardim D, Robba C, Bohdanowicz M, et al. Non-invasive monitoring of intracranial pressure using transcranial Doppler ultrasonography: is it possible? *Neurocrit Care* 2016;**25**:473–91.

12. Rajajee V, Vanaman M, Fletcher JJ, Jacobs TL. Optic nerve ultrasound for the detection of raised intracranial pressure. *Neurocrit Care* 2011;**15**:506–15.

13. Robba C, Santori G, Czosnyka M, et al. Optic nerve sheath diameter measured sonographically as non-invasive estimator of intracranial pressure: a systematic review and meta-analysis. *Intensive Care Med* 2018;**44**:1284–94.

14. Suarez JI, Qureshi AI, Yahia AB, et al. Symptomatic vasospasm diagnosis after subarachnoid hemorrhage: evaluation of transcranial Doppler ultrasound and cerebral angiography as related to compromised vascular distribution. *Crit Care Med* 2002;**30**:1348–55.

15. Vajkoczy P, Roth H, Horn P, et al. Continuous monitoring of regional cerebral blood flow: experimental and clinical validation of a novel thermal diffusion microprobe. *J Neurosurg* 2000;**93**:265–74.

16. Al-Mufti F, Amuluru K, Damodara N, et al. Novel management strategies for medically-refractory vasospasm following aneurysmal subarachnoid hemorrhage. *J Neurol Sci* 2018;**390**:44–51.

17. Ko SB, Choi HA, Parikh G, et al. Real time estimation of brain water content in comatose patients. *Ann Neurol* 2012;**72**:344–50.

18. Lindegaard KF, Nornes H, Bakke SJ, Sorteberg W, Nakstad P. Cerebral vasospasm diagnosis by means of angiography and blood velocity measurements. *Acta Neurochir (Wien)* 1989;**100**:12–24.

19. Robertson CS, Gopinath SP, Goodman JC, et al. SjvO2 monitoring in head-injured patients. *J Neurotrauma* 1995;**12**:891–6.

20. Schell RM, Cole, DJ. Cerebral monitoring: jugular venous oximetry. *Anesth Analg* 2000;**90**:559–66.

21. Siegemund M, van Bommel J, Ince C. Assessment of regional tissue oxygenation. *Intensive Care Med* 1999;**25**:1044–60.

22. Francoeur CL, Pain M, Mayer SA. Multimodality monitoring: illuminating the Comatose Human Brain. *Semin Neurol* 2016;**36**:560–9.

23. Bohman LE, Pisapia JM, Sanborn MR, et al. Response of brain oxygen to therapy correlates with long-term outcome after subarachnoid hemorrhage. *Neurocrit Care* 2013;**19**:320–8.

24. Hlatky R, Valadka AB, Gopinath SP, Robertson CS. Brain tissue oxygen tension response to induced hyperoxia reduced in hypoperfused brain. *J Neurosurg* 2008;**108**:53–8.

25. Nangunoori R, Maloney-Wilensky E, Stiefel M, et al. Brain tissue oxygen-based therapy and outcome after severe traumatic brain injury: a systematic literature review. *Neurocrit Care* 2012;**17**:131–8.

26. Johnston AJ, Steiner LA, Coles JP, et al. Effect of cerebral perfusion pressure augmentation on regional oxygenation and metabolism after head injury. *Crit Care Med* 2005;**33**:189–95; discussion 255–187.

27. Oddo, M, Levine JM, Mackenzie L, et al. Brain hypoxia is associated with short-term outcome after severe traumatic brain injury independently of intracranial hypertension and low cerebral perfusion pressure. *Neurosurgery* 2011;**69**:1037–45; discussion 1045.

28. Naidech AM, Bendok BR, Ault ML, Bleck TP. Monitoring with the somanetics INVOS 5100C after aneurysmal subarachnoid hemorrhage. *Neurocrit Care* 2008;**9**:326–31.

29. Rosenthal G, Furmanov A, Itshayek E, Shoshan Y, Singh V. Assessment of a noninvasive cerebral oxygenation monitor in patients with severe traumatic brain injury. *J Neurosurg* 2014;**120**:901–7.

30. Jaeger M, Dengl M, Meixensberger J, Schuhmann MU. Effects of cerebrovascular pressure reactivity-guided optimization of cerebral perfusion pressure on brain tissue oxygenation after traumatic brain injury. *Crit Care Med* 2010;**38**:1343–7.

31. Jaeger M, Schuhmann, MU, Soehle M, Meixensberger J. Continuous assessment of

cerebrovascular autoregulation after traumatic brain injury using brain tissue oxygen pressure reactivity. *Crit Care Med* 2006;**34**:1783–8.

32. Czosnyka M, Smielewski P, Piechnik S, Steiner LA, Pickard JD. Cerebral autoregulation following head injury. *J Neurosurg* 2001;**95**:756–63.

33. Zeiler FA, Thelin EP, Helmy A, et al. A systematic review of cerebral microdialysis and outcomes in TBI: relationships to patient functional outcome, neurophysiologic measures, and tissue outcome. *Acta Neurochir (Wien)* 2017;**159**:2245–73.

34. Sahuquillo J, Merino MA, Sánchez-Guerrero A, et al. Lactate and the lactate-to-pyruvate molar ratio cannot be used as independent biomarkers for monitoring brain energetic metabolism: a microdialysis study in patients with traumatic brain injuries. *PLoS One* 2014;**9**:e102540.

35. Hlatky R, Valadka AB, Goodman JC, Contant CF, Robertson CS. Patterns of energy substrates during ischemia measured in the brain by microdialysis. *J Neurotrauma* 2004;**21**:894–906.

36. Helbok R, Schmidt JM, Kurtz P, et al. Systemic glucose and brain energy metabolism after subarachnoid hemorrhage. *Neurocrit Care* 2010;**12**:317–23.

37. Hillered L, Vespa PM, Hovda DA. Translational neurochemical research in acute human brain injury: the current status and potential future for cerebral microdialysis. *J Neurotrauma* 2005;**22**:3–41.

38. Vespa, P, Prins M, Ronne-Engstrom E, et al. Increase in extracellular glutamate caused by reduced cerebral perfusion pressure and seizures after human traumatic brain injury: a microdialysis study. *J Neurosurg* 1998;**89**:971–82.

39. Sarrafzadeh AS, Sakowitz OW, Kiening KL, et al. Bedside microdialysis: a tool to monitor cerebral metabolism in subarachnoid hemorrhage patients? *Crit Care Med* 2002;**30**:1062–70.

40. Sarrafzadeh A, Haux D, Kuchler I, Lanksch WR, Unterberg AW. Poor-grade aneurysmal subarachnoid hemorrhage: relationship of cerebral metabolism to outcome. *J Neurosurg* 2004;**100**: 400–6.

41. Skjoth-Rasmussen J, Schulz M, Kristensen SR, Bjerre P. Delayed neurological deficits detected by an ischemic pattern in the extracellular cerebral metabolites in patients with aneurysmal subarachnoid hemorrhage. *J Neurosurg* 2004;**100**:8–15.

42. Ferguson M, Bianchi MT, Sutter R, et al. Calculating the risk benefit equation for aggressive treatment of non-convulsive status epilepticus. *Neurocrit Care* 2013;**18**:216–27.

43. Caricato A, Melchionda I, Antonelli M. Continuous electroencephalography monitoring in adults in the intensive care unit. *Crit Care* 2018;**22**:75.

44. Herman ST, et al. Consensus statement on continuous EEG in critically ill adults and children, part I: indications. *J Clin Neurophysiol* 2015;**32**:87–95.

45. Claassen J, Mayer SA, Kowalski RG, Emerson RG, Hirsch LJ. Detection of electrographic seizures with continuous EEG monitoring in critically ill patients. *Neurology* 2004;**62**:1743–8.

46. Farrokh S, Tahsili-Fahadan P, Ritzl EK, Lewin JJ 3rd, Mirski MA. Antiepileptic drugs in critically ill patients. *Crit Care* 2018;**22**:153.

47. Chang SH, Park YG, Kim DH, Yoon SY. Monitoring of motor and somatosensory evoked potentials during spine surgery: intraoperative changes and postoperative outcomes. *Ann Rehabil Med* 2016;**40**:470–80.

48. Rosenthal ES. The utility of EEG, SSEP, and other neurophysiologic tools to guide neurocritical care. *Neurotherapeutics* 2012;**9**:24–36.

49. Sanchez-Pinto LN, Luo Y, Churpek, MM. Big data and data science in critical care. *Chest* 2018;**154**:1239–48.

50. Yang S, Stansbury LG, Rock, P, Scalea T, Hu PF. Linking big data and prediction strategies: tools, pitfalls, and lessons learned. *Crit Care Med* 2019;47 (6):840–8.

51. *Learning Health Systems | Agency for Healthcare Research & Quality* www.ahrq.gov/professionals/sys tems/learning-health-systems/index.html (2019).

52 Li P, Xie C, Pollard T, et al. Promoting secondary analysis of electronic medical records in China: summary of the PLAGH-MIT critical data conference and health Datathon. *JMIR Med Inform* 2017;**5**:e43.

53. Flechet M, Grandas FG, Meyfroidt G. Informatics in neurocritical care: new ideas for Big Data. *Curr Opin Crit Care* 2016;**22**:87–93.

54. *ICM+ Features | Cambridge Enterprise ICM+.*, https:// icmplus.neurosurg.cam.ac.uk/home/icm-features/ (2018).

55. Johnson AE, Pollard TJ, Shen L, et al. MIMIC-III, a freely accessible critical care database. *Sci Data* 2016;**3**:160035.

56. Saeed M, Villarroel M, Reisner AT, et al. Multiparameter intelligent monitoring in intensive care II: a public access intensive care unit database. *Crit Care Med* 2011;**39**:952–60.

57. Maas AI, Menon DK, Steyerberg EW, et al.
Collaborative European NeuroTrauma Effectiveness
Research in Traumatic Brain Injury (CENTER-TBI):
a prospective longitudinal observational study.
Neurosurgery 2015;**76**:67–80.

58. *Multimodal Data Integration – Moberg ICU
Solutions: Transforming Neurocritical Care.*,
www.moberg.com/solutions/multimodal-data-
integration (2018).

Cerebral Oximetry

Benjamin Salter and Elvera Baron

Introduction

The risk of perioperative neurologic injury has decreased over the years with advances in surgical and anesthetic techniques; however, it remains a significant clinical problem that may result in severe debilitation and death. Of non-neurological surgeries, cardiac surgery is associated with the highest risk of perioperative neurologic injury, including cognitive dysfunction, postoperative visual loss, cerebrovascular accidents (CVA), nonfatal diffuse encephalopathy, and peripheral nerve injury. The incidence of new ischemic lesions following cardiac surgery is 27.6% in coronary artery bypass graft (CABG) surgery, 63% in aortic surgery, and 84% in valve replacement.[1] In particular, the incidence of a stroke in the cardiac surgical population is estimated to range from 1 to 7% and approaches 12% in patients with severe carotid stenosis.[2,3] Most of these events occur during the operation, or at least their genesis begins intraoperatively. Thus, there is a need to better assess for potential neurologic injury, guide hemodynamic therapy, and alert physicians that a neurologic rescue or protective therapy is indicated.

Noninvasive intraoperative monitoring of regional cerebral oxygen saturation ($rScO_2$) by near-infrared spectroscopy (NIRS) is increasingly used in this vein to ensure an adequate balance between cerebral oxygen supply and demand. Since perioperative neurologic injury is not unique to cardiac surgical patients, NIRS technology is increasingly employed in orthopedic, vascular, and neurosurgical procedures too. It is also being utilized in other clinical settings, including trauma, critical care, and cardiopulmonary resuscitation.[4,5] This chapter reviews the basic principles and interpretation of cerebral oximetry, research studies that examine its efficacy, and novel uses of this technology. For the purpose of simplification, the terms "NIRS," "cerebral oximetry," and "$rScO_2$" will be used interchangeably throughout the following discussion.

Cerebral Oximetry

Principles of Near-Infrared Spectroscopy

In 1977, Franz Jabsis presented the concept of a noninvasive real-time measurement of cerebral tissue oxygenation using wavelengths of light in the near-infrared spectrum.[6] His theory was based on the observation that near-infrared light (wavelength range 660–940 nm) passes easily through skull and brain tissue. In this range, light is absorbed by certain biological molecules in the brain, including hemoglobin, and to a much lesser degree by water, lipids, skin, and bone, allowing for little interference.[7–10] Hemoglobin molecules, present in both oxygenated and deoxygenated forms, have different absorption spectra. Deoxygenated hemoglobin absorbs light waves in the 650–1000 nm range, and oxygenated hemoglobin absorbs light waves in the 700–1150 nm range.[10] Using the principles of the Beer–Lambert law and proprietary algorithms, a ratio or percentage of oxygenated hemoglobin to deoxygenated hemoglobin is generated and an $rScO_2$ value is displayed. Cerebral oximeters do not rely on pulsatile flow and assume a fixed proportion (70:30 or 75:25) of venous-to-arterial blood volume. Bilateral cerebral oximetry probes provide information on the regional supply and demand balance of the frontal cortical tissue supplied by the anterior and middle cerebral arteries. This watershed area is the most vulnerable to hypoxemia.[8,11,12] Very basically, the lower the cerebral oximetry value (i.e., $rScO_2$), the greater the likelihood that there is an oxygen delivery–consumption imbalance. Similar to the systemic circulation, oxygen delivery is dependent on both flow and oxygen content of the blood, while consumption is determined by metabolic demand and is most affected by temperature and depth of anesthesia.

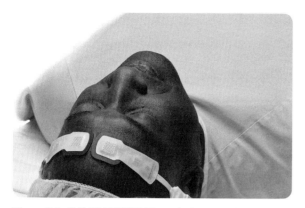

Figure 3.1 CASMED FORESIGHT™ cerebral oximetry adult probe placement. *Printed with permission from the manufacturer.

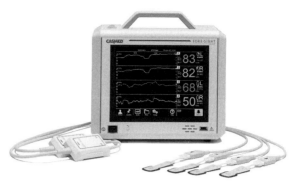

Figure 3.2 CASMED FORESIGHT™ monitor, cables, and oximetry probes. (A black and white version of this figure will appear in some formats. For the color version, please refer to the plate section.) *Printed with permission from the manufacturer.

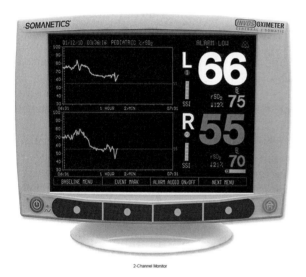

Figure 3.3 Somanetics INVOS™ cerebral oximetry monitor. (A black and white version of this figure will appear in some formats. For the color version, please refer to the plate section.) *Printed with permission from the manufacturer.

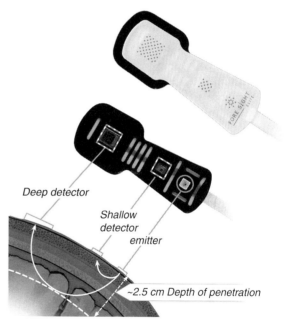

Deep detector

Shallow detector

emitter

~2.5 cm Depth of penetration

Figure 3.4 CASMED FORESIGHT™ oximetry probe and depth of penetration. (A black and white version of this figure will appear in some formats. For the color version, please refer to the plate section.) *Printed with permission from the manufacturer.

Normally, the cerebral oximetry system consists of an oximeter probe (or two) attached to a cable and device monitor (Figures 3.1–3.3). In the United States, a variety of NIRS monitoring devices are commercially available, including the INVOS™ (Somanetics/Covidien, Inc., Boulder, CO), FORESIGHT™ (CAS Medical Systems, Branford, CT), and EQUANOX™ (Nonin Medical Inc., Plymouth, MN).[11] The INVOS and FORESIGHT probes utilize a single light-emitting source and two detectors spaced several centimeters apart, with the proximal detector receiving the reflection from superficial tissues and the more distal detector receiving the reflection from deeper tissues (approximately 2–2.5 cm) (Figure 3.4). The EQUANOX device uses two emitters and two detectors (Figure 3.5). Although all three of the proprietary sensors have some amount of extracranial signal contamination, EQUANOX has the least compared to the other two.[13] Unfortunately, the different proprietary algorithms used by each system make comparisons of the different NIRS technologies difficult.[12]

21

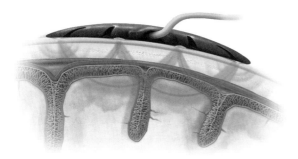

Figure 3.5 Nonin EQUANOX™ cerebral oximetry sensors. (A black and white version of this figure will appear in some formats. For the color version, please refer to the plate section.) *Printed with permission from the manufacturer.

Interpretation

It is important for clinicians utilizing cerebral oximetry to understand factors that influence the values displayed on the monitors. Alterations in the emitter-to-sensor distance by tissue edema and changes in the arterial and venous hemoglobin distribution (e.g., by arterio-venous shunts, hematomas, and hemodilution) do not necessarily affect tissue oxygenation but can impact oximeter readings. Motion artifact, jaundice, and hair pigmentation can all cause decreased oximeter accuracy; however, skin color and melanin content do not appear to have an effect, unlike in pulse oximetry.

In order to establish a reference point for measurements throughout the procedure, it is recommended that baseline oximetry values be determined in the awake, spontaneously breathing patient. Low baseline oximetry values are commonly observed in patients with brain atrophy, diastolic dysfunction, poor left ventricular function, anemia, and hemodialysis,[14–18] and they are associated with higher incidences of morbidity, including postoperative delirium and mortality.[4,19–21] Baseline $rScO_2$ values, however, have significant inter-individual variation and can range from 50% to 80% in healthy patients.[8,10,22] Thus, trending values may be more indicative of the ensuing cerebral supply–demand balance than absolute values. Additionally, cerebral desaturation load (CDL), defined as the product of the duration and severity of desaturations, has been investigated as a trigger for intervention.[4,23]

Cerebral oximetry data reflect the balance between regional tissue oxygen supply and demand. Factors that affect this balance, therefore, will contribute to alterations in the displayed $rScO_2$ value. Supply is directly influenced by cerebral blood flow (CBF) that is autoregulated, cardiac output, and arterial oxygen

content. Oxygen content is determined by the hemoglobin concentration, oxygen saturation, and, to a lesser degree, oxygen tension (which depends on the inspired oxygen concentration and the alveolar-arterial gradient). Common perioperative factors associated with decreased $rScO_2$ values that often are of great concern are low cardiac output, hypoxemia, anemia (e.g., secondary to hemorrhage or hemodilution), hyperventilation that causes cerebral vasoconstriction, extreme perturbations in acid–base balance, increased oxygen demand (e.g., under-anesthetized patients, hyperthermia, convulsions), and circulatory collapse (Box 3.1).[4,7,24] In cardiovascular surgery specifically, unilateral and bilateral cerebral desaturations occur with catastrophic events such as acute dissection, vascular compression, inadequate anterograde cerebral perfusion, and cannula misplacement. By contrast, common perioperative factors associated with increased $rScO_2$ values are usually of lesser concern and include hypoventilation that causes cerebral vasodilation, hypertension, and hypothermia-associated decreased oxygen extraction (Box 3.2).

As $rScO_2$ perturbations often reflect a mismatch between cerebral oxygen supply and demand, they warrant a thorough and systematic evaluation. Once a possible etiology has been identified, interventions should be discussed and considered with all involved team members. Deschamps et al.[4] proposed a

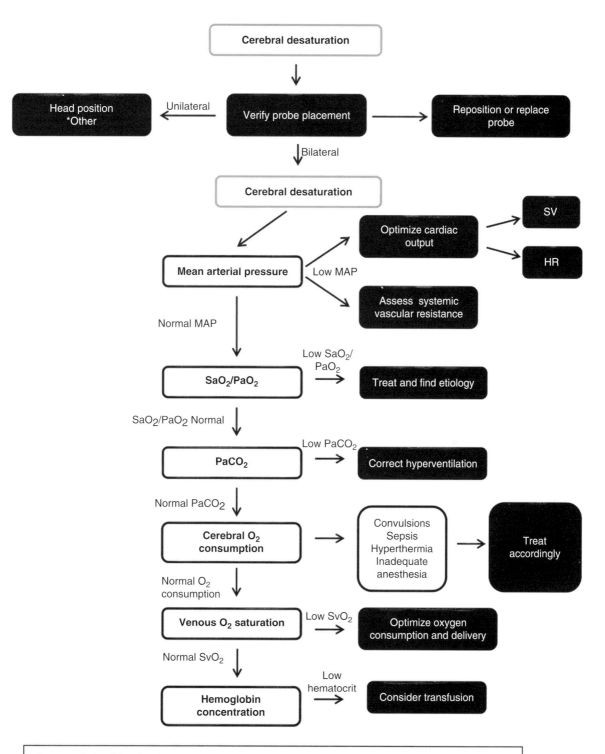

Proposed algorithm for the treatment fo cerebral desaturations
* Correlate Clinically: etiology can include cannula malposition, venous obstruction, dissection, and one-lung ventilation.

Figure 3.6 Proposed algorithm for the treatment of cerebral desaturations.

systematic approach to the correction of cerebral desaturations in patients undergoing high-risk cardiac surgery. A modified version of this intervention protocol is presented here (Figure 3.6).

Near-Infrared Spectroscopy in Clinical Practice

The relationship between cerebral tissue oxygenation and clinical outcomes has been most studied in patients undergoing cardiac surgery due to concerns regarding end-organ perfusion while on cardiopulmonary bypass (CPB).[25] As NIRS technology has become more sophisticated, its clinical use has expanded into other surgical settings such as vascular, orthopedic, and general surgery, as well as nonsurgical settings such as management of cerebral autoregulation, traumatic brain injury (TBI), and cardiopulmonary resuscitation.

Cardiopulmonary Bypass

Cardiac surgery can result in significant complications, including death, stroke, delirium, and respiratory failure. Several studies have shown associations between cerebral oxygen saturation monitoring and these events.[17,20,24,26] As previously mentioned, in patients undergoing cardiac surgery requiring CPB, low baseline and intraoperative $rScO_2$ values are associated with higher rates of mortality and other adverse outcomes, including cardiopulmonary dysfunction.[17,20]

Studies performed in patients undergoing CABG surgery suggest that an algorithmic approach to interventions to increase cerebral oxygenation can result in improved outcomes, including decreased incidence of stroke resulting in permanent loss of function,[27] better cognitive outcomes,[28,29] and less injury to other organs.[30] A retrospective, non-blinded study conducted in patients undergoing aortic arch surgery with anterograde cerebral perfusion demonstrated that cerebral oximetry desaturations predicted perioperative neurological complications.[31]

By contrast, several reviews have found no benefit of NIRS monitoring in the perioperative setting. Serraino et al. conducted a systematic review and meta-analysis involving almost 1,500 adult patients and found that the use of cerebral oximetry did not reduce brain, heart, or kidney injury during CPB.[32] A multicenter randomized controlled trial (PASPORT) did not support the use of an oximetry-based algorithm for optimization of tissue perfusion in adult cardiac surgery, as it showed no evidence of reduction in neurocognitive dysfunction or biomarkers of renal, myocardial, and neurologic injury.[33]

Carotid Endarterectomy

The rate of perioperative stroke associated with carotid endarterectomy (CEA) ranges from 1% to 6%.[34] Intraoperative hypoperfusion is one of the major causes of this devastating complication. Transcranial Doppler (TCD), electroencephalography (EEG), and NIRS have all been utilized to minimize perioperative hypoperfusion, as well as assist in the decision whether to place a carotid shunt. While EEG and TCD can be cumbersome and intrusive, NIRS offers clinicians a simple, affordable, and noninvasive method of monitoring bilateral cerebral supply during CEA. When compared to EEG and TCD, NIRS has been shown to reliably predict changes in intraoperative cerebral supply during carotid cross-clamping.[35,36] Several studies, however, failed to identify reliable $rScO_2$ cutoff values that provide reasonable sensitivity and specificity for the onset of ischemia; some authors proposed that a decrease of 20% from baseline indicates the need for intervention.[35,37] It therefore remains unclear whether cerebral oximetry alone can serve as a reliable clinical monitor during CEA. One must also consider that a false-positive identification of ischemia with $rScO_2$ monitoring may lead to unnecessary treatment with associated risk.[11,38] No well-powered studies have examined the association between NIRS data and stroke in patients undergoing CEA.[25] If cerebral oximetry were shown to have similar predictive values as other modalities, its use would be invaluable.

Orthopedic Surgery

Patients undergoing orthopedic surgery in the beach chair position are more likely to have blunted cerebral autoregulation that can lead to rare but devastating neurologic complications.[39] The use of cerebral oximetry as a monitor of adequate cerebral perfusion has been examined in beach chair positioning.[40,41] Fischer et al. reported that decreases in blood pressure during beach chair positioning were accompanied by episodes of cerebral oxygen desaturation. These desaturations resolved with the administration of phenylephrine and increases in the mean arterial pressure (MAP). The authors proposed that cerebral oximetry monitoring may be of value in the management of patients undergoing surgery in the beach chair position, in order to determine the adequacy of blood pressure at the level of the brain.[40] Murphy et al.

also reported significant reductions of cerebral oxygenation in patients undergoing surgery in the beach chair position compared to the lateral decubitus position.[41] In a literature review, Salazar et al. concluded that accurate intraoperative cerebral perfusion monitoring by cerebral oximetry or other methods (invasive blood pressure monitoring at the brain level, EEG), as well as alternatives to general anesthesia and judicious use of intraoperative blood pressure control, may improve patient safety in this patient population.[42]

General Surgery

The number of elderly patients undergoing surgical procedures requiring general anesthesia has dramatically increased over time. Because this patient population has lower physiologic reserve and more comorbidities, their risk for postoperative complications is significant. Although the brain is particularly at risk in geriatric surgical patients, it is rarely monitored. Investigations have sought to decrease the risk of post-procedural neurocognitive decline by monitoring cerebral supply and demand.[43] Thus, the association between cerebral oximetry monitoring and other outcomes has also been investigated. In a study by Casati et al., 122 elderly patients undergoing major abdominal surgery were randomized into a control group in which the anesthesiologist was blinded to the $rScO_2$ and an intervention group with their $rScO_2$ values visible and maintained above 75%. They concluded that low cerebral saturations were associated with longer post-anesthesia care unit stays and an increased rate of hospital readmissions.[43] Furthermore, the maintenance of cerebral saturations equal to or above 75% was associated with a significant reduction in hospital length of stay. In a prospective observational study, Casati et al. again demonstrated similar results, confirming an association between cerebral desaturation in the elderly undergoing abdominal surgery, postoperative cognitive decline (POCD), and a longer hospital stay.[44] While these findings are encouraging, larger prospective randomized investigations are needed. Given that these mostly observational studies were performed more than a decade ago, however, there seems to be waning enthusiasm.

Cerebral Autoregulation

Cerebral autoregulation is typically maintained between MAPs of 50–150 mmHg. The specific MAP threshold needed to ensure constant CBF for any individual patient, however, is unknown, and some data have suggested that the lower limit of CBF autoregulation is in the range of 45–80 mmHg.[45] Autoregulation is also affected by factors other than the MAP, including intracranial pressure, partial pressure of carbon dioxide, as well as a variety of brain pathologies, including traumatic injury, tumor, stroke, ruptured cerebral aneurysm, and ischemic cerebrovascular disease.[46] Even in patients with neurologic disease, there is still an optimal blood pressure range in which autoregulatory function is intact.[47] By identifying an individual's autoregulatory range, we can provide targeted and patient-specific management in a variety of perioperative settings.

It has been suggested that clinicians can generate an index of autoregulation, known as the cerebral oximetry index (COx),[45,47–49] by plotting cerebral oxygen saturation over blood pressure. More specifically, the COx is a continuous, moving Pearson's correlation coefficient to measure the strength of association between MAP and cerebral oximetry values.[45] A value that approaches zero indicates CBF autoregulation, while values closer to 1 indicate dysregulation. Several authors have concluded that loss of autoregulation due to hypotension can be accurately assessed by the COx for patients with acute brain injury and those undergoing CPB.[45,48,50] The COx potentially has value in traditional intraoperative settings and postoperative critical care settings, but further investigation is needed.

Postoperative Cognitive Decline

Many non-neurosurgical procedures are associated with a risk for POCD, particularly cardiac surgery. Cerebral hypoperfusion is a major risk factor for POCD;[51,52] therefore, as a noninvasive monitor of cerebral supply, NIRS has the potential to be valuable in guiding therapy and possibly preventing POCD. A number of studies have found an association between cerebral desaturation events and POCD in cardiac surgery patients. In an observational study by Yao et al., multivariate data analysis suggested that time spent at cerebral saturations less than 40% predicted cognitive deficits.[53] Several smaller studies have demonstrated that low $rScO_2$ during CPB was associated with POCD[54] and that maintenance with a higher $rScO_2$ during CPB was associated with a lower incidence of POCD.[55] In contrast, Hong et al. found that low intraoperative cerebral saturations were unrelated to POCD in cardiac surgery patients.[56] Furthermore, a review of six studies of 962 patients in total presented moderate-quality evidence that NIRS monitoring is not associated with decreased incidence of POCD at one week post-surgery.[57] The use of perioperative cerebral NIRS monitoring to decrease the occurrence of POCD, therefore, is not supported by the existing evidence.

Cardiopulmonary Resuscitation

Advanced cardiac life support (ACLS) is often delivered without 100% compliance to guidelines. Inadequate rate and depth of chest compressions, combined with errors in medication administration, continue to be problems, despite extensively developed evidence-based guidelines and considerable provider education and training. Methods to improve the quality of ACLS are continually being investigated in an effort to improve patient outcomes.[58] It has been proposed that cerebral oximetry may be used to monitor ACLS adequacy.[59,60] This field is in its infancy, but investigators have demonstrated that higher cerebral oximetry saturations are associated with better neurologic outcomes, and that mean $rScO_2$ values over the course of the ACLS are more strongly correlated with the return of spontaneous circulation than the initial $rScO_2$ values.[61,62] It has been suggested that a sustained inability to achieve cerebral saturations greater than 30% could be included in the criteria for ceasing ACLS efforts.[62] There is no evidence, however, that the cerebral saturation data can be used to successfully guide ACLS, as the studies are primarily observational.

Traumatic Brain Injury

Near-infrared spectroscopy has been used to predict and assess the impact of goal-directed treatment in patients with TBI.[63] Rosenthal et al. compared jugular bulb venous measurements with NIRS in an attempt to provide an accurate estimation of cerebral oxygenation. They concluded that measuring regional cerebral tissue oxygenation by NIRS was feasible in patients with severe TBI and could provide an estimation of cerebral oxygenation status in a noninvasive manner.[63] There is a need for larger-scale studies examining the utility of NIRS monitoring to predict clinical outcomes in the complex physiologic state of TBI.[25,64]

Conclusion

Novel medical technologies need to be investigated and scrutinized prior to their acceptance into clinical practice, and cerebral oximetry is no exception. While many technologies measure variables heretofore impossible to obtain, or may noninvasively measure variables that previously required interventional or impractical complex methods, the standard for acceptance into practice is increasingly an improved outcome driven by use of the technology. Routine NIRS use remains controversial despite a significant market penetrance in cardiac surgery and increasing use in other procedures (e.g., carotid endarterectomy). While some studies suggest that NIRS monitoring and NIRS-guided interventions may decrease cerebral injury and improve neurological outcomes, others do not support its ubiquitous use and officially the "jury is still out."

References

1. Torres J, Ishida K. Neuroprotection after major cardiovascular surgery. *Curr Treat Options Neurol* 2015;**17**(7):28.

2. Costa MA, Gauer MF, Gomes RZ, Schafranski MD. Risk factors for perioperative ischemic stroke in cardiac surgery. *Rev Bras Cir Cardiovasc* 2015;**30**(3):365–72.

3. Andersen ND, Hart SA, Devendra GP, et al. Atheromatous disease of the aorta and perioperative stroke. *J Thorac Cardiovasc Surg* 2018;**155**(2):508–16.

4. Deschamps A, Hall R, Grocott H, et al. Cerebral oximetry monitoring to maintain normal cerebral oxygen saturation during high-risk cardiac surgery. *Anesthesiology* 2016;**124**(4):826–36.

5. Nielsen HB. Systematic review of near-infrared spectroscopy determined cerebral oxygenation during non-cardiac surgery. *Front Physiol* 2014;**5**:93.

6. Jöbsis FF. Noninvasive, infrared monitoring of cerebral and myocardial oxygen sufficiency and circulatory parameters. *Science* 1977;**198**(4323):1264–7.

7. Fischer GW, Silvay G. Cerebral oximetry in cardiac and major vascular surgery. *HSR Proc Intensive Care Cardiovasc Anesth* 2010;**2**(4):249–56.

8. Green DW, Kunst G. Cerebral oximetry and its role in adult cardiac, non-cardiac surgery and resuscitation from cardiac arrest. *Anaesthesia* 2017;**72**:48–57.

9. Smythe PR, Samra SK. Monitors of cerebral oxygenation. *Anesthesiol Clin North Am* 2002;**20**(2):293–313.

10. Tosh W, Patteril M. Cerebral oximetry. *BJA Educ* 2016;**16**(12):417–21.

11. Steppan J, Hogue CW Jr. Cerebral and tissue oximetry. *Best Pract Res Clin Anaesthesiol* 2014;**28**(4):429–39.

12. Ghosh A, Elwell C, Smith M. Cerebral near-infrared spectroscopy in adults. *Anesth Analg* 2012;**115**(6):1373–83.

13. Davie SN, Grocott HP. Impact of extracranial contamination on regional cerebral oxygen saturation: a comparison of three cerebral oximetry technologies. *Anesthesiology* 2012;**116**(4):834–40.

14. Kobayashi K, Kitamura T, Kohira S, et al. Factors associated with a low initial cerebral oxygen saturation value in patients undergoing cardiac surgery. *J Artif Organs* 2017;**20**(2):110–6.

15. Madsen PL, Nielsen HB, Christiansen P. Well-being and cerebral oxygen saturation during acute heart failure in humans. *Clin Physiol* 2000;**20**(2):158–64.

16. Paquet C, Deschamps A, Denault AY, et al. Baseline regional cerebral oxygen saturation correlates with left ventricular systolic and diastolic function. *J Cardiothorac Vasc Anesth* 2008;**22**(6):840–6.

17. Sun X, Ellis J, Corso PJ, et al. Mortality predicted by preinduction cerebral oxygen saturation after cardiac operation. *Ann Thorac Surg* 2014;**98**:91–6.

18. Wen SYB, Peng AZY, Boyle S, et al. A pilot study using preoperative cerebral tissue oxygen saturation to stratify cardiovascular risk in major non-cardiac surgery. *Anaesth Intensive Care* 2017;**45**(2):202–9.

19. Lei L, Katznelson R, Fedorko L, et al. Cerebral oximetry and postoperative delirium after cardiac surgery: a randomised, controlled trial. *Anaesthesia* 2017;**72**(12):1456–66.

20. Heringlake M, Garbers C, Käbler JH, et al. Preoperative cerebral oxygen saturation and clinical outcomes in cardiac surgery. *Anesthesiology* 2011;**114**(1):58–69.

21. Ghosal S, Trivedi J, Chen J, et al. Regional cerebral oxygen saturation level predicts 30-day mortality rate after left ventricular assist device surgery. *J Cardiothorac Vasc Anesth* 2018;**32**(3):1185–90.

22. Thavasothy M, Broadhead M, Elwell C, Peters M, Smith M. A comparison of cerebral oxygenation as measured by the NIRO 300 and the INVOS 5100 near-infrared spectrophotometers. *Anaesthesia* 2002;**57**(10):999–1006.

23. Deschamps A, Lambert J, Couture P, et al. Reversal of decreases in cerebral saturation in high-risk cardiac surgery. *J Cardiothorac Vasc Anesth* 2013;**27**(6):1260–6.

24. Vretzakis G, Georgopoulou S, Stamoulis K, et al. Cerebral oximetry in cardiac anesthesia. *J Thorac Dis* 2014;**6**(Suppl 1):S60–9.

25. Bickler P, Feiner J, Rollins M, Meng L. Tissue oximetry and clinical outcomes. *Anesth Analg* 2017;**124**(1):72–82.

26. Fischer GW, Lin HM, Krol M, et al. Noninvasive cerebral oxygenation may predict outcome in patients undergoing aortic arch surgery. *J Thorac Cardiovasc Surg* 2011;**141**(3):815–21.

27. Goldman S, Sutter F, Ferdinand F, Trace C. Optimizing intraoperative cerebral oxygen delivery using noninvasive cerebral oximetry decreases the incidence of stroke for cardiac surgical patients. *Heart Surg Forum* 2004;**7**(5):E376–81.

28. Slater JP, Guarino T, Stack J, et al. Cerebral oxygen desaturation predicts cognitive decline and longer hospital stay after cardiac surgery. *Ann Thorac Surg* 2009;**87**(1):36–45.

29. Colak Z, Borojevic M, Bogovic A, Ivancan V, Biocina B, Majeric-Kogler V. Influence of intraoperative cerebral oximetry monitoring on neurocognitive function after coronary artery bypass surgery: a randomized, prospective study. *Eur J Cardiothoracic Surg* 2015;**47**(3):447–54.

30. Murkin JM, Adams SJ, Novick RJ, et al. Monitoring brain oxygen saturation during coronary bypass surgery: a randomized, prospective study. *Anesth Analg* 2007;**104**(1):51–8.

31. Olsson C, Thelin S. Regional cerebral saturation monitoring with near-infrared spectroscopy during selective antegrade cerebral perfusion: diagnostic performance and relationship to postoperative stroke. *J Thorac Cardiovasc Surg* 2006;**131**(2):371–9.

32. Serraino GF, Murphy GJ. Effects of cerebral near-infrared spectroscopy on the outcome of patients undergoing cardiac surgery: a systematic review of randomised trials. *BMJ Open* 2017;**7**(9):e016613.

33. Rogers CA, Stoica S, Ellis L, et al. Randomized trial of near-infrared spectroscopy for personalized optimization of cerebral tissue oxygenation during cardiac surgery. *Br J Anaesth* 2017;**119**(3):384–93.

34. Wu TY, Anderson NE, Barber PA. Neurological complications of carotid revascularisation. *J Neurol Neurosurg Psychiatry* 2012;**83**(5):543–50.

35. Cho JW, Jang JS. Near-infrared spectroscopy versus transcranial Doppler-based monitoring in carotid endarterectomy. *Korean J Thorac Cardiovasc Surg* 2017;**50**(6):448–52.

36. Perez W, Dukatz C, El-Dalati S, et al. Cerebral oxygenation and processed EEG response to clamping and shunting during carotid endarterectomy under general anesthesia. *J Clin Monit Comput* 2015;**29**(6):713–20.

37. Mauermann WJ, Crepeau AZ, Pulido JN, et al. Comparison of electroencephalography and cerebral oximetry to determine the need for in-line arterial shunting in patients undergoing carotid

endarterectomy. *J Cardiothorac Vasc Anesth* 2013;**27**(6):1253–9.

38. Pennekamp CWA, Bots ML, Kappelle LJ, Moll FL, de Borst GJ. The value of near-infrared spectroscopy measured cerebral oximetry during carotid endarterectomy in perioperative stroke prevention. A review. *Eur J Vasc Endovasc Surg* 2009;**38**(5):539–45.

39. Laflam A, Joshi B, Brady K, et al. Shoulder surgery in the beach chair position is associated with diminished cerebral autoregulation but no differences in postoperative cognition or brain injury biomarker levels compared with supine positioning: the anesthesia patient safety foundation beach chair study. *Anesth Analg* 2015;**120**(1):176–85.

40. Fischer GW, Torrillo TM, Weiner MM, Rosenblatt MA. The use of cerebral oximetry as a monitor of the adequacy of cerebral perfusion in a patient undergoing shoulder surgery in the beach chair position. *Pain Pract* 2009;**9**(4):304–7.

41. Murphy GS, Szokol JW, Marymont JH, et al. Cerebral oxygen desaturation events assessed by near-infrared spectroscopy during shoulder arthroscopy in the beach chair and lateral decubitus positions. *Anesth Analg* 2010;**111**(2):496–505.

42. Salazar D, Hazel A, Tauchen AJ, Sears BW, Marra G. Neurocognitive deficits and cerebral desaturation during shoulder arthroscopy with patient in beach-chair position: a review of the current literature. *Am J Orthop (Belle Mead NJ)* 2016;**45**(3):E63–8.

43. Casati A, Fanelli G, Pietropaoli P, et al. Continuous monitoring of cerebral oxygen saturation in elderly patients undergoing major abdominal surgery minimizes brain exposure to potential hypoxia. *Anesth Analg* 2005;**101**(3):740–7.

44. Casati A, Fanelli G, Pietropaoli P, et al. Monitoring cerebral oxygen saturation in elderly patients undergoing general abdominal surgery: a prospective cohort study. *Eur J Anaesthesiol* 2007;**24**(1):59.

45. Brady K, Joshi B, Zweifel C, et al. Real-time continuous monitoring of cerebral blood flow autoregulation using near-infrared spectroscopy in patients undergoing cardiopulmonary bypass. *Stroke* 2010;**41**(9):1951–6.

46. Tameem A, Krovvidi H. Cerebral physiology. *Contin Educ Anaesth Crit Care Pain* 2013;**13**(4):113–8.

47. Moerman A, De Hert S. Recent advances in cerebral oximetry. Assessment of cerebral autoregulation with near-infrared spectroscopy: myth or reality? *F1000Research* 2017;**6**:1615.

48. Joshi B, Ono M, Brown C, et al. Predicting the limits of cerebral autoregulation during cardiopulmonary bypass. *Anesth Analg* 2012;**114**(3):503–10.

49. Steiner LA, Pfister D, Strebel SP, Radolovich D, Smielewski P, Czosnyka M. Near-infrared spectroscopy can monitor dynamic cerebral autoregulation in adults. *Neurocrit Care* 2009;**10**(1):122–8.

50. Brady KM, Lee JK, Kibler KK, et al. Continuous time-domain analysis of cerebrovascular autoregulation using near-infrared spectroscopy. *Stroke* 2007;**38**(10):2818–25.

51. Pappa M, Theodosiadis N, Tsounis A, Sarafis P. Pathogenesis and treatment of post-operative cognitive dysfunction. *Electron Physician* 2017;**9**(2):3768–75.

52. Messerotti Benvenuti S, Zanatta P, Longo C, Mazzarolo AP, Palomba D. Preoperative cerebral hypoperfusion in the left, not in the right, hemisphere is associated with cognitive decline after cardiac surgery. *Psychosom Med* 2012;**74**(1):73–80.

53. Yao FS, Tseng CC, Ho CY, Levin SK, Illner P. Cerebral oxygen desaturation is associated with early postoperative neuropsychological dysfunction in patients undergoing cardiac surgery. *J Cardiothorac Vasc Anesth* 2004;**18**(5):552–8.

54. Fudickar A, Peters S, Stapelfeldt C, et al. Postoperative cognitive deficit after cardiopulmonary bypass with preserved cerebral oxygenation: a prospective observational pilot study. *BMC Anesthesiol* 2011;**11**(1):7.

55. Colak Z, Borojevic M, Bogovic A, Ivancan V, Biocina B, Majeric-Kogler V. Influence of intraoperative cerebral oximetry monitoring on neurocognitive function after coronary artery bypass surgery: a randomized, prospective study. *Eur J Cardiothoracic Surg* 2015;**47**(3):447–54.

56. Hong SW, Shim JK, Choi YS, Kim DH, Chang BC, Kwak YL. Prediction of cognitive dysfunction and patients' outcome following valvular heart surgery and the role of cerebral oximetry. *Eur J Cardiothoracic Surg* 2008;**33**(4):560–5.

57. Yu Y, Zhang K, Zhang L, Zong H, Meng L, Han R. Cerebral near-infrared spectroscopy (NIRS) for perioperative monitoring of brain oxygenation in children and adults. *Cochrane Database Syst Rev* 2018;**1**:CD010947.

58. Sutton RM, Nadkarni V, Abella BS. Putting it all together to improve resuscitation quality. *Emerg Med Clin North Am* 2012;**30**(1):105–22.

59. Genbrugge C, Dens J, Meex I, et al. Regional cerebral oximetry during cardiopulmonary resuscitation: useful or useless? *J Emerg Med* 2016;**50**(1):198–207.

60. Ibrahim AW, Trammell AR, Austin H, et al. Cerebral oximetry as a real-time monitoring tool to assess

quality of in-hospital cardiopulmonary resuscitation and post cardiac arrest care. *J Am Heart Assoc* 2015;**4** (8):e001859.

61. Sinha N, Parnia S. Monitoring the brain after cardiac arrest: a new era. *Curr Neurol Neurosci Rep* 2017;**17** (8):62.

62. Cournoyer A, Iseppon M, Chauny JM, Denault A, Cossette S, Notebaert É. Near-infrared spectroscopy monitoring during cardiac arrest: a systematic review

and meta-analysis. *Acad Emerg Med* 2016;**23**(8):851–62.

63. Rosenthal G, Furmanov A, Itshayek E, Shoshan Y, Singh V. Assessment of a noninvasive cerebral oxygenation monitor in patients with severe traumatic brain injury. *J Neurosurg* 2014;**120**(4):901–7.

64. Weigl W, Milej D, Janusek D, et al. Application of optical methods in the monitoring of traumatic brain injury: A review. *J Cereb Blood Flow Metab* 2016;**36**(11):1825–43.

The Oxygen Reserve Index

Andrew B. Leibowitz

The introduction of pulse oximetry into operating room and intensive care units in the early 1980s was revolutionary. In 1986 pulse oximetry became the American Society of Anesthesiologists formal standard for intra-operative monitoring,[1] and in 1988 it was referred to as the "fifth vital sign."[2] Real-time continuous noninvasive measurement of the pulse oxygen saturation (SpO_2) is now so ingrained in our practice that it is hard to imagine an era when physicians relied on patient skin color to assess the adequacy of oxygenation. Intuitively, SpO_2 was so useful that even when a large study published in the journal *Anesthesiology* reported no difference in outcomes in over 20,000 surgical patients randomly assigned to monitoring with versus without oximetry, it did not deter its widespread acceptance.[3]

In brief review, pulse oximetry relies on light-emitting diodes (LEDs) that emit at least two wavelengths of light, typically a red wavelength of 660 nm and an infrared wavelength of 905 or 940 nm. These wavelengths of light are absorbed to different degrees by oxygenated (oxyhemoglobin) and deoxygenated (reduced hemoglobin) hemoglobin. A photodiode used to measure the amount of absorbed light is positioned opposite the LEDs, usually on the other side of a finger or earlobe, and resultant light that reaches it allows for the calculation of the ratio of the two absorbed wavelengths. This ratio is then converted to SpO_2 using a lookup table created by measuring the ratios in volunteers whose saturations were altered from 100% to 70% by breathing increasingly hypoxic gas mixtures. Pulse oximeters are designed to measure the absorbance of these wavelengths in the pulsatile arterial blood by filtering out the signal contributed by venous blood and other tissues, and in many models motion artifact. Additional wavelengths of light may also be incorporated, in order to noninvasively and continuously determine the percent concentration of total hemoglobin ($SpHb^*$),

methemoglobin ($SpMet^*$), and carboxyhemoglobin ($SpCO^*$).

Pulse oximetry, however, has limitations: (1) its accuracy is ± 1.5–4% compared to arterial oxygen saturation (SaO_2) measured by a CO oximeter utilizing multiwavelength spectrophotometry of a blood sample;[4,5] (2) an $SpO_2 \geq 98\%$ may represent arterial oxygen tension (PaO_2) between 75 mmHg and 650 mmHg (e.g., on a FiO_2 of 1.0), so decreases in PaO_2 from 650 mmHg to 75 mmHg may go undetected while the SpO_2 remains in a reassuring $\geq 94\%$–98% range; (3) the relationship between PaO_2 and SaO_2 is not linear but sigmoidal, thus when the PaO_2 is 60 mmHg and the SpO_2 is 90% at the inflection point of the O_2 hemoglobin dissociation curve, the PaO_2 and SpO_2 may decline rapidly without a clinically predictable nadir (see Figure 4.1); and (4) it is difficult to predict the time to significant desaturation to SpO_2 less than 90% during apnea or rapid changes in ventilation and perfusion, particularly in certain high-risk patients.

Use of current monitoring technology to help avoid desaturation has cardiopulmonary physiologic limitations too. In the operating room, measurement of end tidal expired O_2 is used during pre-oxygenation to assess denitrogenation of the functional residual volume and maximize O_2 reserve in order to increase the time to desaturation during apnea. The success of a strategy aimed toward optimizing end tidal expired O_2, however, may be altered by reduced functional residual capacity (FRC), increased closing capacity-FRC ratio, increased O_2 consumption, and decreased O_2-carrying capacity, each of which independently changes the rate of decline in the PaO_2 and SpO_2 during apnea and thereby complicates the accurate estimation of time to desaturation. These perturbations occur quite frequently in obese patients, as well as in emergency intubations and critically ill patients where continuous changes in ventilation

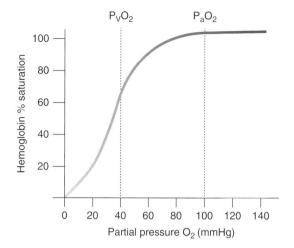

Figure 4.1 Oxygen hemoglobin saturation curve highlighting the typical mixed venous partial pressure of oxygen (PvO$_2$) and arterial oxygen tension (PaO$_2$) ranges.

and perfusion due to extreme and acute respiratory and circulatory compromise are more common.[6,7] Not only do they experience greater risk of rapid decline in PaO$_2$ and SpO$_2$, but they also have an associated increased risk of morbidity and mortality.[8] Children are also at greater risk of rapid decline in PaO$_2$ and SpO$_2$ during apnea because their relative consumption-reserve ratio is greater than that of adults.

A warning that hypoxemia is imminent would potentially be a useful addition to standard pulse oximetry and capnometry. The association between PaO$_2$ and SpO$_2$ decreases and increased morbidity and mortality during emergency intubations suggests that the ability to predict the time to desaturation to a hypoxemic range may result in better real-time management and improved outcomes. This capability would complement the myriad functionality that has been engineered into pulse oximeters since their inception, such as reduction of motion artifact, assessment of pulse pressure variation, detection of dyshemoglobins, and miniaturization.

Newer technology aims to overcome the limitations of pulse oximetry outlined above by measurement of an oxygen reserve index (ORi). The ORi is determined from the very small changes to the absorption pattern of blood in states where the SpO$_2$ is $\geq$ 98%. While the ratio of the difference in absorbance to the traditional red and infrared wavelengths decreases as the oxygen saturation reaches 100%, the moderate hyperoxic region of the oxygen dissociation curve in the PaO$_2$ of 100–200 mmHg range provides a detectable change in absorbance signals utilizing other wavelengths of light in addition to the standard 660 and 905 or 940 nm. Currently, above that range, no usable absorbance signals have been detected.

Masimo pulse CO oximeters use additional wavelengths of light and advanced signal processing to collect optical absorbance information that enables them to resolve extremely small differences in absorbance in the PaO$_2$ 100–200 mmHg range. The signal is then processed and expressed as a unitless ORi value from 0.0 (no reserve) to 1.0 (good or "much" reserve). In the original publication in 2014 the ORi scale was 100–200, reflecting the original focus on the utility of this new index associated with changes in this PaO$_2$ range.[9]

Devices with this functionality do not have FDA 510(k) clearance and are not available for purchase in the United States, but they are commercially available in Japan and countries that require CE marking. In a very recent study, 20 healthy volunteers breathing gas mixtures ranging from hypoxemic to hyperoxic had their ORi and PaO$_2$ simultaneously measured, yielding 1,090 paired data points.[10] The ORi trended the PaO$_2$ within the 100–200 mmHg range with a concordance of 94%, and the ORi predicted a PaO$_2$ less than 100 mmHg with an area under the curve of 0.91.

While avoidance of hypoxemia has been a dominant clinical focus since the advent of arterial blood gas analysis, the ORi potentially may also be used to prevent hyperoxia without the need for arterial blood gas analysis and reduce the exposure to harmful oxygen supplementation, a long-recognized risk in newborns and more recently appreciated risk in post-resuscitative states.

Much of the attention to this technology's potential has focused on the time taken for patients to desaturate to an SpO$_2$ 94%–98%, versus the time to the start of an ORi alarm triggered by either a decrease to an absolute value or a rate of change, or both. The difference in time between the actual desaturation versus the alarm preceding the desaturation is referred to by Masimo as the "increase in the warning time," but alternatively it might be considered as a clinical "window of opportunity" to intervene.

Szmuk et al. tested the hypothesis that the ORi provides warning of impending desaturation during induction of anesthesia.[11] Twenty-five pediatric surgical patients aged 7.6 ± 4.6 years with the American Society of Anesthesiologists physical status I and II

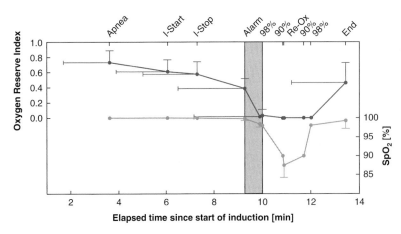

Figure 4.2 The ORi and SpO$_2$ values at different times of study. I-Start = beginning of intubation; I-Stop = end of intubation; Alarm = start of the oxygen reserve alarm; Re-Ox = reoxygenation; End = end of recording. The *points* and *error bars* represent mean (SD) values. Reproduced with permission from Szmuk P, Steiner JW, Olomu PN, Ploski RP, Sessler DI, Ezri T. Oxygen reserve index: A novel noninvasive measure of oxygen reserve – A pilot study. *Anesthesiology* 2016;124(4):779–84.

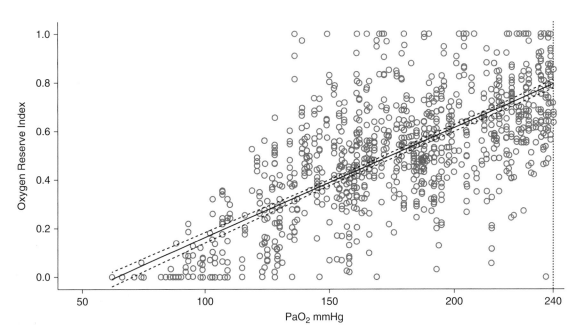

Figure 4.3 Plot of ORi compared with arterial PaO$_2$ obtained from 106 patients undergoing surgery in whom measured PaO$_2$ from 485 arterial blood gas analyses was between 62 and 534 mmHg. Patients had more than one sensor applied, with analysis done using 1,594 ORi values. Locally weighted regression analysis showed a nonlinear relationship overall, with a more positive relationship for PaO$_2$ up to 240 mmHg compared to > 240 mmHg.

Reproduced with permission from Applegate RL II, Dorotta IL, Wells B, Juma D, Applegate PM. The relationship between oxygen reserve index and arterial partial pressure of oxygen during surgery. *Anesth Analg* 2016;123(3):626–33.

were pre-oxygenated, general anesthesia was induced, the trachea intubated, the anesthesia circuit was disconnected, and the oxygen saturation was allowed to decrease to 90% before resuming ventilation. The ORi slowly decreased over a mean apneic period of 5.9 ± 3.1 minutes, from 0.73 ± 0.16 to 0.37 ± 0.11, while the SpO$_2$ remained at 100% (see Figure 4.2). The ORi alarm was triggered by its fractional rate of change

in a median of 31.5 seconds (interquartile range 19–34.3) before the SpO$_2$ decreased to 98%.

Applegate et al. investigated the relationship between the ORi and PaO$_2$ during surgery in 106 patients who had simultaneous arterial blood gas analysis and ORi monitoring, and found a correlation between the ORi and PaO$_2$ of $r^2 = 0.546$ (see Figure 4.3).[12] An ORi > 0.55 indicated a PaO$_2 \geq 150$ mmHg, and an ORi > 0.24 indicated a PaO_2 of about 100 mmHg. The findings also suggested that an ORi decrease to 0.24 may provide an increase in the warning time when the SpO_2 is greater than 98%.

In an abstract presented at the International Anesthesia Research Society (IARS) in 2017, Lee et al. studied 40 critically ill adult patients undergoing elective surgery requiring tracheal intubation; 33 completed the study and had their data compositely analyzed, excluding 4 outliers considered separately.[13] The time from the ORi alarm triggered by a "decrease in the absolute value and rate of change" to the time the SpO_2 was 94% was compared to the time taken for the SpO_2 to decrease from 98% to 94%. The increase in warning time was considered to be the time difference between the ORi alarm start to the time when the SpO_2 was 98%. The average time from the ORi alarm until an SpO_2 of 94% was 80 ± 38 seconds (range 29–227), while the average time for SpO_2 to decrease from 98% to 94% was 46 ± 23 seconds (range 12–108). The increase in warning time was 34 ± 23 seconds (range 4–119), or on a percentage basis 96 ± 92% (range 5%–479%)

These investigations demonstrate that in specific circumstances the ORi may be used to increase the warning time to impending desaturation or, at least, desaturation to $SpO_2 \leq 98\%$. These findings, however, require further consideration of several points before adopting this technology into general practice. Assuming the investigations published thus far are accurate in their findings, it is unclear whether a 30–40 second advanced warning that the SpO_2 will decrease to ≤ 98% is clinically advantageous. It is even conceivable that such an advanced warning may be harmful. Interruption of tracheal intubation (which has a success rate greater than 99%) in order to address the alarm by resumption of mask ventilation or other maneuvers may delay time to intubation, increase the risk of airway management failure, increase time spent in the hypoxemic zone, and increase risk for trauma and aspiration.

Further investigation is necessary by a randomized controlled trial comparing this technology versus standard pulse oximetry in patient groups with high rates of hypoxemia complicating intubation, as is the case for intubations done under emergent conditions and in intensive care units. Outcomes of interest would be incidence and time of SpO_2 less than 90%, hemodynamic instability, morbidity including airway injury and aspiration, and mortality. None of the studies performed thus far have occurred in these environments or evaluated patient outcomes.

Both the fundamental principle of detecting very small changes in light absorption using multiple wavelengths and the new advanced signal processing underlying this technology are enticing. The clinical value of detecting such minimal changes, given the known limitations of SpO_2 measurement (i.e., accurate to ± 1.5–4% in arterial blood), and using that change in a proprietary algorithm to estimate the PaO_2 between 100 mmHg and 200 mmHg, requires more evidence, especially under real-world conditions. Common potential confounding factors include:

(1) Anemia and polycythemia
(2) Shifts in the oxygen–hemoglobin dissociation curve due to acid base balance, temperature, and 2,3-diphosphoglycerate (2,3-DPG) levels
(3) Increased cardiac output states
(4) Increased oxygen consumption
(5) Poor peripheral circulation impacting both SpO_2 and ORi measurement
(6) Skin pigmentation and tissue absorption in the ORi range may be greater sources of error than in the typical SaO_2 range
(7) Pre-oxygenation efforts that do not reliably increase the PaO_2 to ≥ 200 mmHg (a common finding in intensive care patients) would predictably result in a shorter indeterminate warning time and void the potential benefit of this early alarm
(8) The impact of dyshemoglobins on the absorption of these new wavelengths of light has not been reported

Routine use of this technology, however, may lead to a change in customary practice once the warning time is understood in the context of observed results. For example, while the premise of pre-oxygenation was a known physiologic concept, after routine measurement of end tidal oxygen became available, correct application of a face mask and the time needed to achieve optimal denitrogenation were widely appreciated, and even in the absence of the monitor these improved practices would contribute a safety margin. Although studies have not demonstrated a relationship between SpO_2 monitoring and outcomes, simply using SpO_2 monitors may have led to better management in hundreds of millions of anesthetics once previously unobserved phenomena were appreciated and customary practice changed as a result. In essence, using the pulse oximeter was like simulator training that allowed persons to learn from near misses and incorporate changes in management that prevented harm even when the monitor was not used.

In conclusion, the ORi is an interesting innovation with the potential to improve patient care. The literature thus far is preliminary, with only a few small studies that have varied in terms of patient populations and alarm triggers (i.e., an absolute value versus a rate of change, or both) and no study of clinical outcomes. It is necessary to determine if this alarm function results in a reduced incidence or severity of desaturation, particularly in high-risk patients. The underlying physiologic assumptions may be limited by common pathologies, and this also requires investigation. Further, the algorithm and technology require more detailed understanding in order for clinicians to have confidence in a displayed ORi's utility. Nonetheless, development of the ORi is an advance and reveals that the limits of pulse oximeter technology have not yet been reached, despite the fact that they have been a bedside staple for more than 30 years.

References

1. American Society of Anesthesiologists: standards for basic intraoperative monitoring. *Anesth Patient Safety Newslett* 1987;**2**(1):1–8.

2. Neff TA. Routine oximetry: a fifth vital sign. *Chest* 1988;**9**:277.

3. Moller JT, Johannessen NW, Espersen H, et al. Randomized evaluation of pulse oximetry in 20,802 patients. *Anesthesiology* 1993;**78**:436–53.

4. Milner QJ, Mathews RG. An assessment of the accuracy of pulse oximeters. *Anaesthesia* 2012;**67**:396–401.

5. Chan ED, Chan MM, Chan MM. Pulse oximetry: understanding its basic principles facilitates appreciation of its limitations. *Respir Medicine* 2013;**107**:789–99.

6. Peppard PE, Ward NR, Morrell MJ. The impact of obesity on oxygen desaturation during sleep-disordered breathing. *Am J Respir Crit Care Med* 2009;**180**;788–93.

7. Leibowitz AB. Persistent preoxygenation efforts before tracheal intubation in the intensive care unit are of no use: who would have guessed? *Crit Care Med* 2009;**37**(1):335–6.

8. Jaber S, Amraoui J, Lefrant JY, et al. Clinical practice and risk factors for immediate complication of endotracheal intubation in the intensive care unit: a prospective multiple-center study. *Crit Care Med* 2006;**34**;2355–61.

9. Szmuk P, Steiner JW, Olomu PN, Curuz JD, Sessler D. Oxygen reserve index – a new, noninvasive method of oxygen reserve measurement. October 14, 2014 American Society of Anesthesiologists Annual Meeting, New Orleans, LA Abstract BOC12.

10. Vos JJ, Willems CH, Van Amsterdam K, et al. Oxygen reserve index: validation of a new variable. *Anesth Analg* 2019:**129**(s):409–15.

11. Szmuk P, Steiner JW, Olomu PN, Ploski RP, Sessler DI, Ezri T. Oxygen reserve index: a novel noninvasive measure of oxygen reserve – A pilot study. *Anesthesiology* 2016;**124**(4):779–84.

12. Applegate RL II, Dorotta IL, Wells B, Juma D, Applegate PM. The relationship between oxygen reserve index and arterial partial pressure of oxygen during surgery. *Anesth Analg* 2016;**123**(3):626–33.

13. Lee L, Singh A, Applegate R, Fleming N. *Oxygen Reserve Index: An Early Warning for Desaturation in Critically Ill Patients*. Proceedings from the 2017 IARS Annual Meeting, Washington, DC. Abstract #A1406.

Point-of-Care Transesophageal Echocardiography

Ronald A. Kahn

Introduction

Transesophageal echocardiography (TEE) was introduced into anesthesiology practice in the late 1980s before becoming a standard in cardiac anesthesiology within the following decade. Slowly it has spread outside of the cardiac operating rooms and is frequently used in other high-risk operations, in patients with significant cardiac disease undergoing only moderate risk surgery, and in intensive care units. All perioperative physicians, even those not adept at personally performing TEE, should have a working knowledge of the TEE principles and practice.

Technical Concepts

The complex physics of ultrasound may be reviewed in detail elsewhere, but the salient concepts are as follows.[1] An ultrasound beam is a continuous or intermittent train of sound waves emitted by a transducer or wave generator. Ultrasound waves are characterized by their wavelength, frequency, and velocity. *Wavelength* is the distance between the two nearest points of equal pressure or density in an ultrasound beam, and *velocity* is the speed at which the waves propagate through a medium. The number of cycles per second (hertz) is called the *frequency* of the wave. The relationship among the frequency (*f*), wavelength (λ), and velocity (*v*) of a sound wave is defined by the formula:

$$v = f \times \lambda$$

Because the frequency of an ultrasound beam is determined by the properties of the emitting transducer, and the velocity is a function of the tissue density through which the sound travels, wavelengths vary according to the relationship expressed in the above equation.

Ultrasound waves are reflections when the width of the reflecting object is larger than one-fourth of the ultrasound wavelength. To visualize smaller objects, ultrasound waves of shorter wavelengths must be used. Because the velocity of sound in soft tissue is approximately constant, shorter wavelengths are obtained by increasing the frequency of the ultrasound beam. The ultrasonic impedance of a structure (density times the ultrasound velocity through the structure) must be significantly different from the ultrasonic impedance of surrounding structures, otherwise ultrasound cannot distinguish the different structures. The ultrasound impedances of air and bone are significantly different from that of blood. Ultrasound is strongly reflected from air and bone, thereby limiting the ability of ultrasound to visualize structures deep to them.

Most modern echo scanners combine Doppler capabilities with their two–dimensional (2D) imaging capabilities. In pulsed-wave (PW) Doppler, blood flow parameters can be determined at precise locations within the heart by emitting repetitive short bursts of ultrasound at a specific frequency (pulse repetition frequency, or PRF) and analyzing the frequency shift of the reflected echoes at an identical sampling frequency (f_s). The trade-off for the ability to measure flow at precise locations is that ambiguous information is obtained when flow velocity is very high. By contrast, continuous-wave (CW) Doppler technique uses continuous, rather than discrete, pulses of ultrasound waves. As a result, the region in which flow dynamics are measured cannot be precisely localized. Blood flow velocity is measured with great accuracy, however, even at high flows.

During color flow Doppler (CFD) mapping, real-time blood flow within the heart is displayed in colors, along with 2D images in black and white. In addition to showing the location, direction, and velocity of

35

cardiac blood flow, the images produced by these devices allow estimation of flow acceleration and differentiation of laminar and turbulent blood flow. Color flow Doppler echocardiography is based on the principle of multi-gated, PW Doppler where blood flow velocities are sampled at many locations along many lines covering the entire imaging sector. At the same time, the sector is also scanned to generate a 2D image.

Complications and Contraindications

Complications resulting from intraoperative TEE can be separated into two groups: injury from direct trauma to the airway and esophagus, and indirect effects of TEE. In the first group, potential complications include esophageal bleeding, burning, tearing, dysphagia, and laryngeal discomfort. Many of these complications could result from pressure exerted by the tip of the probe on the esophagus and the airway. Although in most patients even maximal flexion of the probe will not result in pressure above 17 mmHg, occasionally, even in the absence of esophageal disease, pressures greater than 60 mmHg will result.[2]

Further confirmation of the low incidence of esophageal injury from TEE is apparent in the few case reports of complications. In a study of 10,000 TEE examinations, there was one case of hypopharyngeal perforation (0.01%), two cases of cervical esophageal perforation (0.02%), and no cases of gastric perforation.[3] Kallmeyer et al. reported overall incidences of TEE-associated morbidity and mortality of 0.2% and 0%, respectively.[4] The most common TEE-associated complication was severe odynophagia (0.1%); other complications were dental injury (0.03%), endotracheal tube malpositioning (0.03%), upper gastrointestinal hemorrhage (0.03%), and esophageal perforation (0.01%). Piercy et al. reported a gastrointestinal complication rate of approximately 0.1%, with a great frequency of injuries among patients older than 70 years and women.[5] If resistance is met while advancing the probe, the procedure should be aborted to avoid these potentially lethal complications.

The second group of complications that result from TEE includes hemodynamic and pulmonary effects of airway manipulation and, particularly for new TEE operators, distraction from patient care.

Fortunately, in the anesthetized patient there are rarely hemodynamic consequences to esophageal placement of the probe, and thus there are no studies that specifically address this question. More important for the anesthesiologist is the problem of distraction from patient care.

Absolute contraindications to TEE in intubated patients include esophageal stricture, diverticula, tumor, recent suture lines, and known esophageal interruption. Relative contraindications include symptomatic hiatal hernia, esophagitis, coagulopathy, esophageal varices, and unexplained upper gastrointestinal bleeding. It should be noted that, despite these relative contraindications, TEE has been used in patients undergoing hepatic transplantation without reported sequelae.[6,7]

Basic American Society of Echocardiography TEE Views

There is general agreement on the echocardiography views that should be obtained during all examinations (Figure 5.1).[8]

Transgastric Mid-Papillary Short-Axis View

While the American Society of Echocardiography recommends multiple views for the definition of cardiac pathology and function, the assessment of preload, function, and pericardial effusions are the most important aspects of the evaluation. All of these parameters may be evaluated in the transgastric (TG) mid-papillary short-axis view. The probe is advanced into the stomach and slightly anteroflexed until the posterolateral and anterolateral papillary muscles are visualized at their attachment to the ventricular wall. It is important to image the insertion of the papillary muscles to insure accurate intra- and interobserver examinations. The left ventricle (LV) is centered on the screen. If the mitral valve apparatus is visualized, the probe should be further advanced or posteroflexed. Similarly, if the ventricular apex is visualized, the probe should be either withdrawn or anteroflexed. All six middle segments of the ventricle are visualized, which represents perfusion from each of the three coronary arteries. The size and function of both the right and left ventricles may be evaluated. Although qualitative evaluation of right ventricular function may be performed, quantitative measurement of left ventricular fractional area of shortening

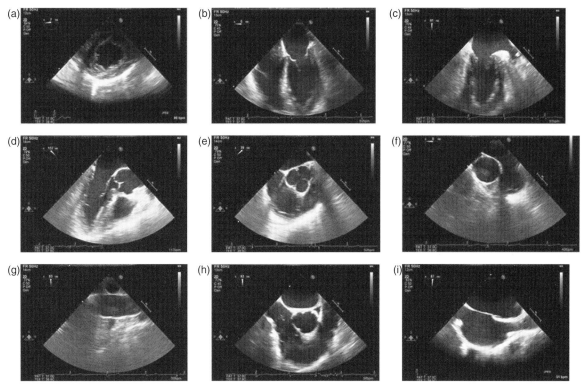

Figure 5.1 American Society of Echocardiography basic TEE views. **(a)** Transgastric mid-papillary short axis. **(b)** Mid-esophageal four chamber. **(c)** Mid-esophageal two chamber. **(d)** Mid-esophageal long axis. **(e)** Mid-esophageal aortic valve short axis. **(f)** Mid-esophageal ascending aortic short axis. **(g)** Mid-esophageal ascending aortic long axis. **(h)** Mid-esophageal right ventricular inflow-outflow. **(i)** Mid-esophageal bi-caval.

may be calculated. Regional wall motion abnormalities may be visualized, which may represent myocardial ischemia.

Mid-Esophageal Four-Chamber View

Maintaining the probe at approximately 0°, the probe is withdrawn into the mid-esophagus. Slight retroflexion is usually necessary to avoid foreshortening of the left ventricle. The array may need to be rotated approximately 10° to avoid imaging the left ventricular outflow tract and optimize visualization of the basal aspect of the inferoseptal left ventricular wall. In this view, the basal, middle, and apical aspects of the anterolateral and inferoseptal left ventricle walls may be evaluated. The presence of left atrial spontaneous echo contrast ("smoke") may be observed in patients with left atrial stasis; the left atrial appendage may be examined for evidence of thrombus. Right ventricular size and function may be evaluated.

Both anterior and posterior leaflets of the mitral valve may be imaged and evaluated for motion and pathology. With the echo probe optimally retroflexed with full visualization of the left ventricular apex, the most posteromedial aspects of the anterior and posterior mitral valve leaflets are usually imaged. As the probe is either slowly anteroflexed or withdrawn, the middle and final anterolateral aspects of these leaflets may be imaged. The septal and posterior tricuspid valve leaflets are usually visualized; however, if the probe is withdrawn too far or is too far anteroflexed, the anterior tricuspid valve leaflet may be visualized instead of the posterior leaflet. Pulsed wave Doppler at the level of the mitral valve leaflet tips may be used to evaluate diastolic function and the severity of mitral stenosis; with moderate to severe mitral stenosis, CW Doppler will probably be required. Color flow Doppler may be used to evaluate the severity of mitral and tricuspid regurgitation (TR) as well as the presence of an atrial septal defect. Because of the small expected gradients between the atria, a lower CFD setting is required in order to appreciate interatrial flow if it is present.

Mid-Esophageal Two-Chamber View

Rotation of the transducer array to 90° will develop the mid-esophageal (ME) two-chamber view. All segments of the anterior and inferior left ventricular walls may be evaluated for thickness and contractility. The anterior and posterior leaflets of the mitral valve are imaged, and evidence of stenosis and regurgitation may be obtained. The left atrial size may be measured, and "smoke" may be imaged if present. The left atrial appendage can be examined for thrombus, which is not uncommon with left atrial stasis.

Mid-Esophageal Long-Axis View

Further rotation to 120° develops the long-axis view. A single axis from the left ventricular apex to the left ventricular outflow tract to the aortic valve to the ascending aorta should be developed; further rotation to 130° or 140° may be necessary to obtain this axis alignment with cardiac rotation. In this view, both segments (basal and middle) of the anteroseptal and inferolateral walls may be evaluated. Posterior leaflet restriction may be seen with ischemic cardiac disease, and systolic anterior motion of the anterior mitral valve leaflet may be easily appreciated with hypertrophic obstructive cardiomyopathy. The severity of mitral regurgitation may be estimated by CFD.

Mid-Esophageal Aortic Valve Short-Axis View

The aortic valve is centered on the screen and the array is rotated to approximately 30°. The three cusps of the aortic valve (right, left, and non-coronary) may be visualized along with its triangular opening. Evidence of pathology on the aortic valve cusps may be appreciated. Aortic valve stenosis may be qualitatively estimated by observing the aortic valve leaflet opening (see section on aortic stenosis). Quantization of aortic stenosis by planimetry may be attempted in this view; however, its use may be limited by shadowing caused by valvular calcification. Color flow Doppler may be used to identify the site of aortic valve regurgitation, but quantification using this view may be

difficult. The left main coronary artery may be imaged as it emerges adjacent to the left coronary cusp. Its bifurcation into the left anterior descending and circumflex artery is occasionally appreciated.

Mid-Esophageal Ascending Aortic Short-Axis View

The array probe is returned to 0° and the aortic valve is once again centered on the screen. The probe is withdrawn through the base of the heart until the pulmonary artery and its bifurcation are imaged. The severity of proximal and middle ascending aortic atherosclerosis and pathology may be evaluated.

Mid-Esophageal Ascending Aortic Long-Axis View

The transducer is rotated to 90–120° to visualize the ascending aorta in its long axis. The proximal and middle section of the aorta can usually be seen and examined for atherosclerotic disease up to the crossing of the right pulmonary artery. The distal ascending aorta, however, usually cannot be visualized because it is interposed between the esophagus and either the trachea or the bronchus.

Mid-Esophageal Right Ventricular Inflow-Outflow View

The transducer array is returned to 0° and the four-chamber view is redeveloped. The tricuspid valve is centered on the screen and the array is rotated to approximately 60°. In addition to the left atrium, the right atrium, tricuspid valve, right ventricle, right ventricular outflow tract, pulmonary valve, and proximal pulmonary artery may be visualized. The septal and anterior leaflet of the tricuspid valve may be seen. Color flow Doppler may be superimposed, evaluating the severity of tricuspid regurgitation. If there is tricuspid regurgitation, CW Doppler may be used to estimate systolic pulmonary artery pressure. Moving the color Doppler field to the pulmonary valve allows estimation of pulmonary regurgitation.

Mid-Esophageal Bi-Caval View

If the array is rotated to approximately 90° and clockwise, the bi-caval view may be obtained. The superior and inferior vena cava may be visualized as they enter the right atrium. The Eustachian valve may be seen as a fibrinous structure at the junction of the inferior vena cava with the right atrium. Septum secundum may be visualized as it extends superiorly into the right atrium, while septum primum may be visualized as it extends from the inferior aspect towards the left atrium. Low-velocity CFD may be used to image either of these two atrial septal defects, which usually are associated with left to right flows.

Descending Aortic Short-Axis View

The probe is turned leftward toward the descending thoracic aorta. Because the probe is severely rotated, the orientation of the images will have changed. From this angle, the top of the image is the antero-medial aortic wall while the bottom of the image is the posterolateral wall. The probe is advanced toward the stomach until the image is lost. It is then withdrawn slowly, imaging the entire descending aorta and observing for atherosclerotic disease. When the probe reaches the level of the upper esophagus, a long-axis view of the aortic arch may be seen.

Descending Aortic Long-Axis View

The probe is returned to the stomach and the array is rotated to 90° to develop a long-axis view of the descending aorta. Once again, the probe is slowly withdrawn. It may be necessary to rotate the probe right and left to optimize this long-axis visualization. The aortic arch is visualized in the upper esophageal area when a cross-sectional image is developed.

Evaluation of Ventricular Size and Function

Left Ventricular Size and Function

The fractional area change (FAC) is the parameter most often requested from the echocardiographer. While this measurement is dependent upon loading conditions, it is frequently used to guide clinical management of patients with cardiovascular disease. This measurement is simple and reproducible. The LV cavity is imaged in a transgastric midpapillary short-axis (SAX) view and the area measured in end-systole and end-diastole (Figure 5.2). The difference between

the areas in end-diastole and end-systole divided by the area in end-diastole, represents the FAC.

$$FAC = (EDA - ESA)/EDA$$

EDA = end-diastolic area

ESA = end-systolic area

Since the biplane disk summation method (modified Simpson's) corrects for shape distortions, it is currently the recommended method of 2D volume measurements (Figure 5.2). With biplane disk summation, the total LV volume is calculated from the summation of a stack of elliptical disks. The height of each disk is calculated as a fraction of the LV long axis, based on the longer of the two lengths from the two- and four-chamber views. The cross-sectional area of the disk is based on the diameters obtained, and the volume of the disk is estimated. The volume is obtained by summing these values.

While in conventional hemodynamics preload is often estimated by measuring left-heart filling pressures (i.e., pulmonary capillary wedge pressure, left atrial pressure, or LV end-diastolic pressure), in echocardiography it can be determined by measuring LV end-diastolic dimensions. There are two main echocardiographic signs of decreased preload. (1) Decreased EDA (< 5.5 cm^2/m^2) invariably reflects hypovolemia. It is, however, difficult to set an upper limit of EDA below which hypovolemia can be confirmed. This is particularly true in patients with impaired contractility where a compensatory baseline increase in preload makes the echocardiographic diagnosis of hypovolemia difficult. (2) Obliteration of the end-systolic area (ESA), also known as the "kissing ventricle" sign, often accompanies a decreased EDA in severe hypovolemia.

Right Ventricular Size and Function

The right ventricle (RV) is a complex structure that pumps venous blood to the normally low pressure/low resistance pulmonary arterial circuit. Owing to the historical focus on the left side of the circulation, lack of geometrical assumptions of RV shape, and the difficulty in imaging the right heart, information regarding the RV has been limited until relatively recently. When right ventricular function and loading conditions are normal, the RV is typically triangular when viewed in the mid-esophageal four-chamber

Diastole   Systole

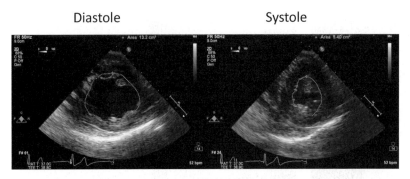

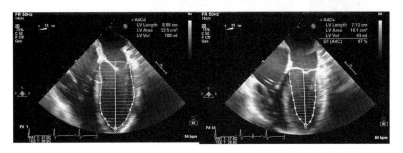

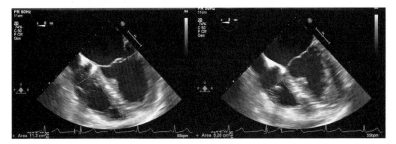

Figure 5.2 Calculation of fractional area of change (FAC) and ejection fraction (EF). The left column is diastole and the right column is systole. The first row illustrates the calculation of left ventricular (LV) FAC using the transgastric mid-papillary view. The second row illustrates the calculation of LV EF using a modified Simpson's method with the mid-esophageal four-chamber view. The third row illustrates the calculation of right ventricular FAC using the mid-esophageal four-chamber view.

view and crescent-shaped when viewed in the transgastric mid-papillary short-axis view.

Right ventricle dilation is readily identified by echocardiography and may be assessed qualitatively or quantitatively. Qualitatively, the RV size is compared to the LV size in the mid-esophageal four-chamber view; its cross-sectional area normally occupies two-thirds of the normal LV cross-sectional area (Figure 5.3). Mild enlargement is defined as an RV size that is more than two-thirds the LV size, moderate enlargement is defined as the chambers being equal in size, and severe enlargement is defined as the RV area greater than the LV area. Quantitatively, the RV is difficult to assess due to its complex shape and the poor interobserver reproducibility of RV chamber size measurements. Current RV chamber quantification guidelines suggest upper reference values of a 4.1 cm diameter at the base and a 3.5 cm diameter in the midlevel of the RV on a transthoracic

RV-focused apical four-chamber view.[9] There are no guidelines specific to TEE. Right ventricle pressure or volume overload may cause distortion or flattening of the interventricular septum that is most easily identified in the TG mid-papillary short-axis view (Figure 5.3). The overload of the RV, as well as the underfilling of the LV from reduced RV output, leads to a leftward deviation of the septum and a "D-shaped" LV chamber appearance.

Right ventricular FAC is another 2D-based method of systolic function evaluation. This measurement may be obtained in an ME four-chamber view, tracing the RV from the lateral tricuspid annulus, down the RV free wall to the apex, and returning along the septum to the tricuspid annulus (Figure 5.2). The change in this area measurement between diastole and systole is calculated as a percentage. An RV FAC less than 35% is indicative of RV dysfunction.[8]

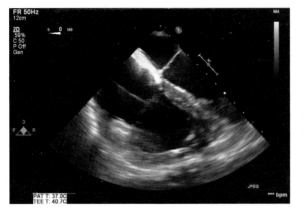 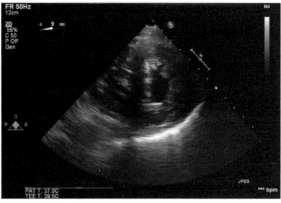

Figure 5.3 Large right ventricle. Mid-esophageal four-chamber view on the left demonstrates a right ventricle that is significantly larger than the left ventricle. A transgastric mid-papillary view demonstrates a "D-shaped" left ventricle because of the increase in right ventricular pressure.

Assessment of Coronary Ischemia

The ability to reliably detect regional wall motion abnormalities (RWMA) is clinically relevant because of its diagnostic and therapeutic implications. Not every RWMA detected by TEE is diagnostic for myocardial ischemia. Myocarditis, ventricular pacing, and bundle branch blocks can easily lead to wall motion abnormalities that can be misinterpreted and potentially lead to clinical mismanagement.

Regional wall motion abnormalities anatomical localization and degree of dysfunction should be described according to the ASE classification, which is based on a 16-segment model of the LV (Figure 5.4).[8] This model subdivides the LV into three zones (basal, mid, and apical). The basal (segments 1–6) and mid-ventricular (segments 7–12) zones are each subdivided into six segments, while the apical zone is subdivided into four (segments 13–16).

The coronary distribution related to the individual segments can be assessed, enabling the echocardiographer to make assumptions regarding the localization of a potential coronary lesion. Segments 1, 2, 7, 13, 14, and 17 are in the distribution territory of the left anterior descending artery. Segments 5, 6, 11, 12, and 16 are associated with the circumflex artery, and segments 3, 4, 9, 10, and 15 are supplied by the right coronary artery (Figure 5.4). This segmental distribution, however, can be variable among patients due to the variability of the coronary arteries.

In addition to defining anatomical segments of the LV, it is important to grade segment thickening and excursion. The simplest assessment is achieved by the echocardiographer "eyeballing" the motion of the ventricle and classifying it as normal, hypokinetic, akinetic, dyskinetic, or aneurysmal. The degree of thickening (i.e., the percentage change in wall thickness during systole) can also be used to assess overall function of the observed segment. A thickening greater than 30% is normal, 10–30% indicates mild hypokinesia, 0–10% indicates severe hypokinesia, no thickening indicates akinesia, and bulging of the segment during systole indicates dyskinesia.

Assessment of Pressures and Flow

Doppler echocardiographic measurements may be used to calculate pressure gradients. The Bernoulli principle states that an increase in the speed of the fluid occurs simultaneously with a decrease in its pressure or a decrease in the fluid's potential energy. When flow acceleration and viscous friction variables of blood are ignored, and flow velocity proximal to a fixed obstruction is significantly less than flow velocity after the obstruction, a simplified modified Bernoulli equation may be defined as:

$$\Delta P = 4(V)^2$$

where ΔP is the pressure difference between two structures and V is the velocity across the structures.

With this formula, the pressure gradient across a fixed orifice can be estimated.

Aortic Valve Evaluation

Two-dimensional transesophageal echocardiographic interrogation provides information on valve area, leaflet structure, and mobility. The valve is composed

41

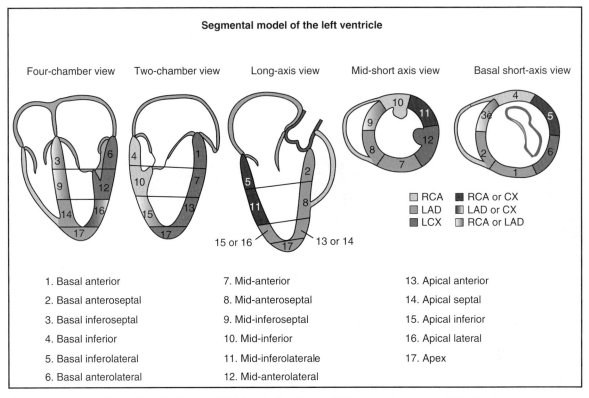

Segmental model of the left ventricle

Four-chamber view Two-chamber view Long-axis view Mid-short axis view Basal short-axis view

15 or 16   13 or 14

RCA   RCA or CX
LAD   LAD or CX
LCX   RCA or LAD

1. Basal anterior	7. Mid-anterior	13. Apical anterior
2. Basal anteroseptal	8. Mid-anteroseptal	14. Apical septal
3. Basal inferoseptal	9. Mid-inferoseptal	15. Apical inferior
4. Basal inferior	10. Mid-inferior	16. Apical lateral
5. Basal inferolateral	11. Mid-inferolaterale	17. Apex
6. Basal anterolateral	12. Mid-anterolateral	

Figure 5.4 was taken from Badano LP, Picano E. (2015) Standardized Myocardial Segmentation of the Left Ventricle. In: *Stress Echocardiography*. Springer, Cham. (A black and white version of this figure will appear in some formats. For the color version, please refer to the plate section).

of three fibrous cusps (right, left, and non-coronary) attached to the root of the aorta. The spaces between the attachments of the cusps are called the "commissures" and the circumferential connection of these commissures is the sinotubular junction. The aortic wall bulge behind each cusp is known as the sinus of Valsalva. The sinotubular junction, the sinuses of Valsalva, the valve cusps, and the junction of the aortic valve with the ventricular septum and anterior mitral valve leaflet comprise the aortic valve complex. The three leaflets of the aortic valve are easily visualized, and vegetations or calcifications can be identified on basal transverse imaging or longitudinal imaging.

Aortic Stenosis

Aortic stenosis may be caused by congenital unicuspid, bicuspid, tricuspid, or quadricuspid valves, rheumatic fever, or degenerative calcification of the valve in the elderly.[10] Valvular aortic stenosis is characterized by thickened, echogenic, calcified,

immobile leaflets and is usually associated with concentric left ventricular hypertrophy and a dilated aortic root. The valve leaflets may be domed during systole; this finding is sufficient for a diagnosis of aortic stenosis.[25]

The quantification of aortic stenosis is summarized in Table 5.1. The aortic valve area may be measured by planimetry (Figure 5.5).[11] A cross-sectional view of the aortic valve orifice may be obtained by TEE, and measurement of the aortic valve area corresponds well to those obtained by transthoracic echocardiography and cardiac catheterization, assuming the degree of calcification is not severe. The severity of aortic stenosis may be quantified using Doppler echocardiography (Figure 5.6).[12] The evaluation of severity, however, may be limited by difficulty aligning the ultrasonic beam with the direction of blood flow through the left ventricular outflow tract. Normal Doppler signals across the aortic valve have a velocity of less than 1.5 m/sec and have peak signals during early

Table 5.1 Summary of aortic stenosis.

	Aortic sclerosis	Mild	Moderate	Severe
Aortic jet velocity (m/s)	≤ 2.5	2.6–2.9	3.0–4.0	> 4.0
Mean gradient (mmHg)		< 20	20–40	> 40
Aortic valve area (cm²)		> 1.5	1.0–1.5	< 1.0

Source: C.M. Otto, Valvular aortic stenosis: disease severity and timing of intervention. *J Am* Coll Cardiol 2006;47:2141–51.

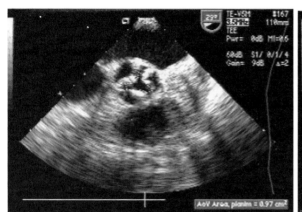
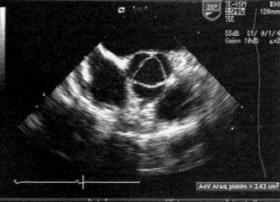

Figure 5.5 Aortic valve stenosis by planimetry. The left panel indicates a normal aortic valve while the right panel indicates an aortic valve with stenosis. Since there is no significant calcification of the valve, planimetry may be used.

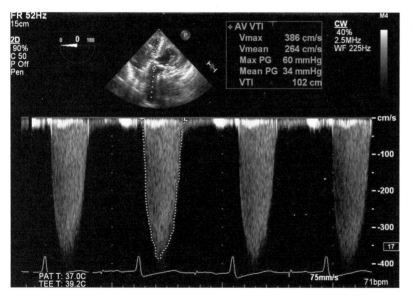

Figure 5.6 Doppler spectrum through a stenotic aortic valve.

systole. With worsening aortic stenosis, the flow velocities increase and the signal's peak is later during systole. These high velocities will limit the use of pulsed wave Doppler and necessitate the use of either CW or high PRF Doppler. Aortic velocity allows classification of stenosis as mild (2.6 to 2.9 m/sec), moderate (3.0 to 4.0 m/sec), or severe (> 4 m/sec).[13]

43

Aortic Regurgitation

Aortic regurgitation or aortic insufficiency (AI) may result from either diseases of the aortic leaflets or the aortic root.[14] Valvular lesions that may result in AI include leaflet vegetations and calcifications, perforation, or prolapse. Aortic insufficiency may be caused by annular dilation secondary to a variety of etiologies, including annulo-aortic ectasia, Marfan's syndrome, aortic dissection, collagen vascular disease, and syphilis.

Cusp pathology (e.g., redundancy, restriction, mobility, thickness, integrity), commissural variations (fusion, splaying, alignment, and attachment site), and root morphology (septal hypertrophy and root dimensions) should be ascertained.[13] Leaflet movement (excessive, restricted, or normal), origin of jet (central or peripheral), and direction of regurgitant jet (eccentric or central) should be determined to provide insight into the underlying pathology. Other signs that may be associated with AI include high-frequency diastolic fluttering of the mitral valve, premature closing of the mitral valve, and reverse doming of the mitral valve.[15,16]

The criteria for qualitative grading of AI are summarized in Table 5.2. Color flow Doppler has traditionally been the major method of assessing the severity of valvular regurgitation. Nyquist limits should provide an aliasing velocity of approximately 50–60 cm/sec and a color gain that just eliminates the random color speckle from nonmoving regions.[17] Aortic regurgitant flow through the outflow tract is characteristically a high-velocity turbulent jet extending through the left ventricular outflow tract and left ventricle during diastole.

The vena contracta is the narrowest portion of a regurgitant jet that usually occurs at or immediately upstream from the valve (Figure 5.7). This jet width is directly proportional to the severity of the AI. It is usually characterized by high velocity and laminar flow and is slightly smaller than the regurgitant orifice.[16] A vena contra diameter less than 0.3 cm is consistent with mild AI, and a diameter greater than 0.6 cm is consistent with severe AI.

Mitral Valve Evaluation

The mitral value consists of two leaflets, chordae tendineae, two papillary muscles, and a valve annulus. The anterior leaflet is larger than the posterior leaflet and is semicircular; the posterior mitral valve leaflet has a longer circumferential attachment to the mitral valve annulus.[18] The leaflets are connected to each other at junctures of continuous leaflet tissue called "commissures." Primary, secondary, and tertiary chordal structures arise from the papillary muscle, subdivide as they extend, and attach to the free edge and several millimeters from the margin on the ventricular surface of both the anterior and posterior valve leaflets.[19] The annulus of the mitral valve primarily supports the posterior mitral valve leaflet, while the anterior mitral valve leaflet is continuous with the membranous ventricular septum, aortic valve, and aorta.

Mitral Stenosis

The most common etiology of mitral stenosis is rheumatic disease; other causes include congenital valvular stenosis, vegetations and calcifications of the leaflets, parachute mitral valve, and annular calcification. In

Table 5.2 Quantification of aortic regurgitation.

	Mild	Moderate	Severe
Left atrial size	Normal	Normal or dilated	Usually dilated
Aortic cusps	Normal or abnormal	Normal or abnormal	Abnormal/flail or wide coaption defect
Jet width in LVOT*	Small in central jets	Intermediate	Large in central jets; variable in eccentric jets
Vena contracta width (cm)*	< 0.3	0.3–0.6	≥ 0.6

* At Nyquist limits of 50–60 cm/sec
CSA = cross-sectional area
LVOT = left ventricular outflow tract

Source: Zoghbi WA, Adams D, Bonow RO, et al. Recommendations for noninvasive evaluation of native valvular regurgitation: a report from the American society of echocardiography developed in collaboration with the society for cardiovascular magnetic resonance. J Am Soc Echocardiogr 2017; 30:303–71.

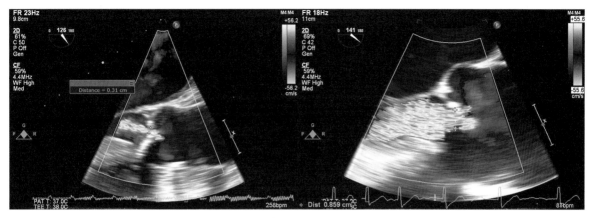

Figure 5.7 Vena contra aortic valve. Mid-esophageal aortic valve long axis. The vena contracta may be used to differentiate among degrees of aortic regurgitation. The image on the left has a narrow vena contracta, which is associated with a mild degree of aortic regurgitation. By contrast, the large vena contracta on the right is associated with a severe degree of aortic regurgitation. (A black and white version of this figure will appear in some formats. For the color version, please refer to the plate section).

addition to structural valvular abnormalities, mitral stenosis may be caused by non-valvular etiologies such as intra-atrial masses (myxomas or thrombus) or extrinsic constrictive lesions.[20,21] Generally, mitral stenosis is characterized by restricted leaflet movement, a reduced orifice, and diastolic doming (Figure 5.8).[22] The diastolic doming occurs when the mitral valve is unable to accommodate all the blood flowing from the left atrium into the ventricle, so the body of the leaflets separates more than the edges. In rheumatic disease, calcification of the valvular and subvalvular apparatus, as well as thickening, deformation, and fusion of the valvular leaflets at the anterolateral and posteromedial commissures, produces a characteristic fish-mouth-shaped orifice.[23] Other characteristics that may be associated with chronic obstruction to left atrial outflow include an enlarged left atrium, spontaneous echo contrast or "smoke" (which is related to low-velocity blood flow with subsequent rouleaux formation by red blood cells[24]), thrombus formation, and RV dilation.

The assessment of the severity of mitral stenosis is summarized in Table 5.3. Because planimetry of the mitral valve orifice is not influenced by assumptions of flow conditions, ventricular compliance, or associated valvular lesions, it is the reference standard for the evaluation of the mitral valve area in mitral stenosis.[25] While at times technically difficult, care should be taken to image the orifice at the leaflet tips. Severe calcification of the mitral valve may interfere with mitral valve area determination and, in patients with significant subvalvular stenosis,

underestimation of the degree of hemodynamic compromise may occur when determining mitral valve area by planimetry.[26]

A transmitral Doppler spectrum is measured along the axis of transmitral blood flow, which may usually be obtained in a mid-esophageal four-chamber view or two-chamber view (Figure 5.8). Transmitral valve flow is characterized by two peaked waves of flow away from the transducer. The first wave (E) represents early diastolic filling, while the second wave (A) represents atrial systole. The transvalvular gradient may be estimated using the modified Bernoulli equation:[27] pressure gradient $= 4 \times$ (maximal velocity)^2. Since peak gradient is heavily influenced by left atrial compliance and ventricular diastolic function, the mean gradient is the relevant clinical measurement.[24] The high velocities that may occur with mitral stenosis limit the use of pulsed wave Doppler echocardiography, thus CW Doppler echocardiography should be utilized.

Mitral Regurgitation

Mitral regurgitation (MR) may be classified as primary or secondary. Primary causes of regurgitation are structural or organic, while secondary causes are functional (i.e., without evidence of structural abnormalities of the mitral valve). The most common causes of primary mitral regurgitation are degenerative (e.g., Barlow's disease, fibroelastic degeneration, Marfan's syndrome, Ehler–Danos syndrome, annular calcification), rheumatic disease, toxic valvulopathies, and endocarditis.[13] Mitral regurgitation may be caused by

Table 5.3 Quantification of mitral stenosis.

	Mild	Moderate	Severe
Valve area (cm²)	> 1.5	1.0–1.5	> 1.0
Mean gradient (mmHg)	< 5	5–10	> 10

Source: Baumgartner H, Hung J, Bermejo J, et al. Echocardiographic assessment of valve stenosis: EAE/ASE recommendations for clinical practice. J Am Soc Echocardiogr 2009;22:1–23.

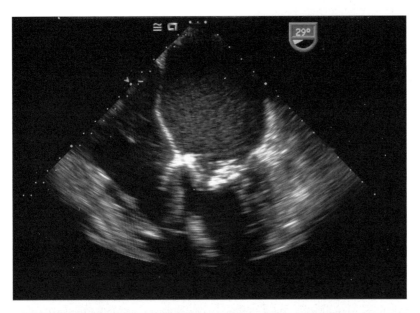

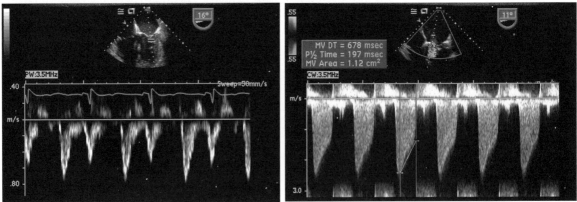

Figure 5.8 Top row: Mid-esophageal four-chamber view. The mitral valve is severely stenotic with severe calcification of the annulus and leaflets. Bottom row: Transmitral Doppler spectrum. The panel on the left is the normal transmitral Doppler flow and the panel on the right is the transmitral flow in the presence of mitral stenosis. (A black and white version of this figure will appear in some formats. For the color version, please refer to the plate section).

disorders of any component of the mitral valve apparatus (i.e., the annulus, the leaflets and chordae, or papillary muscles). With chronic regurgitation the annulus and atrium dilate and the annulus loses its normal elliptical shape, becoming more circular.[28] Annular dilation, in turn, leads to poor leaflet

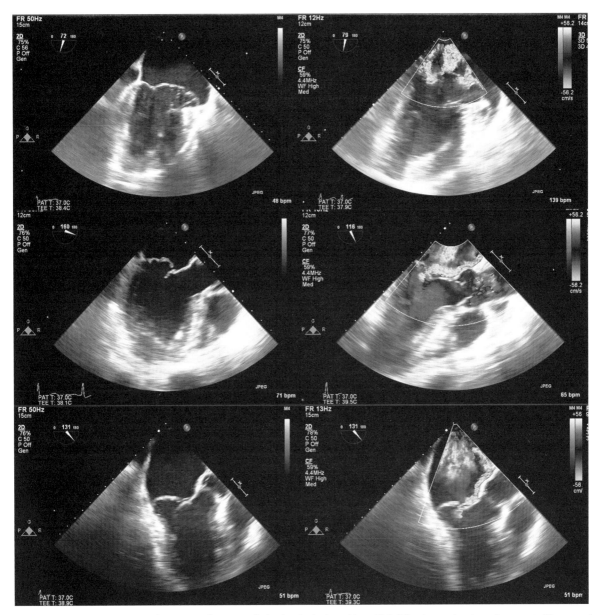

Figure 5.9 Mitral regurgitation. The top row illustrates a Barlow's mitral valve with multiple billowing and prolapsed segments. The second row illustrates a prolapsed posterior leaflet. The posterior leaflet is above the level of the mitral annulus. By contrast, a flail segment is illustrated in the bottom row, with the mitral valve segment pointing toward the atrium. (A black and white version of this figure will appear in some formats. For the color version, please refer to the plate section).

coaptation and worsening mitral regurgitation. Although increased left atrial and ventricular dimensions may suggest severe mitral regurgitation, smaller dimensions do not exclude the diagnosis.[29]

The most common cause of chronic primary MR in developed countries is mitral valve prolapse.[30] Younger individuals present with Barlow's syndrome, while older populations present with fibroelastic deficiency disease. A Barlow's valve is usually characterized by gross redundancy of multiple segments of the anterior or posterior leaflets and chordal apparatus (Figure 5.9). The leaflets are bulky and billowing with multiple areas of prolapse.[31] The chordae are more often elongated rather than ruptured. The leaflets are thickened with severe myxomatous degeneration. The annulus is usually severely dilated and may be calcified.

By contrast, fibroelastic deficiency usually only affects a single segment. The nonaffected leaflets tend to be thin, with a thickening of the affected segment. Elongated chords may produce prolapse of one or both attached leaflets. Excessively mobile structures near the leaflet tips during diastole may represent elongated chords or ruptured minor chords. These structures do not prolapse into the atrium during systole (Figure 5.9). By contrast, ruptured major chords are identified as thin structures with a fluttering appearance in the atrium during systole and are associated with marked prolapse of the affected leaflet. In this instance, the valve segment is termed as "flail." A flail leaflet segment generally points in the direction of the left atrium, and this directionality of leaflet pointing is the principal criterion for distinguishing a flailed leaflet from severe valvular prolapse.[32,33] Flail leaflets are most commonly caused by ruptured chordae and less commonly caused by papillary muscle rupture.

With secondary or functional mitral regurgitation, the mitral valve is structurally normal.[13,29] Left ventricular dilation secondary to another process such as myocardial infarction or idiopathic dilated cardiomyopathies result in papillary muscle displacement and annular dilation with resultant tethering of the mitral valve leaflets with incomplete leaflet coaptation. Since the valvular regurgitation is only one component of the disease process, its progress is worse than primary mitral regurgitation and its treatment is less clear.

Mitral regurgitation is graded semi-quantitatively as mild, moderate, or severe, as summarized in Table 5.4. Regurgitation less than mild may be classified as either trivial or trace. Some authors have suggested the subdividing of moderate regurgitation into mild-moderate and moderate-severe grades.[13,16] The most common method of grading the severity of mitral regurgitation is CFD mapping of the left atrium. With the Nyquist limit set at 50–60 cm/sec, jet areas less than 4 cm^2 or 20% of the left atrial size are usually classified as mild, while jets greater than 10 cm^2 or 40% of the atrial volume are classified as severe.[16] An alternative method of grading mitral regurgitation is based upon the vena contracta width.[34] While the vena contracta is commonly circular, it may be elliptical in shape with secondary etiologies or functional regurgitation.[13] In these cases, multiple views of the vena contra along different axes should be obtained and averaged. A vena contracta width of less than 0.3 cm is associated with mild MR, while a width greater than 0.7 cm is associated with severe MR.[16]

Tricuspid Valve

The tricuspid valve consists of three leaflets, an annular ring, chordae tendineae, and multiple papillary muscles.[35] The anterior leaflet is usually the largest, followed by the posterior and septal leaflets. The septal leaflet of the tricuspid valve is usually further apical than the septal attachments of the mitral valve. Chordae arise from a large single papillary muscle, double or multiple septal papillary muscles, and several small posterior papillary muscles attached to the corresponding walls of the right ventricle.

Intrinsic structural abnormalities of the tricuspid valve that can be well characterized by TEE include rheumatic tricuspid stenosis, carcinoid involvement of the tricuspid valve, tricuspid valve prolapse, flail tricuspid valve, Ebstein's anomaly, and tricuspid endocarditis. Rheumatic involvement of the tricuspid valve, which is typically seen with concomitant mitral valve involvement, is characterized by thickening of the leaflets (particularly at their coaptation surfaces), fusion of the commissures, and shortening of the chordal structures resulting in restricted leaflet

Table 5.4 Summary of mitral regurgitation (data from reference 17).

	Mild	Moderate	Severe
Left atrial size	Normal	Normal or dilated	Usually dilated
Color flow jet area*	Small central jet (< 4 cm^2 or < 20% LA area)		Large central jet (> 10 cm^2 or > 40% LA) or variable-sized wall impinging jet
Vena contracta width (cm)	< 0.3	0.3 – 0.69	≥ 0.7

* At Nyquist limits of 50–60 cm/sec.

Table 5.5 Quantification of tricuspid regurgitation.

	Mild	Moderate	Severe
Right atrial size	Normal	Normal or dilated	Usually dilated
Tricuspid valve leaflets	Usually normal	Normal or abnormal	Abnormal/flail or wide coaption defect
Jet area – central jets (cm²)*	< 5	5–10	> 10
Vena contracta width (cm)*	Not defined	Not defined, but < 0.7	> 0.7

* At Nyquist limits of 50–60 cm/sec.

Source: Zoghbi WA, Adams D, Bonow RO, et al. Recommendations for noninvasive evaluation of native valvular regurgitation: a report from the American society of echocardiography developed in collaboration with the society for cardiovascular magnetic resonance. J Am Soc Echocardiogr 2017;30:303–71.

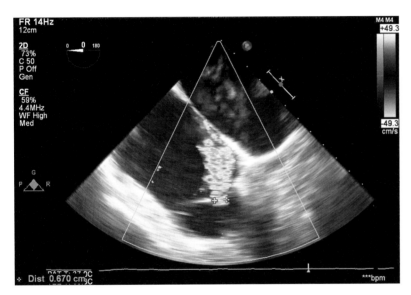

Figure 5.10 Functional tricuspid regurgitation. A mid-esophageal four-chamber view demonstrates a large functional tricuspid regurgitant jet. The vena contracta is measured as the jet emanates from the right ventricle. (A black and white version of this figure will appear in some formats. For the color version, please refer to the plate section).

motion.[36] Carcinoid syndrome results in a diffuse thickening of the tricuspid valve (and pulmonic valve), and endocardial thickening of right-heart structures that may result in restricted tricuspid valve motion (mixed stenosis and regurgitation).[37]

Supravalvular, valvular, or subvalvular restriction may cause tricuspid stenosis. The most common etiology of tricuspid stenosis is rheumatic heart disease, while less common causes include carcinoid syndrome and endomyocardial fibrosis. Tricuspid stenosis is characterized by a domed, thickened valve with restricted movement. Tricuspid regurgitation may be secondary to annular or right ventricular dilation, or pathology of the leaflets or subvalvular apparatus. Continuous wave Doppler measurements of the inflow velocities across the tricuspid valve can be employed to estimate the mean diastolic tricuspid valve gradient with the modified Bernoulli equation.[38]

While tricuspid regurgitation (TR) may have primary etiologies, most causes are secondary or functional as a result of either tricuspid annular dilation (greater than 40 mm) or RV dilation (Figure 5.10).[13] Right ventricle enlargement results in annular dilation and papillary muscle displacement with tethering of the tricuspid valve leaflets. This tethering may result in poor leaflet coaption. This TR results in additional RV enlargement and further leaflet tethering with worsening TR.

The quantification of TR is summarized in Table 5.5. The apparent severity of tricuspid regurgitation is exquisitely sensitive to right-heart loading conditions. A central jet area of less than 5 cm² is consistent with mild regurgitation, while a jet area greater than 10 cm² is consistent with severe regurgitation.[16] Recent guidelines, however, suggest that color flow area of the regurgitant jet should not be used to quantitate the severity of TR.[13] A vena contra width less than 0.3 mm is consistent with mild regurgitation, while a VC greater than 0.7 cm is consistent with severe regurgitation.[39]

Pericardial Disease

The pericardium is a two-layered structure reflecting from a visceral layer to a parietal layer approximately 1–2 cm distal to the origin of the great vessels and around the pulmonary veins. Under normal circumstances 5–10 ml of fluid is contained within the pericardial sack, allowing for practically frictionless motion of the heart during the cardiac cycle. The parietal layer of the pericardium is rich in collagen fibers, making it a low-compliance structure confining the volume of the four cardiac chambers. In other words, a volume increase of one chamber requires a reduction of volume within another. Likewise, if an increase in volume is seen within the pericardial sack, a reduction of chamber volumes must occur.

Pericardial Effusion

Under normal circumstances the echocardiographer is unable to visualize the fluid film between the two

pericardial layers. Under pathological conditions, fluid accumulation can occur, resulting in the development of a pericardial effusion (Figure 5.11). According to the 2013 guidelines, small effusions are usually defined as 50 to 100 mL, moderate as 100 to 500 mL, and large as greater than 500 mL.[40] The size of the effusion correlates poorly with its hemodynamic effect; the rapidity of effusion accumulation has a greater effect on hemodynamics. Different etiologies of pericardial effusions have characteristic sizes and progressions. Idiopathic or viral infections may result in small pericardial effusions, while large effusions may be associated with hypothyroidism, tuberculosis, or neoplasms. Rapid pericardial blood accumulation may be from blunt trauma, ascending aortic dissection, or cardiac rupture (either secondary to myocardial infarction or iatrogenic, such as during invasive cardiac procedures).[41] Free effusions are typically seen in medical conditions leading to pericardial effusions, whereas loculated effusions are seen after surgery or inflammatory processes. In many patients, however, the etiology of pericardial effusions must be classified as idiopathic.

Most echocardiographers use a qualitative grading system to characterize the quantity of pericardial effusion. This qualitative grading uses the diameter of the effusion in two dimensions. The 2013 guidelines are summarized in Table 5.6. Trivial effusions are only seen during systole, mild effusions are less than 1 cm, and large effusions are greater than 2 cm in diameter.

Table 5.6 Severity of pericardial effusions.

Diameter of effusion	Severity
0–1.0 cm	Mild
1.1–2.0 cm	Moderate
> 2.0 cm	Severe

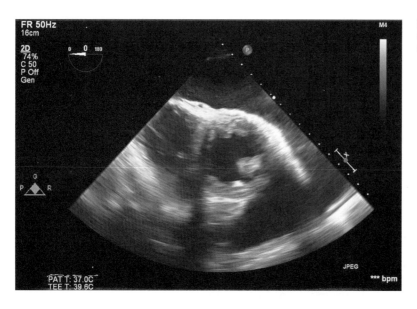

Figure 5.11 Transgastric short-axis view of left ventricle. A large pericardial effusion seen surrounding the LV.

Additionally, the effusion can either encompass the entire heart (free) or be loculated. While transthoracic echocardiography may not be sensitive for the detection of loculated effusions, TEE is an excellent modality for the detection of these effusions. TEE has been demonstrated to be a more sensitive modality for the detection of loculated effusions or intra-pericardial clots, compared with the transthoracic route.[42]

Cardiac Tamponade

Cardiac tamponade and pericardial effusion are not synonymous. A pericardial effusion is an anatomical diagnosis that may or may not lead to hemodynamic alterations. Cardiac tamponade is a pathophysiological diagnosis. Echocardiographically, cardiac tamponade may be identified as right atrial and ventricular collapse during their relaxation phase. This collapse occurs when the intra-pericardial pressure exceeds the intrachamber pressures. The severity and duration of this collapse increase with further increases in the pericardial pressure. Duration of right atrial collapse exceeding one-third of the cardiac cycle is nearly 100% sensitive and specific for clinical cardiac tamponade.[43] Since the right ventricle is thicker than the right atrium, a higher pericardial pressure is required for right ventricular diastolic collapse; right ventricular collapse is a more specific but less sensitive sign of pericardial tamponade.[44] In addition to the presence of a pericardial effusion, other signs of tamponade include a dilated inferior vena cava (IVC), hepatic

venous fullness with systolic blunting of hepatic blood flow velocities, excessive ventricular septal movement with respiration, and a small left ventricle. An IVC greater than 2.1 cm with less than a 50% reduction in diameter during inspiration is indicative of an elevation in systemic venous pressure that accompanies an increased pericardial pressure.[45]

Aortic Disease

The diagnosis of aortic dissection is based on the presence of an intimal flap (Figure 5.12). In the diagnosis of dissection, TEE has overcome some of the major disadvantages of the alternative diagnostic modalities (CT, MRI). In comparison to these other modalities, TEE has been shown to have high sensitivity and specificity.[46,47] According to the 2010 guidelines for the diagnosis and management of aortic disease, TEE, CT, and MRI are all recommended as definitive methods for the identification or exclusion of thoracic aortic dissection.[48] The sensitivity of TEE for the detection of proximal aortic dissection is 88–98%, with a specificity of 90–95%.[49] With further improvement in technology, the sensitivity of TEE in detecting aortic dissections approaches 100%.[50] Ideally the specific locations of the entry and exit sites are also identifiable. The primary tear usually has a diameter of over 5 mm and is frequently located in the proximal part of the ascending aorta in type A dissections and immediately below the origin of the left subclavian artery in type B dissections. Flow in

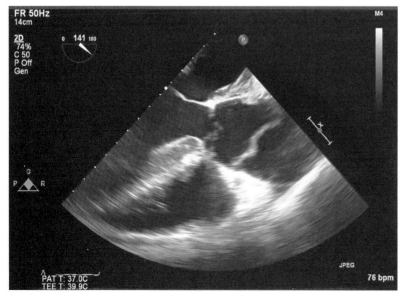

Figure 5.12 Aortic dissection. An aortic long-axis view is presented with an intimal flap from an aortic dissection visualized in the proximal ascending aorta.

both the true and false lumens can be analyzed with Doppler color flow imaging. TEE performed in real time utilizes its unique ability to give functional and hemodynamic information. This enables the detection of the common complications of aortic dissection: aortic valve regurgitation, pericardial tamponade, and left ventricular dysfunction secondary to coronary artery involvement in the dissection process.

Pericardial effusions are commonly seen with acute aortic dissection and may occur as a result of two etiologies.[47] The most common etiology is the transudation of fluid across the thin-walled false lumen into the pericardium. This is usually mild and does not lead to a hemodynamically significant pericardial effusion. Alternatively, the aorta may rupture directly into the pericardium with resultant pericardial tamponade and hemodynamic collapse.

Conclusion

Transesophageal echocardiography is a powerful diagnostic tool that revolutionized the practice of cardiac anesthesia. While its full functionality is most often utilized by cardiac anesthesiologists, its application to other high-risk surgeries (e.g., liver transplantation), high-risk patients with diseases like pulmonary hypertension and aortic stenosis undergoing routine surgery, and as a "rescue" diagnostic method to access hemodynamic collapse is unpatrolled. Perioperative physicians should have a basic knowledge of the principles of TEE, and may enhance their everyday practice by incorporating some of the basic aspects of TEE examination.

References

1. Kahn RA, Fischer GW. Transesophageal echocardiography. In: Reich DL, Kahn RA, Mittnacht AN, et al. eds. *Monitoring in Anesthesia and Perioperative Care*. New York, NY: Cambridge University Press, 2011;105–35.

2. Urbanowicz JH, Kernoff RS, Oppenheim G, et al. Transesophageal echocardiography and its potential for esophageal damage. *Anesthesiology* 1990;72:40.

3. Min JK, Spencer KT, Furlong KT, et al. Clinical features of complications from transesophageal echocardiography: a single-center case series of 10,000 consecutive examinations. *J Am Soc Echocardiogr* 2005;18:925–9.

4. Kallmeyer IJ, Collard CD, Fox JA, et al. The safety of intraoperative transesophageal echocardiography: a case series of 7200 cardiac surgical patients. *Anesth Analg* 2001;92:1126–30.

5. Piercy M, McNicol L, Dinh DT, Story DA, Smith JA. Major complications related to the use of transesophageal echocardiography in cardiac surgery. *J Cardiothorac Vasc Anesth* 2009;23:62–5.

6 Ellis JE, Lichtor JL, Feinstein SB, et al. Right heart dysfunction, pulmonary embolism, and paradoxical embolization during liver transplantation. *Anesth Analg* 1989;68:777.

7 Suriani RJ, Cutrone A, Feierman D, Konstadt S. Intraoperative transesophageal echocardiography during liver transplantation. *J Cardiothorac Vasc Anesth* 1996;10:699–707.

8. Reeves ST, Finley AC, Skubas NJ, et al. Council on Perioperative Echocardiography of the American Society of Echocardiography; Society of Cardiovascular Anesthesiologists. Basic perioperative transesophageal echocardiography examination: a consensus statement of the American Society of Echocardiography and the Society of Cardiovascular Anesthesiologists. *J Am Soc Echocardiogr* 2013;26:443–56.

9. Lang RM, Badano LP, Mor-Avi V, et al. Recommendations for cardiac chamber quantification by echocardiography in adults: an update from the American society of echocardiography and the European association of cardiovascular imaging. *J Am Soc Echocardiogr* 2015;28:1–39.

10. Rapaport E, Rackley CE, Cohn LH. Aortic valve disease. In: Schlant RC, Alexander RW, O'Rourke RA, et al. eds. *Hurst's The Heart: Arteries and Veins*. New York: McGraw Hill, 1994.

11. Stoddard MF, Arce J, Liddell NE, et al. Two dimensional transesophageal echocardiographic determination of aortic valve area in adults with aortic stenosis. *Am Heart J* 1991;122:1415.

12. C.M. Otto, Valvular aortic stenosis: disease severity and timing of intervention. *J Am Coll Cardiol* 2006;47:2141–51.

13. Baumgartner H, Hung J, Bermejo J, et al. Recommendations on the echocardiographic assessment of aortic valve stenosis: a focused update from the European Association of Cardiovascular Imaging and the American Society of Echocardiography. *J Am Soc Echocardiogr* 2017;30 (4):372–92.

14. Lancellotti P, Tribouilloy C, Hagendorff A, et al. Scientific Document Committee of the European Association of Cardiovascular Imaging. Recommendations for the echocardiographic assessment of native valvular regurgitation: an executive summary from the European Association of Cardiovascular Imaging. *Eur Heart J Cardiovasc Imaging* 2013;14(7):611–44.

15. Roberson WS, Stewart J, Armstrong WF, Dillon JC, Feigenbaum H. Reverse doming of the anterior mitral leaflet with severe aortic regurgitation. *J Am Coll Cardiol* 1984;**3**:431.

16. Ambrose JA, Meller J, Teichholz LE, Herman MV. Premature closure of the mitral valve: echocardiographic clue for the diagnosis of aortic dissection. *Chest* 1978;**73**:121.

17. Zoghbi WA, Adams D, Bonow RO, et al. Recommendations for noninvasive evaluation of native valvular regurgitation: a report from the American Society of Echocardiography developed in collaboration with the Society for Cardiovascular Magnetic Resonance. *J Am Soc Echocardiogr* 2017;**30**:303–71.

18. Ranganathan N, Lam JHC, Wigle ED, Silver MD. Morphology of the human mitral valve: II. The valve leaflets. *Circulation* 1970;**41**:459–67.

19. Perloff JK, Roberts WC. The mitral apparatus: functional anatomy of mitral regurgitation. *Circulation* 1972;**46**:227–39.

20. Hammer WJ, Roberts WC, deLeon AC Jr. Mitral stenosis secondary to combined massive mitral annular calcific deposits and small, hypertrophied left ventricles: hemodynamic documentation in four patients. *Am J Med* 1978;**64**:371–6.

21. Pai RG, Tarazi R, Wong S. Constrictive pericarditis causing extrinsic mitral stenosis and a left heart mass. *Clin Cardiol* 1996;**19**:517.

22. Felner JM, Martin RP. The echocardiogram. In: Schlant RC, Alexander RW, O'Rourke RA, et al. eds. *Hurst's The Heart: Arteries and Veins*. New York: McGraw Hill, 1994, 375–422.

23. Roberts WE. Morphological features of the normal and abnormal mitral valve. *Am J Cardiol* 1983;**51**: 1005–28.

24. Chen YT, Kan MN, Chen JS, et al. Contributing factors to formation of left atrial spontaneous echo contrast in mitral valvular disease. *J Ultrasound Med* 1990;**9**:151–5.

25. Baumgartner H, Hung J, Bermejo J, et al. Echocardiographic assessment of valve stenosis: EAE/ ASE recommendations for clinical practice. *J Am Soc Echocardiogr* 2009;**22**:1–23.

26. Feigenbaum H. *Acquired valvular heart disease in Echocardiography*, Philadelphia: Lea & Febiger, 1994, pp. 239–349.

27. Currie PJ, Seward JB, Reeder GS, et al. Continuous- wave Doppler echocardiographic assessment of severity of calcific aortic stenosis: a simultaneous Doppler-catheter correlative study in 100 adult patients. *Circulation* 1985;**71**:1162.

28. Ormiston JA, Shah PM, Tei C, Wong M. Size and motion of the mitral valve annulus in man. *Circulation* 1981;**64**:113.

29. Burwash IG, Blackmore GL, Koilpillai CJ. Usefulness of left atrial and left ventricular chamber sizes as predictors of the severity of mitral regurgitation. *Am J Cardiol* 1992;**15**:774.

30. Nishimura RA, Otto CM, Bonow RO, et al. 2017 AHA/ ACC focused update of the 2014 AHA/ACC guideline for the management of patients with valvular heart disease: a report of the American College of Cardiology/American Heart Association Task Force on Clinical Practice Guidelines. *J Am Coll Cardiol* 2017;**70**(2):252–89.

31. Anyanwu AC, Adams DH. Etiologic classification of degenerative mitral valve disease: Barlow's disease and fibroelastic deficiency. *Semin Thorac Cardiovasc Surg* 2007;**19**:90–6.

32. Mintz GS, Kotler MN, Segal BL, Parry WR. Two dimensional echocardiographic recognition of ruptured chordae tendineae. *Circulation* 1978;**57**:244.

33. Ogawa S, Mardelli TJ, Hubbard FE. The role of cross- sectional echocardiography in the diagnosis of flail mitral leaflet. *Clin Cardiol* 1978;**1**:85.

34. Tribouilloy CB, Shen WF, Quere JP, et al. Assessment of severity of mitral regurgitation by measuring regurgitant jet width at its origin with transesophageal Doppler color flow imaging. *Circulation* 1992;**85**:1248– 53.

35. Silver MD, Lam JHC, Ranganathan N, Wigle ED. Morphology of the human tricuspid valve. *Circulation* 1971;**43**:333–48.

36. Guyer DE, et al. Comparison of the echocardiographic and hemodynamic diagnosis of rheumatic tricuspid stenosis. *J Am Coll Cardiol* 1984;**3**:1135.

37. Lundin L, Landelius J, Andrea B, Oberg K. Transesophageal echocardiography improves the diagnostic value of cardiac ultrasound in patients with carcinoid heart disease. *Br Heart J* 1990;**64**:190–4.

38. Perez JE, Ludbrook PA, Ahumada GG. Usefulness of Doppler echocardiography in detecting tricuspid valve stenosis. *Am J Cardiol* 1985;**55**:601.

39. Tribouilloy CM, Enriquez-Sarano M, Bailey KR, Tajik AJ, Seward JB. Quantification of tricuspid regurgitation by measuring the width of the vena contracta with Doppler color flow imaging: a clinical study. *J Am Coll Cardiol* 2000;**36**:472–8.

40. Klein AL, Abbara S, Agler DA, et al. American society of echocardiography clinical recommendations for multimodality cardiovascular imaging of patients with pericardial disease: endorsed by the Society for Cardiovascular Magnetic Resonance and Society of

Cardiovascular Computed Tomography. *J Am Soc Echocardiogr* 2013;26(9):965–1012.

41. Sagrista-Sauleda J, Merce J, Permanyer-Miralda G, Soler-Soler J. Clinical clues to the causes of large pericardial effusions. *Am J Med* 2000;**109**:95–101.

42. Berge KH, Lanier WL, Reeder GS. Occult cardiac tamponade detected by transesophageal echocardiography. *Mayo Clin Proc* 1992;**67**:667–70.

43. Gillam LD, Guyer DE, Gibson TC, et al. Hydrodynamic compression of the right atrium: a new echocardiographic sign of cardiac tamponade. *Circulation* 1983;**68**:294–301.

44. Wann S, Passen E. Echocardiography in pericardial disease. *J Am Soc Echocardiogr* 2008;**21**: 7–13.

45. Himelman RB, Kircher B, Rockey DC, Schiller NB. Inferior vena cava plethora with blunted respiratory response: a sensitive echocardiographic sign of cardiac tamponade. *J Am Coll Cardiol* 1988;**12**:1470–7.

46. Ballal RS, Nanda NC, Gatewood R, et al. Usefulness of transesophageal echocardiography in assessment of aortic dissection. *Circulation* 1991;**84**:1903–14.

47. Simon P, Owen AN, Havel M, et al. Transesophageal echocardiography in the emergency surgical management of patients with aortic dissection. *J Thor Card Surg* 1992;**103**:1113–8.

48. Hiratzka LF, Bakris GL, Beckman JA, et al.; American College of Cardiology Foundation/American Heart Association Task Force on Practice Guidelines; American Association for Thoracic Surgery; American College of Radiology; American Stroke Association; Society of Cardiovascular Anesthesiologists; Society for Cardiovascular Angiography and Interventions; Society of Interventional Radiology; Society of Thoracic Surgeons; Society for Vascular Medicine. 2010 ACCF/AHA/AATS/ACR/ASA/SCA/SCAI/SIR/STS/SVM guidelines for the diagnosis and management of patients with thoracic aortic disease: executive summary. A report of the American College of Cardiology Foundation/American Heart Association Task Force on Practice Guidelines, American Association for Thoracic Surgery, American College of Radiology, American Stroke Association, Society of Cardiovascular Anesthesiologists, Society for Cardiovascular Angiography and Interventions, Society of Interventional Radiology, Society of Thoracic Surgeons, and Society for Vascular Medicine. *J Am Coll Cardiol* 2010–4;**55**:e27–e129.

49. Shiga T, Wajima Z, Apfel CC, et al. Diagnostic accuracy of transesophageal echocardiography, helical computed tomography, and magnetic resonance imaging for suspected thoracic aortic dissection: systematic review and meta-analysis. *Arch Intern Med* 2006;**166**:1350–6.

50. Goldstein SA, Evangelista A, Abbara S, et al. Multimodality imaging of diseases of the thoracic aorta in adults: from the American Society of Echocardiography and the European Association of Cardiovascular Imaging: endorsed by the Society of Cardiovascular Computed Tomography and Society for Cardiovascular Magnetic Resonance. *J Am Soc Echocardiogr* 2015;**28**:119–82.

Point-of-Care Transthoracic Echocardiography

Julia Sobol and Oliver Panzer

Introduction

Point-of-care transthoracic echocardiography (TTE) has become integral to the practice of acute care medicine. It can help assess patients quickly, accurately, and noninvasively,[1] and allows repeated examinations to evaluate the effects of interventions.[2] The key aspect of this examination is to rapidly provide diagnostic information to the acute care practitioner. Therefore, this examination is focused primarily on differentiating normal from severe cardiac dysfunction as the cause of hemodynamic instability and does not replace a detailed cardiology TTE. Some educators have argued that formal, basic perioperative ultrasound training should be included in anesthesiology residency, with more advanced ultrasound teaching during specific fellowship training.[3] In this chapter, we will first discuss how point-of-care TTE works in terms of logistics and diagnostic capabilities and then examine its effect on patient care.

TTE Views and Possible Assessments in Each View

Point-of-care TTE utilizes a phased-array, low-frequency (2.5–3 MHz) probe with a high frame rate (at least 24 frames/second). Imaging relies on B-mode ultrasonography in which high-density, high-impedance structures appear hyperechoic, and low-impedance, fluid-filled structures appear anechoic.

Other imaging modalities to assess cardiac physiology include M-mode and Doppler ultrasonography. M-mode focuses on one anatomical area over time, whereas Doppler examines the motion of fluid (pulsed-wave, continuous-wave, and color - flow Doppler) or structures (tissue Doppler) in relation to the ultrasound probe, with optimal imaging when movement is parallel to the ultrasound beam.[4] Pulsed-wave Doppler (PWD) sends out ultrasound waves in pulses and is able to measure the velocity of blood flow at a specific site, but it is limited by its inability to measure high velocities (Nyquist limit) due to signal aliasing. Continuous-wave Doppler (CWD) transmits ultrasound waves continuously, allowing measurement of very high velocities without the ability to localize the origin.[5] Color flow Doppler depicts flow velocity and direction, with red moving toward and blue away from the probe; optimal imaging occurs when blood flow is parallel to the ultrasound beam.[4] Pulsed-wave tissue Doppler imaging (TDI) evaluates contraction velocity of myocardial tissue.[6]

Standard views used for the point-of-care TTE examination consist of parasternal long-axis (PLAX), parasternal short-axis (PSAX), apical four- (A4 C) and five-chamber (A5 C), and subcostal long- (SLAX) and short-axis (SSAX). Information that may be acquired from each view is summarized in Table 6.1.

Parasternal Long-Axis View

The PLAX view allows visualization of the left atrium (LA), left ventricle (LV), mitral valve (MV), aortic valve (AV), aortic root and LV outflow tract (LVOT), part of the right ventricle (RV), and the descending aorta (descAO). This view is obtained on the left side of the sternum at or near the third intercostal space along the long axis of the heart.[4]

Left ventricle systolic function may be evaluated in the PLAX view by visual estimation, fractional shortening, and E-point septal separation (EPSS). Visual estimation of the change in volume in the LV between systole and diastole can differentiate normal contractility from mildly, moderately, or severely decreased LV function as well as from hyperdynamic motion.[4] Both endocardial border movement toward the center of the LV cavity and increased wall thickness during systole help assess LV systolic function visually.[2]

Table 6.1 Summary of the information and data acquired from each point-of-care transthoracic echocardiographic view.

		PLAX	PSAX	A4 C	A5 C	Subcostal	IVC
LV Systolic Function							
Visual estimation		++	++	++		++	
Fractional shortening		++	++				
LV FAC			++				
Stroke Volume							
	LVOT	++					
	VTI				++		
EPSS		++					
RWMA		+	++	+	+	+	
LV Diastolic Function							
LVH		++	+	+	+	+	
Mitral E/A				++			
Mitral E/e				++			
RV Function							
Visual estimation		+	+	++	+	++	
TAPSE				++			
RVSP/sPAP			++	++			
RVH		+				++	
RAP of CVP							++
Valves							
Aortic	2 D	++	++		++		
	Doppler				++		
Mitral	2 D	+		++			
	Doppler			++			
Tricuspid	2 D			++	++		
	Doppler			++			
Pulmonary	2 D			++			
	Doppler			++			

AV, aortic valve; CVP, central venous pressure; EPSS, E-point septal separation; FAC, fractional area change; IVC, inferior vena cava; LV, left ventricle; LVH, left ventricular hypertrophy; LVOT, left ventricular outflow tract; MV, mitral valve; PV, pulmonic valve; RAP, right atrial pressure; RV, right ventricle; RVH, right ventricular hypertrophy; RVSP, right ventricular systolic pressure; RWMA, regional wall motion abnormality; sPAP, systolic pulmonary artery pressure; SV, stroke volume; TAPSE, tricuspid annular plane systolic excursion; TV, tricuspid valve; VTI, velocity-time integral.

Left ventricle function may be evaluated semi-quantitatively with the M-mode-based method of fractional shortening (FS), which compares the end-diastolic and end-systolic diameters of the LV cavity.[4] The accuracy of FS may be diminished by misalignment of the M-mode cursor and by any abnormality in the examined LV segment shape or movement,[7] limiting its utility in predicting LV function. Another measurement of LV contractility in the PLAX view is EPSS, which correlates well with LV ejection fraction[8] (Figure 6.1). Normally, the anterior leaflet of the mitral valve (ALMV) approaches the LV septal wall when the valve opens during diastole, but with LV dilation and decreased LV contractility, the distance between the open ALMV and the interventricular septum increases. E-point septal separation is

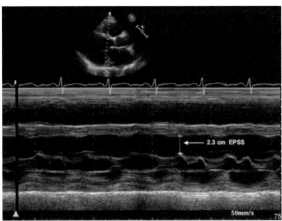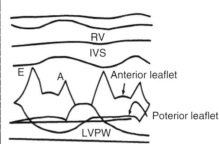

Figure 6.1 E-point septal separation (EPSS) in the parasternal long-axis view of a patient with severe left ventricular systolic dysfunction. EPSS > 8 mm is associated with systolic dysfunction. IVS, interventricular septum; LVPW, left ventricular posterior wall; RV, right ventricle. (A black and white version of this figure will appear in some formats. For the color version, please refer to the plate section.) Reprinted with permission from McKaigney CJ, Krantz MJ, La Rocque CL, et al. E-point septal separation: a bedside tool for emergency physician assessment of left ventricular ejection fraction. *Am J Emerg Med* 2014;32:493–7.

measured with M-mode to evaluate the distance between the E wave (the first wave that shows passive ventricular filling) and the LV septum; EPSS greater than 1 cm is associated with decreased LV contractility. It is inaccurate in cases of mitral stenosis or regurgitation, aortic regurgitation, or severe LV hypertrophy (LVH).[4]

The PLAX view allows assessment of ventricular wall thickness, AV, MV, and LVOT. M-mode or caliper measurements can evaluate LV wall thickness. Left ventricular hypertrophy is associated with LV wall thickness greater than 1 cm,[4] with severe LVH characterized by LV wall thickness greater than 1.5 cm.[7] In the PLAX view, RV-free wall thickness greater than 5 mm implies that RV afterload is likely chronically high.[9,10] The valves should also be examined for leaflet thickness and excursion, as well as calcifications that might suggest aortic stenosis (AS)[11] or mitral valve pathophysiology such as systolic anterior motion of the MV.[12] Mitral and aortic regurgitation can also be detected in this view by color Doppler but should be evaluated in other views as well.[1] The LVOT area may be estimated in this view as part of stroke volume (SV) and cardiac output (CO) calculations. The LVOT diameter is measured between the right and non-coronary cusps of the AV during systole, and the LVOT area is calculated from the diameter (Figure 6.2a). The PLAX view may also show a pericardial effusion appearing as an anechoic region at the pericardial border tracking anterior to the descAO, differentiating the fluid from a pleural effusion, which lies posterior to the descAO.[4]

Parasternal Short-Axis View

By rotating the ultrasound probe 90° clockwise from the PLAX view, the PSAX view will appear with the LV in cross-section. By fanning the probe from the base to the apex of the heart, the ultrasound beam can visualize several levels, including the AV and mid-papillary levels. At the AV level, the AV, both atria, tricuspid valve (TV), RV, pulmonic valve (PV), and pulmonary artery (PA) may be seen.[4] The AV should be assessed visually in this view for leaflet calcification and mobility to evaluate for AS.[11] In addition, as flow through the TV and PV is aligned parallel to the ultrasound beam, tricuspid and pulmonic regurgitant jets may be assessed by Doppler.[9]

At the mid-papillary muscle level, the LV short-axis view can be utilized to estimate LV systolic function visually or by FS. Alternatively, the percentage change between end-diastolic and end-systolic LV area can be measured as the fractional area change (FAC).[13] The formula for FAC is:

FAC(%) = 100 × (LV end-diastolic area – LV end-systolic area)/(LV end-diastolic area)

Normal values are 36–64%.[13] Area measurements, however, assume normal ventricular geometry.[7] In

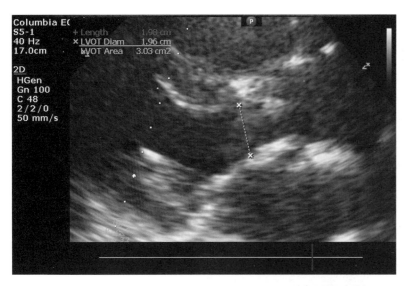

Figure 6.2(a) Close-up of the left ventricular outflow tract (LVOT) in the parasternal long-axis view with the cursor measuring the LVOT diameter during systole. LVOT area is calculated from the diameter by the formula: $LVOT_{area} = \pi \, (diameter/2)^2$.

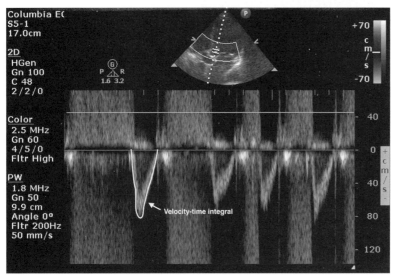

Figure 6.2(b) Apical five-chamber view showing pulsed-wave Doppler (PWD) at the left ventricular outflow tract (LVOT). The velocity-time integral (VTI) function on the ultrasound machine traces the area under the PWD curve, which, when multiplied by the area of the LVOT obtained in the parasternal long-axis view, allows calculation of left ventricular stroke volume. Stroke volume multiplied by heart rate determines cardiac output. (A black and white version of this figure will appear in some formats. For the color version, please refer to the plate section).

case of myocardial ischemia or infarction, regional wall motion abnormalities can be detected as the entire coronary distribution may be seen in this view. The mid-papillary muscle PSAX view is also helpful in assessing RV pressure or volume overload. As RV pressure increases, the interventricular septum (IVS) bows into the LV during systole, and as RV volume increases, the IVS moves toward the LV during diastole. Both of these scenarios lead to a D-shaped LV in the PSAX view.[10]

Apical Four- and Five-Chamber Views

The apical views are obtained by placing the probe at the point of maximal impulse. The A4 C view shows all four chambers and their relative size and function, and this is the best view for Doppler evaluation of the MV and TV as the direction of blood flow is aligned parallel to the ultrasound probe. By angling the probe more superiorly from the A4 C view, the A5 C view is obtained, with the LVOT and AV as the fifth chamber.[4] The apical views are important in assessing LV and RV function as well as in evaluating valvulopathies.

One purpose of the A5 C view is to estimate SV and CO.[4] The SV is calculated by the formula:

$$SV = LVOT_{area} \times VTI$$

The velocity-time integral (VTI) is the area under the PWD curve at the LVOT (Figure 6.2b), representing

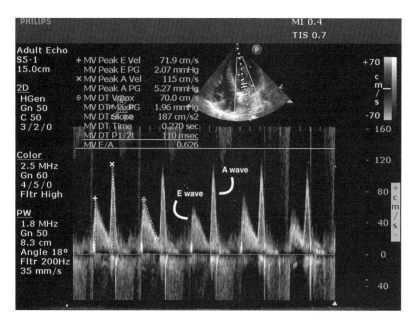

Figure 6.3(a) Apical four-chamber view with pulsed-wave Doppler (PWD) across the mitral valve showing biphasic diastolic flow. The E wave represents early passive filling, whereas the A wave shows atrial contraction during late diastole. Peak E- and A-wave velocities are used to calculate the E/A ratio. (A black and white version of this figure will appear in some formats. For the color version, please refer to the plate section).

blood flow moving through the LVOT in each cardiac cycle.[4] Velocity-time integral measurements should be repeated at least three times to improve accuracy.[13] The LVOT area is obtained from measuring the AV diameter in the PLAX view as described above.[4] Alternatively, Simpson's method is a different way to calculate LV ejection fraction using multiple apical views, but it is time-consuming and requires clear endocardial borders with perfect orientation,[10] limiting its utility in point-of-care TTE.

The A5 C view also allows for the assessment of AV leaflet calcifications and excursion. The degree of AS may be estimated quantitatively by placing the CWD cursor across the AV, which may show elevated peak velocities that indicate moderate (3–4 m/sec) to severe (> 4 m/sec) AS. However, as the peak AV velocity depends on LV contractility, the degree of AS may be underestimated in patients with severe LV dysfunction.[11]

The A4 C view is helpful for assessing LV diastolic function and RV function. Impaired LV relaxation and/or elevated LV stiffness contribute to diastolic dysfunction.[14] The degree of LV diastolic dysfunction can be evaluated using PWD across the MV and TDI at the MV annulus.[10] On PWD, diastolic flow across the MV is biphasic, with the E wave occurring during early passive filling and the A wave during late diastole due to atrial contraction.[6] The PWD is placed between the MV leaflet tips to measure peak E-wave and A-wave velocities[10] (Figure 6.3a). LV relaxation and preload affect the E wave, while LV compliance and LA contraction determine the A wave.[14] By calculating the mitral E/A ratio, different filling patterns may be described. An E/A ratio ≥ 2 in patients older than 40 years usually signifies severe diastolic dysfunction. However, normal and pseudo-normal filling patterns are difficult to distinguish from each other, especially in patients with normal ejection fraction.[6] Furthermore, filling patterns are affected by patient age, hypertrophic or restrictive cardiomyopathy, mitral valve disease, and mitral valve repair/replacement, and they cannot be utilized in patients with atrial arrhythmias.[6,10]

If the E/A ratio is inconclusive or if the patient has normal LV function, it may be helpful to obtain the mitral annular peak velocity via TDI of the mitral annulus[10] (Figure 6.3b). TDI evaluates early (e') and late (a') mitral annular diastolic excursion. Peak e' velocity is due primarily to LV relaxation, independent of preload.[14] The E/e' ratio – a combination of PWD and TDI measurements in early diastole – is less dependent on LV function and age than other indices of diastolic function.[6,14] If E/e' is less than 8, the LV filling pressure is normal, but if the ratio is greater than 14, the LV filling pressure is high.[6] High LV filling pressure identifies patients at risk of cardiogenic pulmonary edema.[10] Other markers of LV diastolic dysfunction may include LA enlargement (a sign of elevated LA pressure in patients without atrial

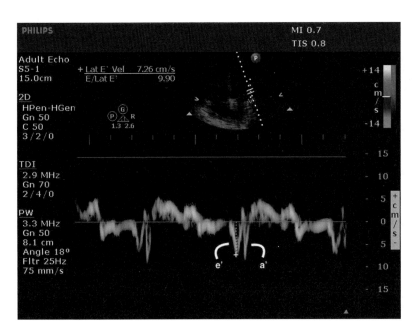

Figure 6.3(b) Apical four-chamber view with tissue Doppler imaging (TDI) of the mitral annulus showing early (e') and late (a') excursion of the mitral annulus during diastole. The E/e' ratio utilizing peak e' velocity is another measure of left ventricular diastolic function. (A black and white version of this figure will appear in some formats. For the color version, please refer to the plate section).

arrhythmias or MV disease) and/or LVH, which is often associated with diastolic dysfunction.[6]

The A4 C view also allows the assessment of the RV. RV pressure or volume overload may lead to RV dilation and dysfunction.[9] RV dilation may be evaluated by comparing LV and RV size.[4] Normally, the end-diastolic RV cavity is 60% of the end-diastolic LV size. RV cavity size greater than 100% the size of the LV denotes severe RV enlargement.[10] While the LV normally occupies the apex of the heart, RV dilation may displace the LV and take over the apex instead.[9] As RV free-wall contraction relies on longitudinal movement, tricuspid annular plane systolic excursion (TAPSE) correlates well with RV systolic function.[10] TAPSE is measured in M-mode, with values less than 16 mm associated with decreased RV systolic function[9] (Figure 6.4).

Tricuspid regurgitation (TR), which is often associated with RV dysfunction, can be assessed by color-flow Doppler and allows estimation of PA systolic pressure (sPAP).[10] The maximal TR jet velocity of blood is converted to a pressure gradient across the TV by the modified Bernoulli equation.[15] The CWD is positioned along the TR jet main axis to calculate blood flow velocity and then pressure across the TV is calculated[10] (Figure 6.5). For greater accuracy of sPAP calculation, the spectral profile should be dense with well-defined borders and the TR jet should be examined from multiple views as angle affects velocity measurements. Peak TR jet velocity estimates RV

systolic pressure (RVSP) using the simplified Bernoulli equation and RA pressure (RAP):

$$RVSP = 4(Vmax)^2 + RAP$$

where Vmax is the peak TR regurgitant jet velocity and RAP is obtained from inferior vena cava (IVC) measurements in the subxiphoid view[9] or from a central venous catheter.[10] RVSP and sPAP are equivalent if there is no gradient across the PV or RVOT.[9]

The apical window is also especially helpful for diagnosing tamponade, as pericardial effusion with diastolic collapse of the RA or RV may be visualized easily in this view.[4]

Subcostal Long- and Short-Axis Views

The subcostal views are particularly useful to evaluate cardiac morphology, the pericardium, and the IVC.[16] They are obtained by pointing the ultrasound beam toward the heart under the sternum by using the liver as an acoustic window, thereby avoiding lung interference. The SLAX view allows visual assessment of both ventricles and atria as well as the pericardial space, similar to the A4 C view. Given its proximity to the ultrasound probe, the RV free wall is easily assessed in this view,[4] with RV free wall thickness greater than 5 mm suggesting RV hypertrophy.[9] By rotating the probe counterclockwise into a sagittal plane, the SSAX view is obtained, which resembles

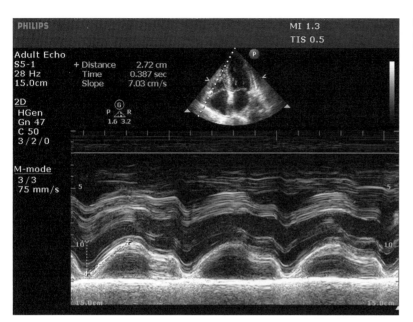

Figure 6.4 Tricuspid annular plane systolic excursion (TAPSE) measured in the apical four-chamber view with M-mode. Values < 16 mm are associated with decreased right ventricular systolic function.

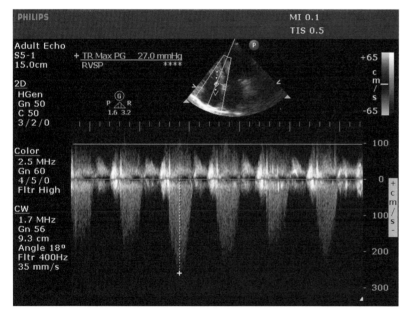

Figure 6.5 Continuous-wave Doppler (CWD) of tricuspid regurgitation (TR) in the apical four-chamber view. Maximal TR jet velocity can be used to calculate right ventricular systolic pressure using the simplified Bernoulli equation and right atrial pressure. (A black and white version of this figure will appear in some formats. For the color version, please refer to the plate section).

the PSAX view.[5] While the subcostal views provide images similar to the A4 C and PSAX views, the ultrasound beam does not align parallel to the direction of blood flow in the subcostal position, limiting its utility in calculating hemodynamic parameters.[16]

In the subcostal position, the IVC may be visualized in short and long axes to measure diameter and respiratory variability, which help estimate central venous pressure (CVP).[4] The IVC should be assessed immediately proximal to the hepatic vein entry,[9] although some recommend measuring it 2 cm caudal to the entry of the hepatic vein.[17] Elevated RAP leads to IVC dilation and reduced IVC collapse with inspiration during spontaneous ventilation. If the IVC diameter is ≤ 2.1 cm with inspiratory collapse greater than 50% with sniffing, RAP is likely 0–5 mmHg, while a diameter greater than 2.1 cm with collapse less than 50% indicates RAP 10–20 mmHg. IVC diameter

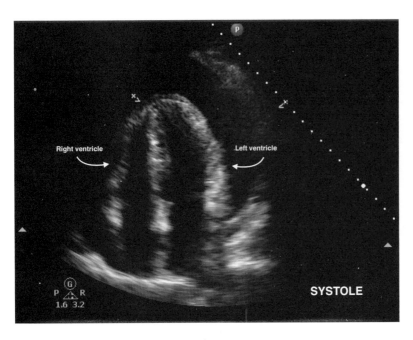

Figure 6.6(a) Apical four-chamber view showing a pericardial effusion during systole.

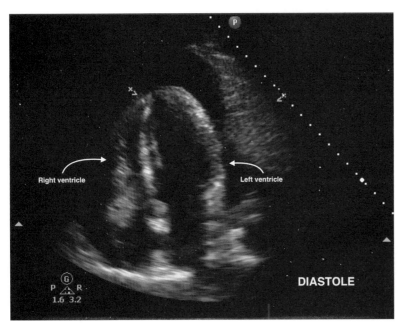

Figure 6.6(b) Apical four-chamber view illustrating a pericardial effusion accompanied by right ventricular diastolic collapse, suggesting tamponade.

should be measured at end-expiration. In mechanically ventilated patients, RAP should be measured by pressure transduction as the IVC may be dilated with no respiratory variation. However, if the IVC diameter is ≤ 1.2 cm in these patients, RAP is probably < 10 mmHg.[9] Inferior vena cava size and collapsibility measures should not be used in patients with elevated intra-abdominal pressure.[2] In addition, the liver may act as an acoustic window for an alternative view of the IVC from a lateral, mid-axillary probe position.[4]

Impact of Point-of-Care TTE on Patient Outcomes

Increased utilization of point-of-care TTE could be of great benefit, particularly in patients at risk of life-threatening shock or cardiac arrest. In non-trauma emergency room patients with undifferentiated hypotension, goal-directed TTE has been shown to help guide treatment interventions, narrow the differential diagnosis,[18] and improve diagnostic accuracy.[19] In the perioperative setting, anesthesiologists performing TTE prior to urgent surgical procedures discovered unexpected pathology that affected anesthetic management in high-risk patients.[20,21] In addition, even brief training of practitioners allows accurate identification of myocardial dysfunction when compared to formal TTE.[22] While data have not shown that point-of-care TTE improves patient outcomes or mortality,[20,21] point-of-care ultrasound can certainly help determine the type and possibly the cause of shock,[23] potentially allowing earlier, more appropriate intervention and treatment.

In patients with hypovolemic or distributive shock, the ventricles are usually both small and sometimes hyperkinetic.[23] Obliteration of the LV cavity at end-systole with vigorous systolic wall motion indicates hyperdynamic function, hypovolemia, and low afterload.[2] As both hypovolemic and distributive shock are associated with an empty LV in systole, the LV size in diastole may help distinguish the two entities: small LV diastolic size suggests hypovolemia, while fuller LV cavity diastolic size may indicate distributive shock due to low afterload.[12] In either type of shock, the diameter of the IVC will likely be small with collapsibility through the respiratory cycle.[24] The subset of patients with hypovolemic and/or distributive shock due to sepsis may exhibit unique findings on point-of-care TTE, such as LV systolic and diastolic dysfunction, as well as RV dysfunction with dilated IVC.[2,23]

Cardiogenic shock presents with poor LV contractility and function as assessed by visual estimation, FS, FAC, EPSS, and calculation of CO.[4] Diastolic heart failure would be associated with changes in flow and motion at the MV, as discussed above.[6] Assessing for regional wall motion abnormality (RWMA) in the LV may identify myocardial ischemia or infarction. The PSAX view is the most suitable for RWMA assessment as it allows visualization of all LV wall segments, which can each be inspected individually. Wall motion may be deemed normal/hyperkinetic, hypokinetic (decreased wall thickening), akinetic (minimal thickening), or dyskinetic (systolic thinning).[7] If the wall thickens less than 50%, or if wall excursion is less

than 5 mm, the segment is contracting abnormally.[10] Evaluation for RWMA should focus on thickening rather than motion, because tethering to nearby wall segments can affect adjacent wall motion.[7]

Point-of-care TTE is also helpful in distinguishing different forms of obstructive shock. Tamponade presents with pericardial effusion plus RA or RV diastolic collapse, often best viewed in the A4 C or subcostal windows (Figures 6.6a and 6.6b). RV diastolic collapse is more specific for tamponade than RA collapse, and progresses with the degree of tamponade from a subtle inward movement of the RV free wall to complete collapse.[4] An increase in intra-pericardial pressure with pericardial fluid accumulation determines whether tamponade physiology occurs, rather than the size of the pericardial effusion itself.[2] The IVC is usually enlarged with no respiratory variation.[24] In the A4 C view, PWD through the MV and TV may identify changes in valvular flow with the respiratory cycle; tamponade physiology is suggested by an increase in flow of greater than 25% across the TV with inspiration, or a decrease in flow of greater than 15% across the MV with inspiration.[4]

Other forms of obstructive shock are primarily due to RV dysfunction. Acute inferior wall myocardial ischemia or infarction could cause RV failure, which might present with RV dilation and dysfunction without elevation of sPAP.[10] The LV posterior or inferior free wall may also show wall motion abnormalities. Acute cor pulmonale with an abrupt increase in RV afterload is most often due to pulmonary embolism (PE) or acute respiratory distress syndrome (ARDS),[25] with an incidence of approximately 30–55% of patients with PE and 25% of patients with ARDS.[15] Acute cor pulmonale due to PE would likely exhibit RV failure, elevated sPAP, and flattening of the interventricular septum, best viewed in the PSAX view[10,24] (Figure 6.7). The IVC is often dilated without respiratory variability, and clot may be visible in the right side of the heart or the PA.[4,24] With a large, acute PE, McConnell's sign may be present, in which the RV base and free wall become hypokinetic, but the apex contracts normally.[24]

To distinguish acute from chronic RV dysfunction, RV wall thickness may be measured; RV wall diameter greater than 6 mm indicates chronic RV strain.[24] Increased RV diastolic wall thickness may occur in response to a sudden rise in RV afterload in as little as 48 hours. In addition, marked trabeculations within the RV cavity often accompany chronic

63

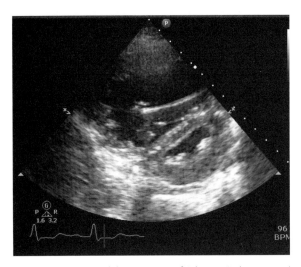

Figure 6.7 Parasternal short-axis view of right ventricular pressure/volume overload with flattening of the interventricular septum in a patient with acute cor pulmonale. The left ventricle appears D-shaped.

cor pulmonale.[25] Chronic conditions that may be associated with RV dysfunction include obstructive sleep apnea, chronic obstructive pulmonary disease, pulmonary hypertension, and chronic pulmonary emboli.[4,24] Pulmonary hypertension would be suggested by sPAP ≥ 35 mmHg, peak TR jet velocity > 2.8 m/sec, TAPSE < 16 mm, RV dilation, and estimated RAP > 15 mmHg.[26] Finally, it is important to remember that the RV may become dilated and dysfunctional due to primary LV dysfunction.[9]

Point-of-care TTE may also be useful in cardiac arrest. An international expert panel in emergency medicine recommends that point-of-care TTE be performed during cardiac arrest while pausing for rhythm checks, thereby minimizing any interruptions of chest compressions. The subcostal view is preferred, with the PLAX view as an alternative window. The initial core views should focus on potentially reversible causes of cardiac arrest such as tamponade, hypovolemia, RV failure, and myocardial dysfunction, as well as evaluation of organized cardiac activity or asystole. Supplementary views including the apical window, the IVC, and the lungs should be performed if time allows and if further information is required.[27]

Performing TTE during cardiac arrest may also help with prognostication. One systematic review showed that cardiac activity detected on point-of-care TTE during cardiac arrest and resuscitation efforts was associated with a much higher rate of

return of spontaneous circulation (ROSC) than no cardiac activity.[28] A recent large, multicenter, prospective observational study showed that non-traumatic cardiac arrest patients who presented to the emergency department with cardiac activity on point-of-care TTE at the beginning of resuscitative efforts had significantly improved odds of survival than those with no cardiac activity.[29] A secondary analysis of this study showed that the type of cardiac activity seen may also be important: patients with disorganized cardiac activity (agonal or twitching myocardial activity on TTE) had significantly lower rates of ROSC compared to those with organized activity (synchronized ventricular wall motion with change in the size of the ventricular cavity).[30] However, utilization of point-of-care TTE in cardiac arrest has not been shown to affect patient outcomes. In a small trial of cardiac arrest patients randomized to TTE or no TTE during resuscitation efforts, those who underwent TTE did not have improved rates of ROSC or survival compared to those without TTE, even though potentially reversible causes of cardiac arrest were found in those who were evaluated by TTE.[31]

Although other disorders may precipitate circulatory failure, the pathophysiologic states described here represent some potentially reversible causes of shock that have widely different therapeutic interventions and management. Point-of-care TTE can help distinguish these causes of shock and expeditiously narrow the differential diagnosis in shock and arrest situations.[2] A focused TTE examination could take as little as 1 minute and may be performed by trained novices.[23] While point-of-care TTE is fast becoming essential to the practice of acute care medicine and anesthesiology,[3] future research in point-of-care TTE should focus on whether patient outcomes are actually improved by its use.

References

1. Shillcutt SK, Bick JS. A comparison of basic transthoracic and transesophageal echocardiography views in the perioperative setting. *Anesth Analg* 2013;**116**:1231–6.

2. Griffee MJ, Merkel MJ, Wei KS. The role of echocardiography in hemodynamic assessment of septic shock. *Crit Care Clin* 2010;**26**:365–82.

3. Mahmood F, Matyal R, Skubas N, et al. Perioperative ultrasound training in anesthesiology: a call to action. *Anesth Analg* 2016;**122**:1794–804.

4. Perera P, Lobo V, Williams SR, et al. Cardiac echocardiography. *Crit Care Clin* 2014;**30**:47–92.

5. Sturgess DJ. Transthoracic echocardiography: an overview. In: Lumb P, Karakitsos D, eds. *Critical Care Ultrasound*. Philadelphia: Elsevier Saunders, 2015;139–45.

6. Nagueh SF, Smiseth OA, Appleton CP, et al. Recommendations for the evaluation of left ventricular diastolic function by echocardiography. *Eur Heart J Cardiovasc Imaging* 2016;**17**:1321–60.

7. Lang R, Badano L, Mor-Avi V, et al. Recommendations for cardiac chamber quantification by echocardiography in adults: an update from the American Society of Echocardiography and the European Association of Cardiovascular Imaging. *Eur Heart J Cardiovasc Imaging* 2015;**16**:233–70.

8. McKaigney CJ, Krantz MJ, La Rocque CL, et al. E-point septal separation: a bedside tool for emergency physician assessment of left ventricular ejection fraction. *Am J Emerg Med* 2014;**32**:493–7.

9. Rudski LG, Lai WW, Afilalo J, et al. Guidelines for the echocardiographic assessment of the right heart in adults: a report from the American Society of Echocardiography. *J Am Soc Echocardiogr* 2010;**23**:685–713.

10. Narasimhan M, Koenig SJ, Mayo PH. Advanced echocardiography for the critical care physician, Part 2. *Chest* 2014;**145**:135–42.

11. Cowie B, Kluger R. Evaluation of systolic murmurs using transthoracic echocardiography by anaesthetic trainees. *Anaesthesia* 2011;**66**:785–90.

12. Zimmerman JM, Coker BJ. The nuts and bolts of performing focused cardiovascular ultrasound (FoCUS). *Anesth Analg* 2017;**124**:753–60.

13. Slama M, Maizel J. Echocardiographic measurement of ventricular function. *Curr Opin Crit Care* 2006;**12**:241–8.

14. Maizel J, El-Dash S, Slama M. Evaluation of left ventricular diastolic function in the intensive care unit. In: Lumb P, Karakitsos D, eds. *Critical Care Ultrasound*. Philadelphia: Elsevier Saunders, 2015;175–8.

15. Krishnan S, Schmidt GA. Acute right ventricular dysfunction. *Chest* 2015;**147**:835–46.

16. Maizel J, Salhi A, Tribouilloy C, et al. The subxiphoid view cannot replace the apical view for transthoracic echocardiographic assessment of hemodynamic status. *Crit Care* 2013;**17**:R186.

17. Wallace DJ, Allison M, Stone MB. Inferior vena cava percentage collapse during respiration is affected by the sampling location: an ultrasound study in healthy volunteers. *Acad Emerg Med* 2010;**17**:96–9.

18. Shokoohi H, Boniface KS, Pourmand A, et al. Bedside ultrasonography reduces diagnostic uncertainty and guides resuscitation in patients with undifferentiated hypotension. *Crit Care Med* 2015;**43**:2562–9.

19. Jones AE, Tayal VS, Sullivan M, et al. Randomized, controlled trial of immediate versus delayed goal-directed ultrasound to identify the cause of nontraumatic hypotension in emergency department patients. *Crit Care Med* 2004;**32**:1703–8.

20. Bøtker MT, Vang ML, Grøfte T, et al. Routine pre-operative focused ultrasonography by anesthesiologists in patients undergoing urgent surgical procedures. *Acta Anaesthesiol Scand* 2014;**58**:807–14.

21. Canty DJ, Royse CF, Kilpatrick D, et al. The impact of pre-operative focused transthoracic echocardiography in emergency non-cardiac surgery patients with known or risk of cardiac disease. *Anaesthesia* 2012;**67**:714–20.

22. Melamed R, Sprenkle MD, Ulstad VK, et al. Assessment of left ventricular function by intensivists using hand-held echocardiography. *Chest* 2009;**135**:1416–20.

23. De Backer D. Ultrasonic evaluation of the heart. *Curr Opin Crit Care* 2014;**20**:309–14.

24. Wu TS. The CORE scan. *Crit Care Clin* 2014;**30**:151–75.

25. Vieillard-Baron A, Prin S, Chergui K, et al. Echo-Doppler demonstration of acute cor pulmonale at the bedside in the medical intensive care unit. *Am J Respir Crit Care Med* 2002;**166**:1310–9.

26. Hellenkamp K, Unsöld B, Mushemi-Blake S, et al. Echocardiographic estimation of mean pulmonary artery pressure: a comparison of different approaches to assign the likelihood of pulmonary hypertension. *J Am Soc Echocardiogr* 2017;**31** (1):89–98.

27. Atkinson P, Bowra J, Milne J, et al. International Federation for Emergency Medicine Consensus Statement: Sonography in hypotension and cardiac arrest (SHoC): an international consensus on the use of point of care ultrasound for undifferentiated hypotension and during cardiac arrest. *CJEM* 2017;**19**:459–70.

28. Blyth L, Atkinson P, Gadd K, et al. Bedside focused echocardiography as predictor of survival in cardiac arrest patients: a systematic review. *Acad Emerg Med* 2012;**19**:1119–26.

29. Gaspari R, Weekes A, Adhikari S, et al. Emergency department point-of-care ultrasound in out-of-hospital and in-ED cardiac arrest. *Resuscitation* 2016;**109**:33–9.

65

30. Gaspari R, Weekes A, Adhikari S, et al. A retrospective study of pulseless electrical activity, bedside ultrasound identifies interventions during resuscitation associated with improved survival to hospital admission. *Resuscitation* 2017;**120**:103–7.

31. Chardoli M, Heidari F, Rabiee H, et al. Echocardiography integrated ACLS protocol versus conventional cardiopulmonary resuscitation in patients with pulseless electrical activity cardiac arrest. *Chin J Traumatol* 2012;**15**:284–7.

Point-of-Care Lung Ultrasound

Zachary Kuschner and John M. Oropello

Introduction

Lung ultrasound was initially thought to be impossible due to the acoustic impedance of air. In the 1960s it was demonstrated that ultrasound could be used to image pleural effusions due to their fluid composition and proximity to the chest wall and diaphragm.[1,2] Subsequent work in the 1980s established that in a normal thoracic cavity the air–fluid interface and the presence of two mobile opposing pleural surfaces generated stereotypical imaging artifacts. Deviations from these normal artifacts correspond to specific pathologic processes,[3,4] and a systematic approach to assessing and monitoring these pathologies in critically ill patients has been developed.[5] Bedsides, lung sonography can be adapted for use by anesthesiologists in the perioperative care setting,[6] where pulmonary complications occur in 5–13% of patients and significantly increase mortality and the cost of care.[7–9]

The standard method of assessing pulmonary pathology in the perioperative setting remains the chest x-ray. Chest x-rays, especially when performed portably, have significant diagnostic limitations and take significantly longer to obtain than bedside sonography.[10,11] Lung ultrasound may yield information not obtained by, and in some situations may even substitute for, a chest x-ray. Lung ultrasound can also be used to determine volume status and guide management.[12,13] This chapter describes the techniques involved in the application of lung ultrasound to the monitoring and management of perioperative patients.

Techniques

Medical diagnostic ultrasound technologies transmit frequencies in the 1–20 megahertz (MHz) range. Low ultrasound frequencies result in lower resolution images than higher frequencies, but have greater penetration and permit evaluation of structures that lie deep within the thorax.[14] The three most common ultrasound transducers are the phased array, linear, and curvilinear probes. They differ with respect to their piezoelectric crystal arrangement, aperture (footprint), and frequency range. Lung ultrasound is performed with phased array or linear probes. The curvilinear (curved linear) probe is generally not used in thoracic ultrasound; because the crystals are organized in an arc, it results in a wide footprint that makes it difficult to find adequate sonographic windows between the ribs.[14]

There are several modes of processing and displaying the ultrasonic echo reflections, including A-mode (amplitude mode), B-mode (brightness mode, also known as 2D mode), and M-mode (motion mode).

The phased array probe emits low ultrasound frequency waves in the 2–8 MHz range.[14] The grouping of crystals in the phased array probe yields a fan-shaped footprint (Figure 7.1a). A variant of the phased array probe is the rectangular-shaped "cardiac" phased array probe. This probe can be used to image lung as well as other structures, such as heart, abdomen, and inferior vena cava; utilizing this single probe permits easy transition between examinations of multiple sites.

The linear probe contains crystals arrayed in a straight line and emits acoustic waves in higher frequencies ranging from 5 to 13 MHz.[14] The grouping of crystals in the linear probe yields a rectangular-shaped footprint (Figure 7.1b). The higher frequencies result in better resolution but have less tissue penetration. The linear probe can occasionally clarify superficial artifacts if the phased array probe images are indeterminate. It is also the best probe for imaging the trachea, as when performing percutaneous tracheostomies.

Lung sonographic exams, similar to other noncardiac sonographic exams, are performed with the probe marker oriented cephalad when scanning in longitudinal orientation, and toward the patient's

(a)   (b)

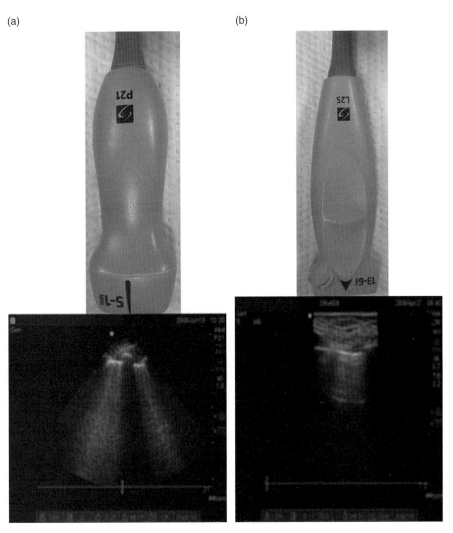

Figure 7.1 (a) Phased array with fanned output. (b) Linear probe with rectangular output.

right side when scanning in transverse orientation. When using M-mode, the provider should set the scan speed to slow, because sonographic studies using the medium or fast speeds may produce repeating horizontal lines that give the erroneous impression of pneumothorax (Figure 7.2).[14] The gain should be adjusted to permit visualization of the artifacts without obscuring the adjacent pulmonary tissue.

The thorax may be divided into superior and inferior zones, each of which are further divided into anterior, lateral, and posterior regions defined by the anterior and posterior axillary lines (Figure 7.3).[5] The probe should be placed in a longitudinal (sagittal) orientation in the midclavicular line, producing an image in which both the superior and inferior ribs are in view, as well as the soft tissue and air–pleural

interface in between the two ribs.[12] This should be repeated in the midaxillary line in both the superior and inferior hemithorax. The diaphragm should be visualized when examining the inferior hemithorax in the midaxillary line.

Artifacts

Unlike traditional sonography in which structures and pathology are visualized directly, pulmonary sonography relies on ultrasonic artifacts created by the interface between air contained within the lungs and fluid within tissue. This interface, in combination with the phasic sliding between the visceral and parietal pleura that accompanies respiration, creates stereotypical artifacts when imaging normal lung.

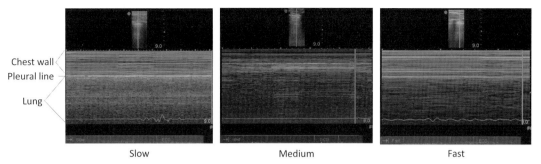

Chest wall
Pleural line
Lung

Slow   Medium   Fast

Figure 7.2 M-mode sweep speed settings. As the sweep speed is increased from slow to medium and then from medium to fast, more horizontal lines are generated giving the false appearance (at medium and fast sweep speeds) of absent pleural sliding (bar-code sign). On the proper slow sweep setting, horizontal lines appear only in the chest wall, not below the pleural line where the lung has a sandy appearance indicating pleural sliding (seashore sign).

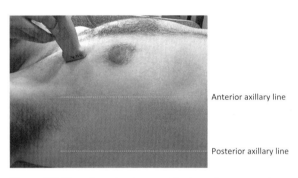

Anterior axillary line

Posterior axillary line

Figure 7.3 Thoracic probe placement for lung ultrasonography. The thorax may be divided into regions: superior (width of patient's hand beginning from right below the clavicle), inferior (another hand's breadth below the superior hand), anterior (anterior to the anterior axillary line), lateral (in between the anterior and posterior axillary lines), and posterior (posterior to the posterior axillary line). Probe placement in the superior anterior region below the midclavicular line is the first place to look for a pneumothorax in a supine patient. As a pneumothorax enlarges, it moves laterally and then posteriorly. Pleural effusions usually begin posteriorly, moving laterally and anteriorly as they enlarge. In critically ill patients with abdominal distension, or on expiration, most of the lung may be close to or above the nipple level. Begin to search for the diaphragm laterally and at the nipple line.

Identification of these normal artifacts can be used to rule out pathology. Absence of normal artifacts and identification of abnormal artifacts can be used to rule in pathology.

Normal Artifacts

The normal artifacts that are indicative of healthy lung tissue are lung sliding (also known as pleural sliding), A-lines, the bat sign, and the seashore sign.

Lung sliding (also known as pleural sliding) and A-lines can both be visualized using the longitudinal orientation in the 2D mode (see Figure 7.4 and video link 1: https://static1.squarespace.com/static/549b0

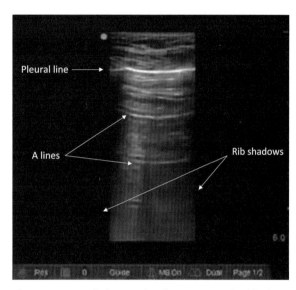

Pleural line

A lines

Rib shadows

Figure 7.4 Normal ultrasound artifacts present in healthy lung tissue. 2D lung still image captured by a linear probe in the sagittal plane, midclavicular line, 2nd interspace. The pleural line consists of the parietal and visceral pleura. The A-lines are reverberation artifacts off the pleural line at a distance equal to the distance between the ultrasound probe and the pleural line. A-lines indicate "air." The anechoic borders are produced by rib shadows. If this were a video, the pleural line would twinkle or shimmer, indicating pleural sliding.

d5fe4b031a76584e558/577dba7a1b631b1456316e53/577dba7a37c581b33317e898/1467857682349/normallungslide.gif?format=500w).

The lung sliding artifact is a shimmering appearance of the lung-chest wall border caused by movement of the visceral and parietal pleurae against one another.[3,15] A-lines are repeating, equidistantly spaced horizontal lines that appear deep to the pleural line (i.e., the most anterior and brightest line seen on

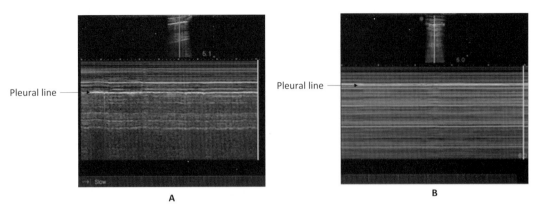

Figure 7.5 (a) M-mode applied to normal lung parenchyma creates an artifact known as "seashore sign" in which horizontal lines corresponding to superficial chest wall tissue appear above the pleural line and pulmonary tissue below the pleura produces a granular pattern. Make sure the sweep speed is set to slow. (b) M-mode in the absence of lung sliding: stratosphere sign or barcode sign in which horizontal lines corresponding to superficial chest wall tissue appear above the pleural line and the air or nonmoving pulmonary tissue below the pleura.

ultrasound) and are the acoustic mirror of the air–fluid interface between apposed pleurae.[12,13]

The bat sign, also seen in the longitudinal 2D mode, is visualization of the pleura of normal lung in which lung sliding and A-lines are flanked by the two ribs' (a superior rib and an inferior rib) acoustic shadows. An image obtained via an abdominal window where there are no ribs will not show a bat sign; thoracentesis or chest tube insertion should not be performed in that location.

In M-mode, normal lung parenchyma creates the seashore sign in which horizontal lines corresponding to superficial chest wall tissue appear superficial to the pleural line and pulmonary tissue deep to the pleura produces a granular pattern (Figure 7.5a).[16] The sign is so named because the horizontal lines of the superficial tissue resemble ocean waves and the granular pattern of the pleural tissue resembles a sandy beach. The M-mode seashore sign is used to augment evaluations where lung sliding is subtle and the shimmer of the opposing pleurae is difficult to perceive in the standard 2D view. Note that M-mode captures lung sliding in a static image that may be printed, whereas video is required to demonstrate lung sliding in 2D mode.

Abnormal Artifacts

Abnormal artifacts that identify lung pathology are due to deviations from the normal air–pleural interface. These deviations may be generated by the pathologic interposition of air or fluid in the pleural space, or by the accumulation of fluid within the lung tissue.

The main principle that governs interpretation of these images is that air rises to occupy the most ascendant point of a body cavity while fluid falls to dependent locations. As with the normal pulmonary artifacts, since fluid has greater acoustic impedance than air, fluid-filled tissue and compressed tissue will better conduct the ultrasound signal.

Pneumothorax

Ultrasound can only rule out a pneumothorax in the thoracic interspace where lung sliding is seen. Given that free air within the pleural cavity rises to the most superior regions if there are no adhesions to trap it, a pneumothorax can only definitively be ruled out when the ultrasound is applied to the most superior region for the patient's position. Several adjacent superior thoracic interspaces should be imaged to assure a sufficiently thorough exam and maximize specificity.

The main abnormal artifacts produced by pneumothorax are abnormal A-lines and the barcode sign. In addition, there are several complementary artifacts that can be used to augment indeterminate exams; these are lung point, heart point, lung pulse and B-lines.

Under 2D ultrasound, absence of lung sliding produces A-lines throughout the entire sonographic field and may reflect a pneumothorax, depending on the clinical scenario.[12] (video link 2: https://static1.square space.com/static/549b0d5fe4b031a76584e558/577dba7 a1b631b1456316e53/577dba7c37c581b33317e8a2/146 7857674242/noslide.gif?format=1000w).

In M-mode, absence of lung sliding produces a stereotypical finding known as the barcode sign (also known as the stratosphere sign). Horizontal lines corresponding to the chest wall tissue appear superficial to the pleural line, and air in the lung deep to the pleura produces a pattern of thin straight repeating horizontal lines and thicker A-lines extending throughout the depth of the sonographic field (Figure 7.5b).[17] The absence of lung sliding on 2D is 100% sensitive and 78% specific for pneumothorax; specificity increases to 94% when absence of lung sliding on 2D is accompanied by the M-mode barcode sign.[12] Conditions other than pneumothorax that may eliminate or reduce lung sliding include apnea, mainstem intubation, phrenic nerve palsy (in spontaneously breathing patients), pleural effusion, consolidation, atelectasis, acute respiratory distress syndrome (ARDS), peripheral bullae, asthma or COPD exacerbation with hyperinflation, pulmonary fibrosis, and pleural adhesions.[4,15,17–19] Most of these conditions can be differentiated on the basis of lung ultrasound in combination with clinical exam (Table 7.1).

In 2D mode the lung point sign (also referred to simply as lung point) is highly specific for pneumothorax. It represents the junction between normal lung that slides with respiration and abnormal lung that does not slide due to the pneumothorax; the point at which lung sliding disappears moves with respiration because an incomplete pneumothorax moves with lung expansion and collapse. This artifact is produced by the edge of an incomplete pneumothorax where intrapleural air abuts the normally apposed visceral and parietal pleura[20] (video link 3: https://images.readcube-cdn.com/publishers/wiley/videos/67a52e479d133bf0d91b95983681a10db66ea507425852f67226dd89ba54e53d/2.mp4). Lung point may also be imaged in M-mode; the seashore sign will appear where the visceral and parietal pleurae are opposed, and the barcode sign will appear at the point where they are separated (Figure 7.6). In M-mode, as in 2D mode, the lung point moves with respiration. When lung point is visualized, it can be used to define the approximate size of a pneumothorax and serial sonographic exams may be performed to monitor its progress.[21,22] Lung point, however, will not be seen in cases of a very large pneumothorax because the air completely surrounds the lung and there is no point where the visceral and parietal pleura meet.[20] Conversely, lung point can be mimicked by pulmonary blebs since air within the bleb generates a sonographic appearance that is similar to pneumothorax.[23]

The heart point sign is a transient visualization of the heart in diastole that is seen in cases of incomplete pneumothorax in the left hemithorax. Heart point, imaged in 2D posterior to the left parasternum, is caused by the intermittent displacement of air anterior to the pericardium by the expanding diastolic heart. As the heart contracts in systole, the interposing air moves away from the chest wall and the heart point sign disappears (video link 4: https://images.readcube-cdn.com/publishers/wiley/videos/67a52e479d133bf0d91b95983681a10db66ea507425852f67226dd89ba54e53d/1.mp4).[24]

Left hemithorax M-mode ultrasound may also reveal a lung pulse sign caused by transmitted impulses of the heart beat through consolidated or atelectatic lung.[25] These transmitted impulses appear as linear, vertical ripples that travel from the lung to the pleural line simultaneous with systole. If the ripples extend above the pleural line into the chest wall, then they are artifacts due to probe movement and do not represent a true lung pulse.

Increased Lung Water

Fluid content of the lungs can be assessed by examining for B-lines (also known as comet tails), vertical hyperechoic rays that emanate from the pleura and radiate into the lung tissue (Figure 7.7). B-lines are indicative of interstitial and/or alveolar edema, and the sonographic effect is generated by fragmentation of the air–fluid interface at the pleura by fluid within inter-lobular septa.[26] The difference in acoustic impedance at the air–fluid interface produces internal reverberations that result in this streaking artifact that crosses through A-lines and can obliterate them.[26] This finding correlates with the chest x-ray finding of Kerley B-lines, after which it is named.[27] B-lines occur not only in cases of cardiogenic (e.g., left heart dysfunction) and non-cardiogenic pulmonary edema (e.g., ARDS), but also in cases of interstitial lung diseases (e.g., idiopathic pulmonary fibrosis) that cause similar changes in acoustic impedance.

B-lines detect alveolar-interstitial syndrome due to congestive heart failure (CHF), noncardiogenic edema, or interstitial thickening, (e.g., interstitial lung diseases, pulmonary fibrosis, inflammatory disease), with a sensitivity of 92.5% and specificity 86.7%.[26] The number of B-lines and the width between each B-line correlate with the degree of

Table 7.1 Sonographic findings that may mimic a pneumothorax.

Condition	Etiology of sonographic findings	Diagnosis and differentiation from pneumothorax
Apnea	Lack of diaphragmatic movement.	Bilateral absence of lung sliding, absence of diaphragmatic contraction in the lower axillary views, clinical absence of chest wall movement, loss of respiratory waveform on end-tidal capnography.
Esophageal Intubation/Absence of Ventilation	Displacement or misplacement of the endotracheal tube, disconnection with the respiratory circuit.	Loss of expired tidal volume, bilateral absence of lung sliding, presence of two sources of A-line artifact in a trans-tracheal view, loss of respiratory waveform on end-tidal capnography.
Mainstem Intubation	Isolation of the unintubated bronchus from ventilation with loss of ventilation of the non-intubated lung.	Noted distal displacement of endotracheal tube from initial depth, increased peak and plateau pressures, return of lung sliding with withdrawal of endotracheal tube.
COPD/Asthma exacerbation	Limited lung excursion due to profound hyperinflation.	Clinical history, return of lung sliding with "sigh" induced by allowing prolonged expiration or temporary removal from vent.
Consolidation	Alveolar filling results in hepatization of tissue with spared bronchi producing internal areas of air-fluid interface resulting in sonographic air bronchograms. Peripheral consolidations may focally reduce or eliminate pleural sliding.	Focal areas of involvement that correlate with lobar distribution. May or may not be stratified by gravity. Presence of sonographic air-bronchograms within hepatized pulmonary tissue. Subpleural consolidations seen as shredded pleural border (shred sign) and focally absent pleural sliding.
Atelectasis	Collapsed pulmonary tissue results in increased local concentration of fluid and decreased local air. Hepatization without sonographic air bronchograms.	Focal areas of involvement correlate with pulmonary anatomy. Do not always respect gravity, although tend to occur in dependent lung regions. Hepatization with lack of air bronchograms. Reduced or absent pleural sliding. May improve with recruitment maneuvers.
ARDS	Patchy and diffuse loss of respirophasic movement with scattered areas of increased extravascular lung water.	B-lines persist in areas even if lung sliding has been lost. There are no B-lines with a pneumothorax.
Pleural Adhesions	Focal restriction of respirophasic movement due to local "tacking" of the lung to the pleura.	History of previous thoracic surgery or inflammatory disease, absence of lung sliding noted on pre-procedural sonographic exam prior to interventions.
Pleural Effusion	Interposition of fluid between the parietal and visceral pleura prevents lung sliding by separating the pleurae.	Loss of lung sliding is gravity dependent, echolucent fluid can be seen in the pleural space and may permit the visualization of thoracic structures, the lung tip may be seen moving within the pleural fluid.
Pulmonary Bleb	Focal restriction of respirophasic movement at the site of the bleb.	History of COPD, noted on pre-procedural scan, remains stable when observed over time.
Phrenic Nerve Palsy	Loss of respirophasic movement due to diaphragmatic paralysis.	Clinical history, loss of diaphragmatic contraction in lower axillary view, return of lung sliding with positive pressure ventilation.

extravascular pulmonary fluid.[26] The presence of multiple confluent B-lines is 97% sensitive for pulmonary edema.[5,28–30] Conversely, in cases where there are fewer than three B-lines per field, pulmonary edema is unlikely.[26,30–33] In volume overload and cardiogenic pulmonary edema, as fluid accumulates in inferiorly located dependent portions of the lung due to the effect of gravity, B-lines are first seen in inferior lung fields. With greater degrees of edema, B-lines become apparent in superior lung fields.[26] Interstitial lung diseases usually can be differentiated from pulmonary edema by clinical history and

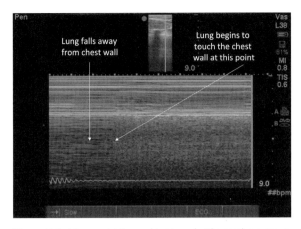

Figure 7.6 A lung point imaged in M-mode. The seashore sign is visualized over a point on the chest where the apposed visceral and parietal pleura touch and the stratosphere (or barcode) sign appears over the point where the lung contracts and air interposes between the visceral and parietal pleura.

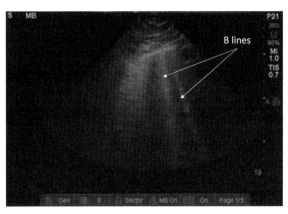

Figure 7.7 B-lines are vertical hyperechoic rays based from the pleural line radiating down into the pulmonary tissue to the end of the screen (regardless of the depth setting, which in this case is 19 cm) that correlate with interstitial thickening (e.g., edema, inflammation, fibrosis) and alveolar edema.

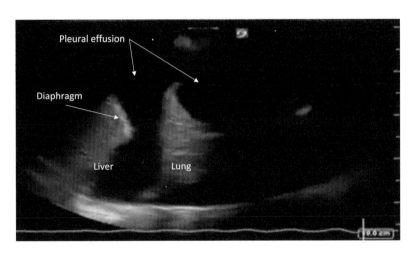

Figure 7.8 Pleural effusions appear anechoic and are visualized as an echolucent space between the diaphragm and pulmonary tissue, or chest wall and pulmonary tissue. The compressed lung edge may be seen swimming in fluid (called jellyfish sign, elephant trunk sign, or simply lung flapping), a dynamic finding that indicates fluid versus an anechoic mimic such as peripheral consolidation, lipoma, or mass that is static without lung flapping.

imaging. In any case, B-lines always rule out pneumothorax.[4,34]

Pleural Effusions

Pulmonary sonography can also be used to diagnose pleural effusions and add to the determination of volume status. The sonographic evaluation of pleural effusions was first described in 1964 and confirmed by thoracentesis in 1967.[2,35] Pleural effusion and hemothorax appear as an echolucent (hypoechoic or anechoic) space between the diaphragm and lung.[36] With large effusions, the compressed lung edge may be seen floating in fluid (Figure 7.8). Modern ultrasound machines can reliably visualize effusions

greater than 100 ml with 100% sensitivity.[37,38] However, pleural thickening may mimic small pleural effusions and subcutaneous emphysema may obscure small pleural effusions.[39]

In indeterminate cases, two other findings should be considered. Normally, vertebral bodies are obscured by the lung in all thoracic views. In an effusion, vertebral bodies appear as saw-toothed hyperechoic lines known as V-lines through the acoustic window created.[40] Pleural effusions can also be verified using M-mode that detects the cyclic movement of collapsed lung parenchyma within the effusion during respiration and reveals a sinusoidal pattern.[13]

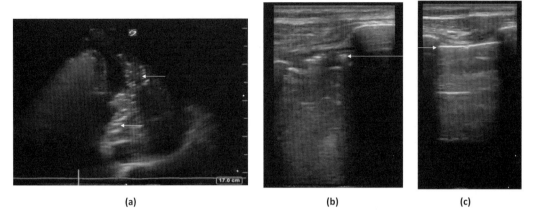

| (a) | (b) | (c) |

Figure 7.9 (a) Consolidation appears as a granular, tissue-like transformation of the lung termed hepatization for its resemblance to the sonographic appearance of liver parenchyma. The hyperechoic white dots and linear structures represent air bronchograms cut in transverse and longitudinal planes respectively. There is also a pleural effusion indicated by the surrounding anechoic area. (b) Subpleural (peripheral) consolidation is identified by an irregular pleural border (arrow) on ultrasound, termed "shred sign". (c) One interspace away from this focal peripheral consolidation the pleural line can be seen and is sharp and smooth (arrow).

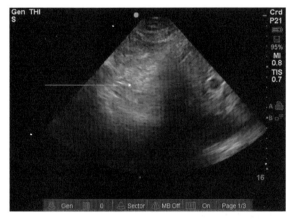

Figure 7.10 Atelectasis. Lung hepatization with rare or absent air bronchograms (indicated by arrow). If there were more hyperechoic white dots and linear structures representing air bronchograms (shown in Figure 7.9), this would be termed "consolidation."

Consolidation and Atelectasis

The alveolar filling that occurs with pulmonary consolidation alters the acoustic impedance of lung tissue. These areas with adjacent patent hyperechoic air bronchi[41,42] appear granular and are similar to ultrasound images of liver parenchyma, an effect known as hepatization (Figure 7.9a).[43] Subpleural consolidation may be identified by an irregular border, termed shred sign, with 90% sensitivity and 98% specificity (Figures 7.9b, 7.9c).[43] Lung ultrasound also can be used to detect atelectasis with 88% accuracy.[41] Atelectasis (Figure 7.10) typically appears as juxtapleural

consolidation without sonographic air bronchograms. Depending on the size of the atelectatic area, lung sliding may be present, reduced, or absent.

Role of Lung Ultrasound in Perioperative Care

The Preoperative Exam

Preoperative pulmonary sonography should be considered if placement of a central venous catheter is planned, there is suspected cardiopulmonary disease, volume status is unclear, or there is underlying thoracic pathology. ASA IV and V status usually confers some or all of these indications.

Preoperative sonographic evaluation can assess volume status and establish a baseline that can be used for comparison to later intraoperative and postoperative studies. When performing a preoperative exam, the bilateral upper and lower thorax should be evaluated in the midclavicular and midaxillary lines at the same points the anesthesiologist might perform intraoperative sonography. Marking these points can ensure fidelity with subsequent studies. The lung apex in the midclavicular line and the diaphragm in the midaxillary line should also be visualized bilaterally. In patients with known lung pathology or prior thoracic surgery, a more thorough exam visualizing all interspaces may identify pleural adhesions and avoid later confusion when considering potential pneumothorax.

Pleural adhesions will appear as areas of absent lung sliding with pleural thickening and can occur in otherwise healthy patients.[44,45] Locations with absent lung sliding and without B-lines may indicate pleural adhesions or bullae, and should be noted or marked when detected to avoid confounding later intra-operative exams. Other imaging (e.g. chest x-ray, CT scan) may be sought in select cases.

A preoperative sonographic study can also be used to assess volume status and predict how fluid administration might be tolerated by establishing the presence or absence of B-lines and pleural effusions.[28] Patients with confluent B-lines may require further workup by electrocardiogram and or echocardiogram, further preoperative optimization (e.g., diuresis, dialysis), or, if the case is emergent, limited fluid administration and invasive monitoring.

Atelectasis detected by preoperative sonography should prompt incentive spirometry, administration of bronchodilators, careful preoxygenation, and aggressive pulmonary toilet before and after intubation. While preoperative pneumonia is unlikely in elective cases, patients requiring emergency operations, especially inpatients, often have comorbidities such as undiagnosed pneumonia. Establishing this diagnosis preoperatively will help guide antibiotic administration, sepsis workup, and postoperative management.

Sonography for Intubation

Sonography can confirm tracheal tube placement. The current standard of care is auscultation and end-tidal capnography.[46,47] Auscultation in morbidly obese patients and those with COPD or acute bronchospasm may result in a false negative exam (suspicion that the tracheal tube is NOT in the trachea when it is), and transmission of sounds from an esophageal intubation may result in a false positive exam (confirmation that the tracheal tube is in the trachea when it is not). Erroneous capnographic findings can occur in low cardiac output states, especially cardiac arrest, or by occlusion of the end-tidal tubing and monitor by debris.

Transthoracic and transtracheal views can be used to confirm tracheal tube placement. Transthoracic imaging may be performed with either a linear probe or the phased array probe, but a linear probe is required to obtain the transtracheal view. After tracheal intubation, thoracic ultrasound that demonstrates bilateral lung sliding or a seashore sign confirms that both lungs are effectively ventilated and localizes the tracheal tube tip to between the carina and the vocal cords. Esophageal intubation will result in absence of lung sliding that is a highly sensitive and specific finding.[48,49] Unilateral lung sliding may indicate a mainstem intubation, and correction can be visualized if withdrawing the tube demonstrates sliding or a comet tail (B-line) artifact.[49–51]

Esophageal intubation can be detected by transtracheal ultrasound that is quite sensitive and specific.[52–54] In this technique the trachea is examined by placing the ultrasound probe in transverse orientation at the level of the cricothyroid membrane, where the trachea appears as a single well-defined column of A-lines produced by the tracheal mucosa-air interface. A tracheal tube will not alter this artifact.[55] While the esophagus also has the potential for a mucosa-to-air interface, it remains masked behind the trachea and an esophageal tube will displace the esophagus, resulting in a second, adjacent A-line. Thus, the presence of a single anatomically normal A-line confirms tracheal tube placement in the trachea, while the presence of a second non-anatomical A-line is evidence that the tube is in the esophagus.[55] The esophagus is displaced leftward in most esophageal intubations, but may occasionally be displaced to the right or posterior to the trachea.[55] When the esophagus is posterior to the trachea, esophageal intubation may be identified by tilting the probe at an oblique angle to the left or right to reveal the presence of two adjacent A-line artifacts.[53,55]

Intraoperative Exam

Unlike routine preoperative lung ultrasound, the intraoperative sonographic exam is performed in response to changes in the patient's clinical condition and/or the need to make a management decision. The issues usually prompting an intraoperative lung ultrasound exam are hypoxemia, hypotension, questionable tracheal tube position, and volume status. The study should first rule out tension pneumothorax. The most superior portion of thorax for the patient's current position should be imaged immediately. This often entails imaging the patient's anterior chest wall, but in certain seated positions may require imaging the lung apex. The presence of bilateral anterior lung sliding effectively rules out tension pneumothorax. Smaller or loculated pneumothoraces might be present, but they should not cause severe hypoxemia or hypotension. After tension pneumothorax has been ruled out, the exam should continue with views obtained in the midaxillary and midclavicular lines in the superior and inferior thorax and visualize the diaphragm to the extent that the operative field allows.

If a pneumothorax is found and the patient is hemodynamically stable, the size of the pneumothorax can be approximated utilizing the lung point.[22] Conservative management of a stable pneumothorax with serial sonography may permit avoidance of chest tube placement.[21] Ultrasound significantly outperforms supine portable chest x-ray for the detection of pneumothorax.[11,56] The presence of B-lines also rules out a pneumothorax, suggests the alternative diagnosis of pulmonary edema, and expands the differential to include volume overload and new left ventricular failure. Pulmonary edema can be further confirmed by the presence of a pleural effusion.

Atelectasis is a significant risk factor for perioperative complications and mortality. Ultrasound can rapidly detect atelectasis as a cause of hypoxemia and other etiologies of increased peak airway pressure.[9] The presence of juxtapleural infiltrates indicates atelectasis as the etiology of hypoxemia, and the patient may be responsive to recruitment maneuvers and bronchodilators. There are case reports of direct visualization of the resolution of atelectasis by ultrasound while performing recruitment maneuvers, and real-time imaging can guide the recruitment maneuver.[57] In hypoxemic patients the presence of a completely unremarkable pulmonary sonographic exam, including bilateral lung sliding, A-lines, and no B–lines, raises the possibility of pulmonary embolus.

If there is concern that the endotracheal tube has been displaced during a procedure, this can be evaluated by repeating the intubation exam described above and may be accompanied by a complementary chest x-ray.

As with hypoxemia, the sonographic evaluation for hypotension begins with ruling out tension pneumothorax. Pulmonary ultrasound can then be paired with cardiac ultrasound, clinical assessment, and IVC examination to distinguish between hypovolemic and cardiogenic shock due to left ventricular failure.[58] The presence of B-lines and pleural effusion should prompt a search for cardiac failure, reduces the likelihood that hypovolemia is the source of hypotension, and increases suspicion for cardiogenic shock.[58,59] In

any case, B-lines and pleural effusions indicate that fluid administration may be contraindicated and that vasopressors and inotropes may optimize hemodynamic status. The absence of B-lines supports a diagnosis of hypovolemic shock, distributive shock, or right heart failure.[58,59] As with hypoxemia, in patients with hypotension and an unremarkable lung ultrasound exam, pulmonary embolus should be considered.

The presence or absence of B lines helps determine the safety of a fluid bolus[58] when combined with cardiac and IVC examinations. A unique benefit of pulmonary ultrasound is that the midclavicular and midaxillary thorax can be reached during most operative procedures without disturbing the sterile field, and images can be obtained even if cardiac and IVC views are not available.

Postoperative Exam

Postoperative pulmonary ultrasound should be considered in patients who develop hypoxemia, become hypotensive, or are having difficulty weaning from mechanical ventilation. When a patient with difficulty weaning from mechanical ventilation has B-lines, diuresis may be indicated. Sonographic evidence of atelectasis suggests that bronchodilators and recruitment maneuvers might be effective; incentive spirometry and optimization of pain relief may also be helpful. These interventions, provided in a timely fashion, should result in more rapid extubation and avoidance of prolonged mechanical ventilation – a source of significantly increased morbidity and mortality in postoperative patients.[60] If sonography demonstrates a shred sign, hepatization, air bronchograms, reduced pleural sliding, or diffuse pathology, then simple atelectasis or overload is unlikely and aspiration, developing pneumonia, or ARDS should be considered.[43,61]

Pulmonary ultrasound can differentiate ARDS from volume overload, which is usually associated with B-lines only. The ultrasound hallmarks of ARDS include dyshomogenous distribution of the increased extravascular water, scattered pleural thickening, reduced pleural sliding, and the presence of a lung pulse.[62] These findings also suggest that in mechanically ventilated patients weaning will be difficult, and in spontaneously breathing patients close observation and preparation for tracheal intubation is warranted. On mechanical ventilation, any new hypoxemia or hypotension can be evaluated by pulmonary ultrasound to rule out pneumothorax due to barotrauma. In conjunction with cardiac and inferior vena cava studies, pulmonary ultrasound can be used to assess volume status and fluid responsiveness.[58]

Conclusion

Lung ultrasound is a point-of-care test particularly well suited to diagnose pneumothorax, pleural effusion, pulmonary edema, and consolidation. In the operating room setting, imaging can establish a baseline for comparison to maximize confidence in later examinations displaying new pathology. In conjunction with cardiac and IVC ultrasound the etiology of hypotension can be ascertained as hypovolemic, distributive, or cardiac. In addition, even more basic assessment regarding volume status and fluid responsiveness is improved. Ultrasound can be used to guide, confirm, and localize tracheal tube placement. In the postoperative setting pulmonary ultrasound can facilitate clinical decisions regarding weaning patients from mechanical ventilation and the need for ICU admission.

References

1. Joyner CR, Jr., Herman RJ, Reid JM. Reflected ultrasound in the detection and localization of pleural effusion. *JAMA* 1967;**200**(5):399–402.

2. Pell R. Ultrasound for routine clinical investigations. *Ultrasonics* 1964;**2**(2):87–9.

3. Rantanen NW. Diseases of the thorax. *Vet Clin North Am Equine Pract* 1986;**2**(1):49–66.

4. Wernecke K, Galanski M, Peters PE, Hansen J. Pneumothorax: evaluation by ultrasound–preliminary results. *J Thorac Imaging* 1987;**2**(2):76–8.

5. Lichtenstein DA, Meziere GA. Relevance of lung ultrasound in the diagnosis of acute respiratory failure: the BLUE protocol. *Chest* 2008;**134**(1): 117–25.

6. Mittal AK, Gupta N. Intraoperative lung ultrasound: a clinicodynamic perspective. *J Anaesthesiol Clin Pharmacol* 2016;**32**(3):288–97.

7. Shander A, Fleisher LA, Barie PS, et al. Clinical and economic burden of postoperative pulmonary complications: patient safety summit on definition, risk-reducing interventions, and preventive strategies. *Crit Care Med* 2011;**39**(9):2163–72.

8. Abstracts of the 30th International Symposium on Intensive Care and Emergency Medicine. Brussels, Belgium. March 9–12, 2010. *Crit Care* 2010;**14** Suppl 1: P1–602.

9. Restrepo RD, Braverman J. Current challenges in the recognition, prevention and treatment of perioperative pulmonary atelectasis. *Expert Rev Respir Med* 2015;**9** (1):97–107.

10. Zieleskiewicz L, Fresco R, Duclos G, et al. Integrating extended focused assessment with sonography for trauma (eFAST) in the initial assessment of severe trauma: Impact on the management of 756 patients. *Injury* 2018;**49**(10):1774–80.

11. Blaivas M, Lyon M, Duggal S. A prospective comparison of supine chest radiography and bedside ultrasound for the diagnosis of traumatic pneumothorax. *Acad Emerg Med* 2005;**12**(9):844–9.

12. Lichtenstein DA, Meziere G, Lascols N, et al. Ultrasound diagnosis of occult pneumothorax. *Crit Care Med* 2005;**33**(6):1231–8.

13. Lichtenstein D, van Hooland S, Elbers P, Malbrain ML. Ten good reasons to practice ultrasound in critical care. *Anaesthesiol Intensive Ther* 2014;**46**(5):323–5.

14. Koh DM, Burke S, Davies N, Padley SP. Transthoracic US of the chest: clinical uses and applications. *Radiographics* 2002;**22**(1):e1.

15. Lichtenstein DA, Menu Y. A bedside ultrasound sign ruling out pneumothorax in the critically ill. Lung sliding. *Chest* 1995;**108**(5):1345–8.

16. Husain LF, Hagopian L, Wayman D, Baker WE, Carmody KA. Sonographic diagnosis of pneumothorax. *J Emerg Trauma Shock* 2012;**5**(1):76–81.

17. Targhetta R, Bourgeois JM, Chavagneux R, et al. Ultrasonic signs of pneumothorax: preliminary work. *J Clin Ultrasound* 1993;**21**(4):245–50.

18. Slater A, Goodwin M, Anderson KE, Gleeson FV. COPD can mimic the appearance of pneumothorax on thoracic ultrasound. *Chest* 2006;**129**(3):545–50.

19. De Luca C, Valentino M, Rimondi MR, et al. Use of chest sonography in acute-care radiology. *J Ultrasound* 2008;**11**(4):125–34.

20. Lichtenstein D, Meziere G, Biderman P, Gepner A. The "lung point": an ultrasound sign specific to pneumothorax. *Intensive Care Med* 2000;**26**(10):1434–40.

21. Sato I, Kanda H, Kanao-Kanda M, Kurosawa A, Kunisawa T. A case of iatrogenic pneumothorax in which chest tube placement could be avoided by intraoperative evaluation with transthoracic ultrasonography. *Ther Clin Risk Manag* 2017;**13**:843–5.

22. Aspler A, Pivetta E, Stone MB. Double-lung point sign in traumatic pneumothorax. *Am J Emerg Med* 2014;**32** (7):819e81–2.

23. Gelabert C, Nelson M. Bleb point: mimicker of pneumothorax in bullous lung disease. *West J Emerg Med* 2015;**16**(3):447–9.

24. Stone MB, Chilstrom M, Chase K, Lichtenstein D. The heart point sign: description of a new ultrasound finding suggesting pneumothorax. *Acad Emerg Med* 2010;**17**(11):e149–150.

25. Lichtenstein DA, Lascols N, Prin S, Meziere G. The "lung pulse": an early ultrasound sign of complete atelectasis. *Intensive Care Med* 2003;**29**(12):2187–92.

26. Lichtenstein D, Meziere G, Biderman P, Gepner A, Barre O. The comet-tail artifact. An ultrasound sign of alveolar-interstitial syndrome. *Am J Respir Crit Care Med* 1997;**156**(5):1640–6.

27. Kerley P. Radiology in Heart Disease. *Br Med J* 1933;**2** (3795):594–612.3.

28. Jambrik Z, Monti S, Coppola V, et al. Usefulness of ultrasound lung comets as a nonradiologic sign of extravascular lung water. *Am J Cardiol* 2004;**93** (10):1265–70.

29. Baldi G, Gargani L, Abramo A, et al. Lung water assessment by lung ultrasonography in intensive care: a pilot study. *Intensive Care Med* 2013;**39** (1):74–84.

30. Platz E, Lewis EF, Uno H, et al. Detection and prognostic value of pulmonary congestion by lung ultrasound in ambulatory heart failure patients. *Eur Heart J* 2016;**37**(15):1244–51.

31. Theerawit P, Touman N, Sutherasan Y, Kiatboonsri S. Transthoracic ultrasound assessment of B-lines for identifying the increment of extravascular lung water in shock patients requiring fluid resuscitation. *Indian J Crit Care Med* 2014;**18**(4):195–99.

32. Aras MA, Teerlink JR. Lung ultrasound: a "B-line" to the prediction of decompensated heart failure. *Eur Heart J* 2016;**37**(15):1252–4.

33. Dietrich CF, Mathis G, Blaivas M, et al. Lung B-line artefacts and their use. *J Thorac Dis* 2016;**8**(6):1356–65.

34. Lichtenstein D, Meziere G, Biderman P, Gepner A. The comet-tail artifact: an ultrasound sign ruling out pneumothorax. *Intensive Care Med* 1999;**25**(4):383–8.

35. Joyner CR Jr, Miller LD, Dudrick SJ, Eskin DJ, Bloom P. Reflected ultrasound in the study of diseases of the chest. *Trans Am Clin Climatol Assoc* 1967;**78**:28–37.

36. Kataoka H, Takada S. The role of thoracic ultrasonography for evaluation of patients with decompensated chronic heart failure. *J Am Coll Cardiol* 2000;**35**(6):1638–46.

37. Kalokairinou-Motogna M, Maratou K, Paianid I, et al. Application of color Doppler ultrasound in the study of small pleural effusion. *Med Ultrason* 2010;**12**(1):12–16.

38. Rothlin MA, Naf R, Amgwerd M, Candinas D, Frick T, Trentz O. Ultrasound in blunt abdominal and thoracic trauma. *J Trauma* 1993;**34**(4):488–95.

39. Hasan AA, Makhlouf HA, Mohamed ARM. Discrimination between pleural thickening and minimal pleural effusion using color Doppler chest ultrasonography. *Egyptian Chest Diseases Tuberculosis* 2013;**62**:429–33.

40. Atkinson P, Milne J, Loubani O, Verheul G. The V-line: a sonographic aid for the confirmation of pleural fluid. *Crit Ultrasound J* 2012;**4**(1):19.

41. Acosta CM, Maidana GA, Jacovitti D, et al. Accuracy of transthoracic lung ultrasound for diagnosing anesthesia-induced atelectasis in children. *Anesthesiology* 2014;**120**(6):1370–9.

42. Weinberg B, Diakoumakis EE, Kass EG, Seife B, Zvi ZB. The air bronchogram: sonographic demonstration. *AJR Am J Roentgenol* 1986;**147**(3):593–5.

43. Lichtenstein DA, Lascols N, Mezière G, Gepner A. Ultrasound diagnosis of alveolar consolidation in the critically ill. *Intensive Care Med* 2004;**30**(2):276–81.

44. Cassanelli N, Caroli G, Dolci G, et al. Accuracy of transthoracic ultrasound for the detection of pleural adhesions. *Eur J Cardiothorac Surg* 2012;**42**(5):813–18; discussion 818.

45. Wei B, Wang T, Jiang F, Wang H. Use of transthoracic ultrasound to predict pleural adhesions: a prospective blinded study. *Thorac Cardiovasc Surg* 2012;**60**(2):101–4.

46. Grmec S. Comparison of three different methods to confirm tracheal tube placement in emergency intubation. *Intensive Care Med* 2002;**28**(6):701–4.

47. Neumar RW, Otto CW, Link MS, et al. Part 8: adult advanced cardiovascular life support: 2010 American Heart Association guidelines for cardiopulmonary resuscitation and emergency cardiovascular care. *Circulation* 2010;**122**(18 Suppl 3):S729–767.

48. Weaver B, Lyon M, Blaivas M. Confirmation of endotracheal tube placement after intubation using the ultrasound sliding lung sign. *Acad Emerg Med* 2006;**13** (3):239–44.

49. Rajan S, Surendran J, Paul J, Kumar L. Rapidity and efficacy of ultrasonographic sliding lung sign and auscultation in confirming endotracheal intubation in overweight and obese patients. *Indian J Anaesth* 2017;**61**(3):230–4.

50. Sim SS, Lien WC, Chou HC, et al. Ultrasonographic lung sliding sign in confirming proper endotracheal intubation during emergency intubation. *Resuscitation* 2012;**83**(3):307–12.

51. Sustic A, Protic A, Cicvaric T, Zupan Z. The addition of a brief ultrasound examination to clinical assessment increases the ability to confirm placement of double-lumen endotracheal tubes. *J Clin Anesth* 2010;**22**(4):246–9.

52. Ma G, Davis DP, Schmitt J, Vilke GM, Chan TC, Hayden SR. The sensitivity and specificity of

transcricothyroid ultrasonography to confirm endotracheal tube placement in a cadaver model. *J Emerg Med* 2007;**32**(4):405–7.

53. Chou HC, Chong KM, Sim SS, et al. Real-time tracheal ultrasonography for confirmation of endotracheal tube placement during cardiopulmonary resuscitation. *Resuscitation* 2013;**84**(12):1708–12.

54. Ma Gene, Hayden SR, Chan Theodore C, et al., Using ultrasound to visualize and confirm endotracheal intubation. *Academic Emergency Medicine* 1999;**6**(5):515.

55. Werner SL, Smith CE, Goldstein JR, Jones RA, Cydulka RK. Pilot study to evaluate the accuracy of ultrasonography in confirming endotracheal tube placement. *Ann Emerg Med* 2007;**49**(1):75–80.

56. Ball CG, Ranson K, Dente CJ, et al. Clinical predictors of occult pneumothoraces in severely injured blunt polytrauma patients: a prospective observational study. *Injury* 2009;**40**(1):44–7.

57. Du J, Tan J, Yu K, Wang R. Lung recruitment maneuvers using direct ultrasound guidance: a case study. *Respir Care* 2015;**60**(5):e93–96.

58. Lichtenstein D. FALLS-protocol: lung ultrasound in hemodynamic assessment of shock. *Heart Lung Vessel* 2013;**5**(3):142–7.

59. Kajimoto K, Madeen K, Nakayama T, et al. Rapid evaluation by lung-cardiac-inferior vena cava (LCI) integrated ultrasound for differentiating heart failure from pulmonary disease as the cause of acute dyspnea in the emergency setting. *Cardiovasc Ultrasound* 2012;**10**(1):49.

60. Smetana GW. Postoperative pulmonary complications: an update on risk assessment and reduction. *Cleve Clin J Med* 2009;**76** Suppl 4:S60–65.

61. Lichtenstein D, Goldstein I, Mourgeon E, et al. Comparative diagnostic performances of auscultation, chest radiography, and lung ultrasonography in acute respiratory distress syndrome. *Anesthesiology* 2004;**100**(1):9–15.

62. Copetti R, Soldati G, Copetti P. Chest sonography: a useful tool to differentiate acute cardiogenic pulmonary edema from acute respiratory distress syndrome. *Cardiovasc Ultrasound* 2008;**6**:16.

Chapter

8

Point-of-Care Ultrasound: Determination of Fluid Responsiveness

Subhash Krishnamoorthy and Oliver Panzer

Introduction

Hypotension and shock in the perioperative setting may arise from a variety of etiologies that require different therapies for successful treatment. A common initial intervention is administration of a fluid bolus to increase the cardiac stroke volume and mean arterial blood pressure; however, fluid responsiveness is absent in up to 50% of all hypotensive patients, and if they receive excessive fluid without the desired hemodynamic response, morbidity and mortality may result. Therefore, there is a clinical need to determine the likelihood that an individual patient will respond to fluid administration. Advances in understanding the physiologic response to fluid administration have led to the development of dynamic predictors of the hemodynamic response. The respiratory variation of stroke volume associated with positive pressure ventilation (*heart–lung interaction model*) and the passive leg raise (PLR) (*endogenous fluid challenge model*) are the two best-validated means to quickly augment stroke volume. The respiratory variation model is most applicable during mechanical ventilation and is useful in the operating room, postoperative arenas, and intensive care units (ICUs). Passive leg raise is only possible in nonoperating room settings when there is no contraindication to moving the lower extremities or pelvis. This chapter will review ultrasound-based parameters such as inferior vena cava diameter change and velocity time integral variation utilizing these two methods of stroke volume augmentation to predict fluid responsiveness.

Shock

It is a challenge to manage hypotension in its most extreme form when it is accompanied by symptoms and signs of hypoperfusion (i.e., shock). Oftentimes management must proceed without knowledge of the patient's pertinent medical history, prior physical status, baseline laboratories, or imaging, in which case rapid, efficient diagnosis and initiation of treatment can be difficult, if not impossible. The most common initial intervention is fluid administration with blood pressure monitoring. Different types of shock, however, require different therapies, and it is therefore helpful to classify shock on the basis of etiology as hypovolemic, distributive, obstructive, or cardiogenic. The underlying etiology may also be mixed, increasing the difficulty in deciding on treatment that may include a combination or permutation of administration of fluids, vasopressors, inotropes, and interventions, including thrombolysis and pericardiocentesis.

Fluid administration is the most common intervention for shock, gaining favor after the 2001 publication of the Early Goal Directed Therapy (EGDT) trial by Rivers et al., one of the most cited references in critical care medicine.[1] The study protocol emphasized fluid administration to target central venous pressure (CVP) ≥ 8–12 mmHg, mean arterial pressure (MAP) ≥ 65 mmHg, urine output ≥ 0.5 ml/kg/hr, and central venous oxygen saturation ($ScvO_2$) ≥ 70%, resulting in patients receiving upwards of 10 liters of fluid over 72 h. More recent trials such as PROCESS[2] and ARISE,[3] however, did not replicate the EGDT trial findings. In addition, there is strong evidence that CVP is not a good marker of volume status and is a poor predictor of fluid responsiveness.[4,5] Central venous pressure may actually decrease with volume resuscitation secondary to the release of vasodilatory substances like nitrous oxide (NO) and atrial natriuretic peptide (ANP).[6] Furthermore, excess fluid administration may harm patients. Monnet et al. suggest that excess fluid may decrease oxygen delivery to the patient's tissues.[7] In fact, only 50% of ICU patients in septic shock will respond to fluid administration with an increase in their MAP.[8] Excessive fluid has been associated with increased mortality in sepsis patients,[9] and pulmonary edema and the need for mechanical ventilation support in acute respiratory distress syndrome (ARDS) patients.[10] The appropriate amount and timing of fluid administration, therefore, has become a key goal of hemodynamic resuscitation and management of hypotension and shock, and requires the accurate prediction of fluid responsiveness prior to the administration of large quantities of fluid in order to prevent iatrogenic harm.

Fluid Responsiveness

Fluid responsiveness is defined as an increase in stroke volume (SV) and cardiac output (CO) that results from a fluid bolus, leading to an increase in the MAP and improved perfusion and oxygen delivery. Most of the literature defines fluid responsiveness as an increase in SV by 10–15% from baseline.[11] As $CO = SV \times Heart\ Rate$ (HR), for the sake of simplicity SV will be the variable discussed. Stroke volume is dependent on preload, contractility, and afterload. Common surrogates for preload are central venous pressure (CVP), pulmonary artery occlusion pressure (PAOP), left or right ventricular end-diastolic pressure (LVEDP, RVEDP), and left or right ventricular end-diastolic volume (LVEDV, RVEDV). The effect of a preload increase on SV depends on the myocardium's position on the Frank Starling Curve (FSC). Generally, an increase in preload will have a significant effect on SV if the myocardium is operating on the steep (ascending) portion of the curve and, therefore, will be preload-dependent and fluid-responsive. The patient is preload-independent and fluid-nonresponsive when the attempt to increase preload has only a minimal effect. This will occur when the myocardium's position is on the flat portion of the FSC and an increase in SV is not possible, or with impaired contractility when the curve is flattened (Figure 8.1). Most hemodynamic parameters, however, cannot assess where a patient's cardiac function lies on the FSC. Furthermore, these static parameters are measured at a single point in time and cannot predict a significant SV increase in response to fluid administration, and therefore cannot discern if a patient may benefit or be harmed by the administration of fluid. Surprisingly, even in normal volunteers, cardiac filling pressures are not reflective of volume status and cannot determine the likelihood of fluid responsiveness.[6]

A dynamic assessment of the likely SV response to a preload challenge allows for a precise determination

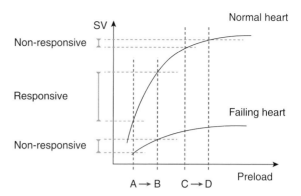

Figure 8.1 FSC of two different hearts, a normal heart versus a failing heart with decreased contractility. The diagram illustrates how both hearts start with the same preload (point A). If the preload is increased to point B, only the normal heart has a significant increase in SV (preload-dependent state), but the failing heart only has a small increase in SV and therefore is not volume-responsive (pre-load independent state). However, if the normal heart is challenged at point C, it also only shows a minimal increase in SV (i.e., is not volume-responsive as it is working on the flat part of the FSC). A hypotensive patient in that state would not benefit from fluid boluses; instead, vasopressors or other interventions should be considered.

of fluid responsiveness (i.e., is the heart in a preload-dependent or preload-independent state), preferably before fluid is administered so that excessive fluid administration can be avoided in patients who are predictably nonresponsive. This chapter focuses on ultrasound techniques for determining fluid responsiveness, including inferior vena cava diameter change in response to ventilation and the velocity time integral of the left ventricular outflow tract (VTI_{LVOT}); arterial waveform interrogation and pulse pressure variation are reviewed in Chapter 11.

Most dynamic measurements are performed using one of two common models to augment SV: (1) the heart–lung interaction during positive pressure ventilation (PPV) model, and (2) the PLR endogenous fluid challenge model. The concepts behind these models are key to understanding all fluid responsiveness tests and avoiding errors in interpretation.

Heart–Lung Interaction Model

The heart–lung interaction model (HLIM) rests on the fact that SV is dependent on the interactions between the heart and thoracic cavity during PPV. In a hypovolemic patient, changes in intrathoracic pressure cause very noticeable variations in SV. In an arterial pressure tracing, the area under the curve is directly proportional to SV, and variations in this area

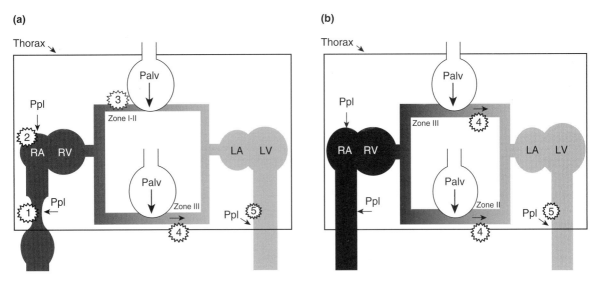

Figure 8.2 Illustration of the heart–lung interaction with positive pressure ventilation in **(a)** a hypovolemic patient, and **(b)** a normo- or hypervolemic patient. Ppl = pleural pressure; Palv = alveolar pressure; RA = right atrium; RV = right ventricle; LA = left atrium; LV = left ventricle. **(a)** In a hypovolemic patient, (1) Ppl compresses IVC, decreasing RV preload; (2) Ppl increases RA intramural pressure decreasing RV preload; (3) Palv compresses pulmonary capillaries in West Zones I and II; (4) capillary pressure exceeds Palv in West Zone III; and (5) an increase in Ppl decreases LV intramural pressure and therefore afterload. **(b)** In a normo- or hypervolemic patient, (4) capillary pressure exceeds Palv in West Zones I, II and III, and (5) an increase in Ppl decreases LV intramural pressure, and therefore afterload is no different than in hypovolemia.

Source: Michard F. Changes in arterial pressure during mechanical ventilation. *Anesthesiology* 2005;103(2):419–28.

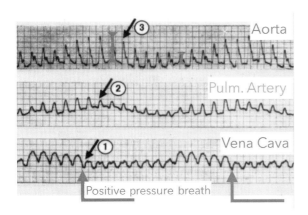

Figure 8.3 Illustration of the heart–lung interaction with positive pressure ventilation in a hypovolemic patient. **(1)** As the pressure increases with the initiation of a mechanical breath, the flow to the RA through the vena cava decreases significantly. **(2)** With a minimal delay the flow in the main pulmonary artery decreases as well, secondary to both an afterload increase and preload decrease. **(3)** The LV SV initially increases as the pulmonary capillaries are drained by the increased intrathoracic pressure and increase the LV preload transiently, however, thereafter preload drops significantly and LV SV drops (red bars). (A black and white version of this figure will appear in some formats. For the color version, please refer to the plate section).

Source: Michard F. Changes in arterial pressure during mechanical ventilation. *Anesthesiology* 2005;103(2):419–28.

are easily detected. Positive pressure breaths increase intrathoracic pressure, which compresses the right atrium (Figure 8.2) and impedes flow from the low-pressure abdominal venous system, and thereby decreases right ventricular preload and right ventricular SV.

In the hypovolemic patient's West lung zones I and II, alveolar pressure is greater than pulmonary capillary pressure, the pulmonary capillaries have lower filling pressure and are easily compressed, and RV afterload increases and right ventricular SV decreases. In West zone III, where alveolar pressure is less than pulmonary capillary pressure, the brief increase in alveolar pressure accompanying positive pressure pushes the blood contained in the capillaries toward the left heart, causing an increase in LV preload and SV for a few heartbeats (Figure 8.3) before the decreased right ventricular SV decreases the left ventricle's preload and SV.

Normovolemic and hypervolemic patients have normal to high filling pressures, the RV is less compressible, the pulmonary capillaries are less compressible, and there is no significant variation in SV over the course of the respiratory cycle (Figures 8.2 and 8.3).

The HLIM has been studied extensively with various LV SV surrogates, such as calculation of the area under an arterial pressure tracing and the more easily

Table 8.1 Summary of established limitations of the HLIM and the associated type of error.

	Limitations	Mechanisms for failure	Type of error
1	Spontaneous breathing activity	Irregular variations in intrathoracic pressure and thus variation in stroke volume do not correlate with preload dependency	False positive (may occasionally be false negative depending on the type of breathing)
2	Cardiac arrhythmias	The variation in stroke volume is related more to the irregularity in diastolic time than to the heart-lung interaction	False positive
3	Mechanical ventilation using low tidal volume ventilation (< 8 ml/kg)	The small variations in intrathoracic pressure secondary to the low tidal volume are insufficient to produce significant changes in intrathoracic pressure	False negative
4	Low lung compliance	The transmission of changes in alveolar pressure to the intrathoracic structures is attenuated	False negative
5	Open thorax	No changes in intrathoracic pressure occur	False negative
6	Increased intra-abdominal pressure	Threshold values for PPV will be elevated	False positive
7	HR/RR ratio < 3.6 (e.g., severe bradycardia or high frequency ventilation)	If the RR is very high, the number of cardiac cycles per respiratory cycle may be too low to cause variation in stroke volume	False negative

Source: Myatra SN, Monnet X, Teboul JL. Use of "tidal volume challenge" to improve the reliability of pulse pressure variation. *Crit Care.* 2017; 21(1):6.

measured pulse pressure variation and systolic pressure change.[11] In most studies the threshold for fluid responsiveness has been found to be between 10 and 15%; if with positive pressure breaths the calculated SV, pulse pressure variation, or systolic pressure change varies more than that, there is about a 90% chance that the administration of fluid will raise the SV and MAP.

This model has several limitations, the two most common being that it requires mechanical ventilation with relatively high tidal volumes (e.g., ≥ 10 ml/kg versus the standard 6 ml/kg) and it is not applicable in the presence of cardiac arrhythmias (Table 8.1). Additionally, this method only assesses the LV for fluid responsiveness, thus patients with isolated RV failure may have a false positive fluid-responsive state because the LV preload is decreased when the RV is failing. Fluid administration in this case would worsen RV function and overall hemodynamics. Ideally, when using the HLIM, SV surrogates for the RV and LV would both be measured.[11]

Reversible Fluid Challenge

The second model utilizing dynamic parameters for fluid responsiveness is the reversible fluid challenge. The best validated method of assessment resting on this model is the PLR "test" in which an endogenous fluid bolus is delivered by gravitationally draining blood from the lower extremities back to the heart by rapidly lifting the legs straight up. The patient is usually first placed in a semi-recumbent position with the head elevated to 45 degrees, and a baseline measurement of the SV or surrogate parameter is taken. Subsequently, by manipulating the patient's bed, their legs are elevated passively to 30–45 degrees as the upper body is lowered into a horizontal plane, and a second measurement of the SV surrogate is performed immediately after the position is reached. This maneuver mobilizes approximately 300–500 mL of venous blood from the extremities and splanchnic circulation toward the heart (Figure 8.4), which increases preload to the RV and then the LV, and results in a significant increase in SV in patients who are fluid-responsive. The effect wears off in about 60–90 seconds,[12] so it is important to perform the PLR and SV measurement rapidly. The advantages of this test are that the fluid challenge is completely reversible and is not dependent on the presence of mechanical ventilation or sinus rhythm. It is, however, limited in that it should not be performed in patients who may not tolerate a change in position, have intra-abdominal hypertension, or have increased intracranial pressure.[13,14]

As an alternative to the PLR test, a small fluid bolus can be administered over a very short period of time.

(a)

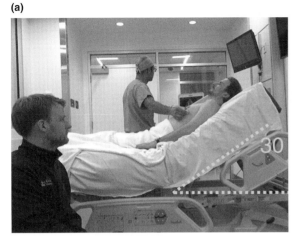

(b)

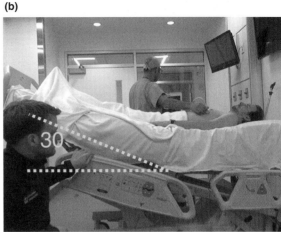

Figure 8.4 Two people are required to perform the passive leg raise test, while ultrasound is performed continuously. **(a)** The first set of SV surrogates are recorded after the patient is placed into a semi-recumbent position, with the torso at a 30–45 degree angle and the legs in a horizontal position. **(b)** The patient's legs are placed at a 30–45 degree angle and the torso moved in a horizontal position. Approximately 300–500 ml of venous blood will be mobilized toward the heart. Preload increases rapidly, therefore the second set of measurements must be obtained quickly.

There is little agreement, however, on the minimal fluid bolus size that may increase the SV, and repeated administration of small boluses of fluid in an effort to increase SV may result in fluid overload.[15]

Ultrasound Techniques to Detect Fluid Responsiveness

The concepts behind fluid responsiveness can be applied to ultrasound-based techniques. The advantages of ultrasound are that it is noninvasive, it does not require arterial line or stand-alone noninvasive cardiac output monitoring devices, it is easily portable, and it is repeatable.

A historical controlled trial compared outcomes in 220 consecutive shock patients treated with standard management versus limited echocardiography (LE)-guided therapy after initial resuscitation. Fluid prescription during the first 24 hours was significantly lower in LE patients (49 [33–74] versus 66 [42–100] mL/kg, $p = 0.01$), although more LE patients received dobutamine (22% versus 12%, $p = 0.01$). The patients treated using LE had better 28-day survival (66% versus 56%, $p = 0.04$), less stage 3 acute kidney injury (20% versus 39%), and more days alive and free of renal support (28 [9.7–28] versus 25 [5–28], $p = 0.04$). Thus, an exam that took only 10 minutes to perform provided four main echocardiographic views

(parasternal long axis, parasternal short axis, four-chamber apical, subcostal) and was adequate to drive therapy that improved outcome.

Inferior Vena Cava Diameter Evaluation

The most basic ultrasound technique to assess fluid responsiveness is measurement of the IVC diameter and its variation during respiration. The IVC is very compliant and as such its diameter is dependent on transmural pressure. During positive pressure inspiration intrathoracic pressure increases and venous return to the heart decreases as blood flow from the IVC into the right atrium (RA) is reduced. Increased blood volume in the IVC causes distension and a measurable increase in diameter. During expiration the opposite occurs; venous blood in the IVC returns to the RA, decreased blood volume contracts the IVC, and the diameter is measurably decreased.[16] During spontaneous breathing the opposite reactions occur and variations in the IVC diameter are just as demonstrable and clinically significant.

Inferior Vena Cava Image Acquisition

Ultrasound assessment of IVC diameter requires a subcostal long axis (i.e., sagittal plane) view. The probe is placed to the right of the xiphoid process with the index marker pointing to the head (Figure 8.5).

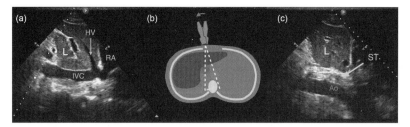

Figure 8.5 Subcostal view required for measurement of the IVC diameter. IVC= inferior vena cava, RA = right atrium, HV = hepatic vein, L = Liver, Ao = aorta, ST = soft tissue layer. **(a)** Subcostal long axis view of the IVC: The IVC is directly attached to the liver parenchyma, receives blood from the hepatic vein (blue arrow) just distal to the diaphragm, and clearly drains into the right atrium; the measurement of the diameter is performed within 3 cm distal to the diaphragm and distal to the HV inlet. **(b)** It is important to differentiate the IVC (blue dot) from the descending aorta (red dot). This is done by tilting the ultrasound beam to the patient's right. **(c)** The resulting view is a subcostal long-axis view of the descending aorta. The aorta is clearly separated from the liver by a soft tissue layer and is not connected to a cardiac chamber at this level. (A black and white version of this figure will appear in some formats. For the color version, please refer to the plate section).

The M-mode is activated and the cursor is placed 1 cm caudal to the branch of the hepatic vein, cutting the IVC perpendicularly. The IVC diameter is then recorded at end-expiration and end-inspiration.

There is no universally agreed upon single location that is ideal to measure the IVC diameter. A study in healthy volunteers assessed the percentage collapse at three locations along the IVC – the diaphragm, the hepatic vein inlet, and the left renal vein. Analysis of the minimum and maximum IVC diameters showed that the percentage of IVC collapse was equivalent at the level of the left renal vein and the hepatic inlet, and were different from the diameter measured at the level of diaphragm.[17] We therefore suggest measuring the IVC just below the hepatic vein inlet, as it is reproducible and the view is easy to obtain.

The subcostal view may not result in an adequate image, particularly in patients after abdominal surgery or recent ingestion of a large meal. In these cases the IVC may be imaged using a lateral view along the right mid-axillary line, with the probe marker pointing cephalad and the probe angled horizontally (i.e., coronal plane). The image obtained should be similar to the subcostal view, although the IVC collapses asymmetrically in an elliptical form and therefore assessment of fluid responsiveness based upon distensibility requires a different guidance that has only recently been investigated.[18]

Inferior Vena Cava Distensibility Index

The respiratory variation in the IVC diameter (ΔIVC) during PPV can be used to evaluate fluid responsiveness; preload-dependent (i.e., fluid-responsive) patients have a large variation in IVC diameter while preload-independent (i.e., fluid nonresponsive) patients have only minimal variation. As described above for the HLIM, the patient must be mechanically ventilated with tidal volumes of at least 8 mL/kg and in sinus rhythm in order for this approach to have reasonable sensitivity and specificity. The IVC distensibility index (IVC DI) can be calculated using the formulas:

$$IVC\ DI = (IVC_{max} - IVC_{min})\ /IVC_{min}$$

or

$$IVC\ DI = (IVC_{max} - IVC_{min})\ /[(IVC_{max} + IVC_{min})/2]$$

Depending on the study, an IVC DI greater than 12–18% signals fluid responsiveness.[19,20] An example of this is provided in Figure 8.6.

Inferior Vena Cava Collapsibility Index

The respiratory variation in IVC diameter can also be used in spontaneously breathing patients to gauge fluid responsiveness; however, the driving force for the IVC diameter change is very different during spontaneous ventilation and PPV. During a positive pressure breath the IVC is "distended" during inspiration secondary to the increasing intrathoracic pressure, whereas during a spontaneous breath the IVC actually "collapses" because it contains less blood as the pressure decreases within the chest. This pressure decrease can vary significantly between breaths depending on the patient's effort and can be exaggerated in a patient who is short of breath, especially in the case of airway obstruction or bronchospasm. This is a significant disadvantage compared to the patient on PPV, where the change in inspiratory

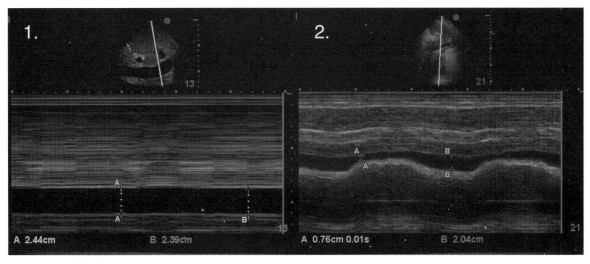

Figure 8.6 M-mode IVC examination.: **(1)** Patient with minimal change form inspiration (A) to expiration (B), therefore unlikely to be fluid responsive. **(2)** Patient with large change from inspiration (A) to expiration (B), therefore likely to be fluid responsive.

intrathoracic pressure is the same for every breath. The IVC collapsibility index (IVC CI) is calculated using the following formula:

$$IVC\ CI = (IVC_{max} - IVC_{min})/IVC_{max}$$

IVC_{max} occurs during expiration and IVC_{min} occurs during inspiration. Studies suggest that a subcostal long-axis IVC CI greater than 40% signals fluid responsiveness with a sensitivity of 70% and specificity of 80%.[21] Zhang et al. performed a systematic review pooling eight studies involving 235 patients determining the ΔIVC prediction of fluid responsiveness under both spontaneous breathing and mechanical ventilation. The respiratory variation in the IVC varied from 12 to 40%, with a pooled sensitivity and specificity of 0.76 and 0.86, respectively. The prediction of fluid responsiveness based upon ΔIVC was better in mechanically ventilated than in spontaneously breathing patients.[22] Similar findings were reported in a larger meta-analysis including both pediatric and adult patients, although the sensitivity and specificity were lower.[23] Overall, the ΔIVC should be interpreted cautiously within the clinical context, especially if the patient is breathing spontaneously.

Use of IVC images has the same limitation as the HLIM. In addition, these measurements only evaluate RV fluid responsiveness. ΔIVC may result in a false positive if the RV is preload-dependent and the LV is functioning on the plateau of the FSC and preload-

independent. Ideally, the test is combined with an LV fluid responsiveness test or at least interpreted with knowledge of the underlying LV function at baseline.

Left Ventricular Outflow Tract/Aortic Valve Velocity Time Integral Evaluation

Another technique to evaluate preload responsiveness involves measuring the variation in the velocity time integral (VTI) of the left ventricular outflow tract (VTI_{LVOT}) or aortic valve (VTI_{AV}), as both closely correlate with stroke volume. Conceptually, the stroke volume in echocardiography is calculated using the same formula in both the LVOT and through the aortic valve (AV):

$$SV = Area_{LVOT} \times VTI_{LVOT}$$

where SV is stroke volume, $Area_{LVOT}$ is the area of the LVOT, and VTI_{LVOT} is the volume time integral of the LVOT. As the areas of the LVOT and AV remain constant during systole across varying preload conditions, the SV is directly proportional to the VTI. Therefore, this single echocardiographic parameter may be used to determine fluid responsiveness.

Image Acquisition

The LVOT image is captured in the five-chamber apical view. Once the view is achieved, the pulsed

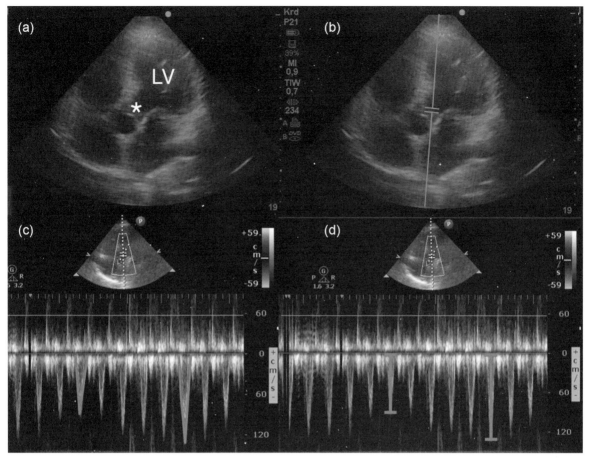

Figure 8.7 Acquisition of the LVOT VTI/ Vmax. **(a)** The apical five-chamber view is obtained with the LVOT (*) positioned in the center of the image. **(b)** The pulsed wave Doppler function is activated and the sample volume (SVol) is placed into the LVOT just above the aortic valve. **(c)** The LVOT is represented by the yellow quadrangle and the aortic valve is highlighted in blue. Once in pulsed wave Doppler mode, the envelopes below the time axis (red dotted line) can be highlighted and the area under the curve can be measured at the point of expiration and inspiration. (A black and white version of this figure will appear in some formats. For the color version, please refer to the plate section).

wave Doppler mode is activated and the cursor is placed to sample the volume in the LVOT. The Doppler signals appear under the time axis and should have an intense (bright white) border with a sharp delineation. The VTI_{LVOT} is obtained by tracing the circumference of the signal, as demonstrated in Figure 8.7.

VTI_{LVOT} Variation: Heart–Lung Interaction Model

Using the HLIM, the VTI_{LVOT} tracing can be used to assess fluid responsiveness. The maximal VTI of the Doppler signal traced during early inspiration (VTI_{max}) and the minimal VTI during expiration (VTI_{min}) are measured; VTI variation (ΔVTI_{LVOT}) is then calculated by the formula:

$$\Delta VTI_{LVOT} = (VTI_{max} - VTI_{min})/[(VTI_{max} + VTI_{min})/2]$$

Studies suggest that a ΔVTI_{LVOT} greater than 20% indicates preload responsiveness.[24] It has been proposed that the variation of the maximal velocity (V_{max}) may also be used as a surrogate for preload responsiveness. By simply measuring the difference in the inspiratory and expiratory LVOT V_{max} by pulsed wave Doppler, the variation may be calculated using the same formula as for the VTI (Figure 8.7). If the change in V_{max} is greater than 12%, the patient is likely fluid-responsive.[25]

Just as IVC assessment does not account for the possible presence of LV dysfunction that may impair potential fluid responsiveness, VTI measurements do not account for the possible presence of RV dysfunction that may impair the potential LV responsiveness to a fluid bolus. Therefore, when using the HLIM it is advisable to perform fluid responsiveness assessments of both the RV and LV simultaneously (i.e., IVC and VTI assessment) to reduce false positive results. As these calculations are dependent on heart–lung interactions, all of the limitations of the HLIM apply.

VTI$_{LVOT}$ Variation: Passive Leg Raise Test

The limitations of the HLIM are avoided by using the VTI$_{LVOT}$ while performing a PLR test. To properly perform this exam, the LVOT view must be maintained throughout the PLR. Several heartbeats must be averaged (minimum of three in sinus rhythm and 5 in an atrial arrhythmia) on the pre- and post-PLR Doppler tracing, and then compared using the same formula presented for calculation of the respiratory VTI variation. If the difference is greater than 12.5–15%, the patient is likely preload-responsive, with a sensitivity range of 77–81% and specificity range of 93–100%.[26]

VTI$_{LVOT}$ Variation: Mini-Fluid Bolus

The focus of this chapter has thus far been on PLR and respiration to augment preload, and measurement of a hemodynamic variable in an attempt to predict fluid responsiveness, usually to a fluid bolus of ≥ 500 ml. A less well-established method for predicting fluid responsiveness is to administer a smaller bolus of fluid (e.g., 100 ml) and measure the VTI$_{LVOT}$ variation, diminishing the risk of fluid overload. In a small study, 39 mechanically intubated patients received a 100 mL hydroxyethyl starch bolus over 1 min to assess pre- and post-bolus VTI$_{LVOT}$, followed by an additional 400 mL and repeated measurement. In response to this mini-fluid challenge, an increase in VTI variation ≥ 10% predicted fluid responsiveness to a total volume of 500 ml ≥ 15%, with a sensitivity of 95% and specificity of 78%.[21] The literature supporting this approach, however, is quite scant.

Carotid Velocity Time Integrals

Obtaining the apical five-chamber view is often difficult in acutely ill patients, especially in the operating room. Therefore, evaluation of more accessible vasculature such as the central arteries close to the aortic arch is of interest. There is increasing evidence that common carotid artery (CCA) Doppler assessment may be a valuable alternative to LVOT flow

assessment. Most of the studies evaluating carotid artery imaging for this purpose have used the corrected flow time (FTc) or the Vmax as an SV surrogate.

Image Acquisition

To obtain a Doppler tracing of the CCA a linear transducer is used. The patient's anterior neck is scanned lateral to the trachea and the CCA is visualized medial to the internal jugular vein (IJV), usually on the medial side of the triangle formed by the medial and lateral heads of the sternocleidomastoid muscle. Subsequently, the transducer is rotated 90 degrees to visualize the CCA in its long axis. The transducer is then moved cranially until the carotid bifurcation is seen. The pulsed wave Doppler is activated, and the cursor and sample volume are placed in the middle of the CCA approximately 2 cm distal to the bifurcation. The insonation angle between blood flow and the pulsed wave cursor should be less than 60 degrees. The orientation of the cursor can be either cephalad or caudal, but should remain the same throughout the assessment (Figure 8.8).

Carotid Doppler Evaluation: Heart–Lung Interaction Model

In mechanically ventilated patients in septic shock, the respiratory variation of the common carotid maximal velocity (CCV$_{max}$) may be used to determine fluid responsiveness. In a study of 59 unstable patients, fluid responsiveness was determined using a CO from a pulmonary artery catheter and compared to the change in CCV$_{max}$. CCV$_{max}$ change was superior to stroke volume variation and pulse pressure variation in differentiating fluid responders from nonresponders; a change of 14% was the cutoff value.[27] In a similar study of 40 coronary artery bypass grafting patients with a normal LVEF, CCV$_{max}$ was the most accurate predictor of fluid responsiveness, with a cutoff value of 11%.[28]

Carotid Doppler Evaluation: Passive Leg Raise Test

Different carotid parameters have been evaluated in conjunction with the PLR test. One study assessed the change of carotid blood flow (carotid area x carotid VTI x HR) and found it to be a very accurate predictor of fluid responsiveness; with a cutoff value of 20% the sensitivity was 94% and the specificity was 86%.[29] This was confirmed by other studies, with similar cutoff values ranging from 22.6 to 24.6% the sensitivity was

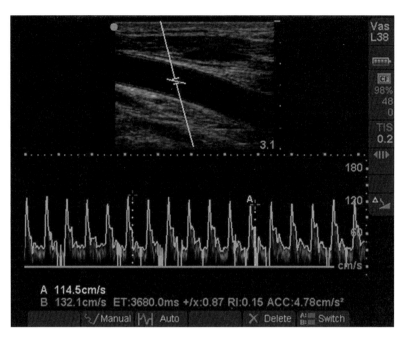

Figure 8.8 Acquisition of the CCA V_{max}. As indicated in the 2D image at the top of the image, the sample volume is placed in the middle of the artery and at an angle less than 60 degrees to the blood flow. Once the Doppler signal has been recorded the maximal and minimal flow velocities are measured, in this case 114.5 cm/s and 132 cm/s.[27] (A black and white version of this figure will appear in some formats. For the color version, please refer to the plate section).

60–76% and specificity was 88.7–92%.[30,31] While these studies have all been small (e.g., 20–40 patients) the results are nevertheless promising.

Conclusions

Hypotension is common in hospitalized patients and delineating the etiology is vital to successful treatment. The long-standing practice of administering large volumes of fluid to target the static parameters of heart rate, blood pressure, and CVP have greater potential risk than previously recognized, as it is now appreciated that fluid overload may cause morbidity and mortality. Echocardiography can be used to elucidate the causes of shock, determine fluid responsiveness, identify patients who likely will respond to fluid administration, and spare nonresponders the increased risk of morbidity and mortality that is associated with fluid overload.

It is known that stroke volume variations occur secondary to heart–lung interactions, and that LVOT VTI variation and PPV are the most accurate methods of assessing preload responsiveness. There are several limitations to acquiring reliable data, including the need for mechanical ventilation with tidal volume greater than 8 ml/kg, which is not the current standard of care. In patients undergoing general anesthesia, some of the limitations can be overcome. For example, the tidal volume can be increased to greater than 8 ml/kg for 1 minute, which will improve the accuracy of the HLIM without worsening lung function.[32] Assessing SV variation via the CCA is especially appealing, since the anesthesiologist frequently has access to the CCA, while access to the chest for performing TTE is often limited. In situations in which the HLIM is not applicable, the PLR test can be used as an alternative. This method has fewer limitations with regard to determining fluid responsiveness, with LVOT VTI measurements being the most accurate. Limitations of the PLR test are that it requires two people to perform quickly, and can be difficult to perform in the OR as the necessary positional changes are prohibitive during most surgical procedures. User skill in acquiring and interpreting the images is variable, but with widespread training and availability of ultrasound, these tests can provide guidance in fluid resuscitation and help prevent unnecessary fluid overload.

References

1. Rivers E, Nguyen B, Havstad S, et al. Early goal-directed therapy in the treatment of severe sepsis and septic shock. *N Engl J Med* 2001;**345**(19):1368–77.

2. ProCESS Investigators, Yealy DM, Kellum JA, et al. A randomized trial of protocol-based care for early septic shock. *N Engl J Med* 2014;**370**(18):1683–93.

3. Peake SL, Bailey M, Bellomo R, et al. Australasian resuscitation of sepsis evaluation (ARISE): a multi-centre, prospective, inception cohort study. *Resuscitation* 2009;**80**(7):811–8.

4. Eskesen TG, Wetterslev M, Perner A. Systematic review including re-analyses of 1148 individual data sets of central venous pressure as a predictor of fluid responsiveness. *Intensive Care Med* 2016;**42**(3):324–32.

5. Osman D, Ridel C, Ray P, et al. Cardiac filling pressures are not appropriate to predict hemodynamic response to volume challenge. *Crit Care Med* 2007;**35**(1):64–8.

6. Kumar A, Anel R, Bunnell E, et al. Pulmonary artery occlusion pressure and central venous pressure fail to predict ventricular filling volume, cardiac performance, or the response to volume infusion in normal subjects. *Crit Care Med* 2004;**32**(3):691–9.

7. Monnet X, Julien F, Ait-Hamou N, et al. Lactate and venoarterial carbon dioxide difference/arterial-venous oxygen difference ratio, but not central venous oxygen saturation, predict increase in oxygen consumption in fluid responders. *Crit Care Med* 2013;**41**(6):1412–20.

8. Michard F, Teboul J-L. Predicting fluid responsiveness in ICU patients: a critical analysis of the evidence. *Chest* 2002;**121**(6):2000–8.

9. Boyd JH, Forbes J, Nakada T-A, Walley KR, Russell JA. Fluid resuscitation in septic shock: a positive fluid balance and elevated central venous pressure are associated with increased mortality. *Crit Care Med* 2011;**39**(2):259–65.

10. National Heart, Lung, and Blood Institute Acute Respiratory Distress Syndrome (ARDS) Clinical Trials Network, Wiedemann HP, Wheeler AP, et al. Comparison of two fluid-management strategies in acute lung injury. *N Engl J Med* 2006;**354**(24):2564–75.

11. Marik PE, Cavallazzi R, Vasu T, Hirani A. Dynamic changes in arterial waveform derived variables and fluid responsiveness in mechanically ventilated patients: a systematic review of the literature. *Crit Care Med* 2009;**37**(9):2642–7.

12. Monnet X, Teboul J-L. Assessment of volume responsiveness during mechanical ventilation: recent advances. *Crit Care* 2013;**17**(2):217.

13. Monnet X, Rienzo M, Osman D, et al. Passive leg raising predicts fluid responsiveness in the critically ill. *Crit Care Med* 2006;**34**(5):1402–7.

14. Boulain T, Achard J-M, Teboul J-L, et al. Changes in BP induced by passive leg raising predict response to fluid loading in critically ill patients. *Chest* 2002;**121**(4):1245–52.

15. Mallat J, Meddour M, Durville E, et al. Decrease in pulse pressure and stroke volume variations after mini-fluid challenge accurately predicts fluid responsiveness. *Br J Anaesth* 2015;**115**(3):449–56.

16. Jue J, Chung W, Schiller NB. Does inferior vena cava size predict right atrial pressures in patients receiving mechanical ventilation? *J Am Soc Echocardiogr* 2014;**5**(6):613–9.

17. Wallace DJ, Allison M, Stone MB. Inferior vena cava percentage collapse during respiration is affected by the sampling location: an ultrasound study in healthy volunteers. *Acad Emerg Med* 2010;**17**(1):96–9.

18. Shah R, Spiegel R, Lu C, Crnosija I, Ahmad S. Relationship between the subcostal and right lateral ultrasound views of inferior vena cava collapse: implications for clinical use. *Chest* 2018;**153**(4):939–45.

19. Barbier C, Loubi Res Y, Schmit C, et al. Respiratory changes in inferior vena cava diameter are helpful in predicting fluid responsiveness in ventilated septic patients. *Intensive Care Med* 2004;**30**(9):1–7.

20. Feissel M, Michard F, Faller J-P, Teboul J-L. The respiratory variation in inferior vena cava diameter as a guide to fluid therapy. *Intensive Care Med* 2004;**30**(9):1834–7.

21. Muller L, Bobbia X, Toumi M, et al. Respiratory variations of inferior vena cava diameter to predict fluid responsiveness in spontaneously breathing patients with acute circulatory failure: need for a cautious use. *Crit Care* 2012;**16**:R188.

22. Zhang Z, Xu X, Ye S, Xu L. Ultrasonographic measurement of the respiratory variation in the inferior vena cava diameter is predictive of fluid responsiveness in critically ill patients: systematic review and meta-analysis. *Ultrasound Med Biol* 2014;**40**(5):845–53.

23. Long E, Oakley E, Duke T, Babl FE, Paediatric research in emergency departments international collaborative (PREDICT). Does respiratory variation in inferior vena cava diameter predict fluid responsiveness: a systematic review and meta-analysis. *Shock* 2017;**47**(5):550–9.

24. Slama M, Masson H, Teboul J-L, et al. Monitoring of respiratory variations of aortic blood flow velocity using esophageal Doppler. *Intensive Care Med* 2004;**30**(6):1182–7.

25. Feissel M, Michard FDR, Faller J-P, Teboul J-L. The respiratory variation in inferior vena cava diameter as a guide to fluid therapy. *Intensive Care Med* 2004;**30**(9):1–4.

26. Lamia B, Ochagavia A, Monnet X, et al. Echocardiographic prediction of volume responsiveness in critically ill patients with spontaneously breathing activity. *Intensive Care Med* 2007;**33**(7):1125–32.

27. Ibarra-Estrada MÁ, López-Pulgarín JA, Mijangos-Méndez JC, Díaz-Gómez JL, Aguirre-Avalos G. Respiratory variation in carotid peak systolic velocity predicts volume responsiveness in mechanically ventilated patients with septic shock: a prospective cohort study. *Crit Ultrasound J* 2015;**7**(1):12.

28. Song Y, Kwak YL, Song JW, Kim YJ, Shim JK. Respirophasic carotid artery peak velocity variation as a predictor of fluid responsiveness in mechanically ventilated patients with coronary artery disease. *Br J Anaesth* 2014;**113**(1):61–6.

29. Marik PE, Levitov A, Young A, Andrews L. The use of bioreactance and carotid Doppler to determine volume responsiveness and blood flow redistribution following passive leg raising in hemodynamically unstable patients. *Chest* 2013;**143**(2):364–70.

30. Jalil B, Thompson P, Cavallazzi R, et al. Comparing changes in carotid flow time and stroke volume induced by passive leg raising. *Am J Med Sci* 2018;**355** (2):168–73.

31. Taggu A, Darang N, Patil S. Carotid artery flow time corrected (FTc) changes induced by passive leg raise (PLR) can predict fluid responsiveness in mechanically ventilated (MV) patients. *Chest* 2016;**150**(4):294A.

32. Myatra SN, Prabu NR, Divatia JV, et al. The changes in pulse pressure variation or stroke volume variation after a "Tidal Volume Challenge" reliably predict fluid responsiveness during low tidal volume ventilation. *Crit Care Med* 2017;**45**(3):415–21.

33. Michard F. Changes in arterial pressure during mechanical ventilation. *Anesthesiology* 2005;103 (2):419–28.

34. Myatra SN, Monnet X, Teboul JL. Use of "tidal volume challenge" to improve the reliability of pulse pressure variation. *Crit Care* 2017;21(1):6.

Point-of-Care Abdominal Ultrasound

Shaun L. Thompson and Daniel W. Johnson

Introduction

Ultrasonography is an indispensable imaging modality that is increasingly utilized by perioperative physicians at the bedside. Abdominal ultrasound should be performed when patient instability in settings that suggest abdominal pathology may be the cause. The focused assessment with sonography in trauma (FAST) examination is the most common Point-of-Care Ultrasound (PoCUS) approach utilized in trauma and is applicable in both ICUs and PACUs. Abdominal sonography may be used to evaluate details of the kidneys, aorta, liver, spleen, gallbladder, bowel, bladder, and intrauterine pregnancy.[1] This chapter will describe various ultrasound techniques and protocols for examining the abdomen in critical care and perioperative medicine that are of interest to anesthesiologists.

Types and Performance of Abdominal Ultrasound

Transducer Selection

Most modern ultrasonography machines can be used to perform abdominal ultrasonography. There are several types of ultrasound transducers, but only two types allow for appropriate imaging of the abdominal structures. These are the phased array transducer (the ideal transducer for transthoracic echocardiography) and the curvilinear transducer, both of which emit ultrasound waves at frequencies from 1 to 5 MHz.[2,3] These low frequencies provide deep tissue penetration up to 30 cm and allow the sonographer to obtain ultrasound views of the abdominal viscera and vasculature, although imaging at increased depths comes at the expense of image resolution. Abdominal imaging usually is not of the same image quality as more superficial imaging with high-frequency linear transducers that have ultrasound frequencies of 5–15 MHz and a

depth limited to 5–10 cm; these higher-frequency linear probes are best used for vascular ultrasound and peripheral nerve blocks.

Focused Assessment with Sonography in Trauma

The FAST exam was most commonly performed to detect free fluid following abdominal trauma. This modality was first described by Asher et al. in 1976, when it was used specifically to assess possible splenic injury after blunt abdominal trauma (BAT);[4,5] it came into common use in the United States in the 1990s and is now routine in this setting.[2,4] Numerous studies have shown that the FAST exam has high sensitivity and specificity for detecting free fluid in the abdomen.[1,4–7]

The original purpose of the FAST exam was to guide trauma surgeons to opt for immediate surgical intervention in BAT patients with ultrasound evidence of free fluid that is likely hemoperitoneum secondary to splenic injury. While BAT patients go to the operating room far less frequently now than in the past decades (for a variety of reasons), the imaging techniques of the FAST exam remain useful. It is a valuable tool for anesthesiologists, as it can be used to detect abdominal bleeding in perioperative and critical care settings.[2] Additionally, serial FAST exams allow anesthesiologists and intensivists to evaluate persistent hypotension. For example, in a patient with multiple traumatic injuries undergoing emergency craniotomy for intracranial hemorrhage, the anesthesiologist can concurrently perform periodic FAST exams to rule out intra-abdominal bleeding.

Because the FAST examination enables rapid, noninvasive detection of free fluid in the abdomen,[1] it reduces the need for computed tomography (CT) scans and diagnostic peritoneal lavages that were the prior standard,[8–13] and thereby decreases the time to initiate potentially life-saving interventions and surgical procedures.[9] Reduced need for CT scans decreases transportation time and its associated risk, radiation exposure, and cost.[8,14–17]

The classic FAST examination involves imaging four regions: perihepatic, perisplenic, pelvic, and pericardial (known as the 4 Ps).[9,18,19] The extended FAST (e-FAST) exam includes lung ultrasound to evaluate for possible pneumothorax or hemothorax in the unstable patient.[3] The e-FAST exam will not be discussed in detail in this chapter, as lung ultrasound is discussed in Chapter 7.

It is important to perform each component of the FAST exam in the same order every time to ensure that all areas are examined thoroughly. In the perioperative arena the exam order should be right upper quadrant (RUQ), left upper quadrant (LUQ), pelvis, and subcostal. In order to rule out the presence of free fluid, multiple planes must be viewed within each window of the examination. This is accomplished by "fanning" the ultrasound sector through organs to ensure the entire space has been examined. Consistency in exam performance between examiners reduces variation and increases interobserver reliability.

Right Upper Quadrant View (Perihepatic)

Beginning the FAST exam in the RUQ (the perihepatic view) has many advantages. In comparison to the other windows, it is easiest to perform and is the most sensitive for detecting free peritoneal fluid following BAT.[2,6,20–22] In this view, the clinician seeks to rule out free fluid in three spaces: (1) the subphrenic space (i.e., between the diaphragm and the dome of the liver); (2) the hepato-renal space; and (3) the inferior pole of the right kidney. In this quadrant free fluid most commonly accumulates in the hepato-renal space (also known as Morrison's pouch).[1,2,6,22,23] Recent literature, however, has shown that free fluid in the abdomen may initially be seen at the caudal edge of the liver, prior to its appearance in the hepato-renal space.[23] If free fluid is found in the RUQ then it is treated as a positive examination and patient status will determine the course of action from that point onward.[2] The sensitivity with a single view FAST exam using only the RUQ ranges from 51 to 82%.[20]

To perform the RUQ exam the transducer is placed in a longitudinal orientation with the probe indicator directed cephalad in the mid-axillary line.[2] The superior aspect of the transducer should be at the

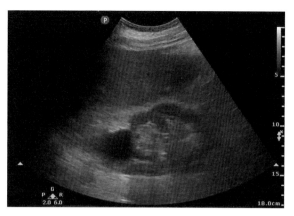

Figure 9.1 Free fluid in the RUQ: note the black (hypoechoic) area in Morrison's pouch, between the liver and the kidney.

level of the xiphoid process in order to visualize both the liver and the right kidney. Image depth should be adjusted to ensure simultaneous visualization of the liver and the right kidney.[2,9] Once the liver and the right kidney are visualized, the transducer should be fanned through this area to ensure that the entire space is imaged.[2,22] The transducer should also be moved cephalad to visualize the right diaphragm in order to detect fluid in the subphrenic space or in the right pleural space.[3] Placing the patient in Trendelenberg position can increase the sensitivity of the FAST examination in the RUQ by moving free fluid up into this area.[2,3,22,24] A common pitfall in the RUQ view is failure to fan the transducer caudad in order to rule out free fluid adjacent to the inferior pole of the right kidney. In upright patients, this area is a frequent site for accumulation of blood (Figure 9.1).

Left Upper Quadrant View (Perisplenic)

The left upper quadrant (LUQ) contains the spleno-renal space, left subphrenic space, and left paracolic gutter. Of the four FAST examination views, this view is the most difficult to acquire.[21] The view is obtained by placing the probe along the posterior axillary line with the superior edge of the probe at the level of the xiphoid process. Starting with the "knuckles to the bed" and aiming the ultrasound beam 45 to 60 degrees anteriorly increases the likelihood of obtaining adequate LUQ views. The probe is fanned in an anterior to posterior fashion in order to completely scan the LUQ to include the spleno-renal and subphrenic space.[2] The subphrenic space can be difficult to

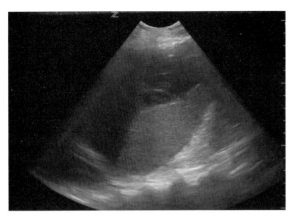

Figure 9.2 Free fluid in the LUQ: note the black (hypoechoic) area between the diaphragm and the spleen.

visualize due to artifact from aerated lung and rib shadows.[2]

The left paracolic gutter located inferior to the spleen is the area where free fluid is most commonly found in the LUQ view.[21] The paracolic gutter can be most easily visualized by moving the probe caudad until this space is found.[3] Cephalad movement of the probe will allow for visualization of the left pleural space.[3] Free fluid is typically not isolated to the LUQ, and if it is seen in the LUQ it is usually found in other areas.[21] If free fluid is isolated to the LUQ, it is most commonly seen in the left paracolic gutter.[21] Because fluid is generally not isolated to this area, if free fluid is found within the LUQ, full visualization of the other areas of the FAST examination are warranted and an exam limited to the LUQ would be inadequate (Figure 9.2).[21,25]

Pelvic View

Following ultrasound of the right and left upper quadrant, the pelvic scan should be performed. This view is obtained by placing the transducer about 1–2 cm superior to the pubic symphysis. The probe is first placed in the transverse plane with the probe marker toward the patient's right side. Subsequently the probe is placed in the sagittal plane with the probe marker toward the patient's head.[3] Again, fanning of the probe to visualize all areas of the pelvis is important to be sure that free fluid is not overlooked. Care must be taken not to mistake normal fluid collections or anatomy in the pelvis as pathological. Normal observations that potentially may be misinterpreted as pathological include the prostate gland and seminal vesicles in males and the small amount of common benign fluid present in females.[2,26,27]

The urinary bladder is the main anatomic landmark to be visualized.[2,3,20] Visualization of the bladder ensures that the image depth will include the common sites of free fluid collection. The rectovesical pouch is the most common area where free fluid is seen in males in the pelvic view.[2,3,20] In females free fluid can collect in both the uterovesicular pouch and the rectouterine space (also known as the pouch of Douglas).[2] A full bladder is helpful for visualization, as it allows not only for proper anatomic guidance but also for ease of visualizing free fluid in the pelvis.[2,3,20] If the urinary bladder is not full, a Foley catheter can be placed and fluid instilled into the bladder to assist in visualization.[3] In comparison with the RUQ view, smaller volumes of fluid are detectable in the pelvic view.[6]

Subcostal View

The final window to be examined in the FAST examination is the pericardial window or the subcostal view. Two main questions must be answered by the subcostal view: (1) Does the patient have cardiac activity? (2) Is there fluid within the pericardial space?

This view is obtained by placing the transducer just below the xiphoid process and tilting the ultrasound beam cephalad almost parallel to the skin surface in order to visualize the heart. The marker of the transducer should be oriented toward the patient's left side. The liver acts as an acoustic window and is found in the near field in this view.[2] The right ventricle occupies the majority of the border with the liver and is well visualized in this window.[3] In this view the left ventricle lies beneath the right ventricle, and the atria are well visualized. Global ventricular function can be assessed to determine whether this may be contributing to hemodynamic compromise.

The subcostal view readily detects the presence of significant pericardial effusion.[1–3,22] The pericardium normally appears as a brightly echogenic line directly adjacent to the myocardium. Pericardial fluid will appear as a hypoechoic or anechoic stripe between the myocardium and the pericardium.[20] The echo texture of the fluid can appear complex when clot begins to form in the pericardial space (Figure 9.3).[28]

While formal diagnosis of pericardial tamponade, pulmonary embolism, and fluid responsiveness is beyond the scope of the traditional FAST exam,

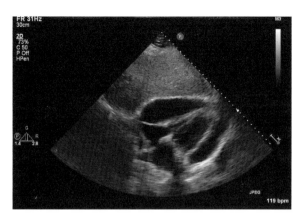

Figure 9.3 Massive pericardial effusion: note the black (hypoechoic) area below the liver, between the pericardium, and the extremely compressed right ventricle. This patient had sustained a knife wound to the anterior chest and required emergency cardiac surgery.

anesthesiologists should be familiar with their ultrasound appearance. Pericardial tamponade should be in the differential diagnosis if a significant pericardial effusion is detected during a state of shock. Right atrial collapse (during ventricular systole) followed by right ventricular collapse (during ventricular diastole) typically is the first ultrasound sign of cardiac tamponade.[28] In severe states of tamponade, the left atrium and left ventricle will show signs of collapse. These findings generally appear late in the course of pericardial fluid accumulation, just prior to a cardiac arrest.[28]

Pulmonary embolism is a common cause of acute hemodynamic collapse in critically ill patients. The subxiphoid view can assess right ventricular size, function, and systolic pressure. Since right ventricular dilation and dysfunction can be associated with other pathologies, these must be ruled out.[28] McConnell's sign is an echocardiographic finding associated with acute pulmonary embolism, consisting of normal function of the right ventricular apex and right ventricular free wall hypokinesis or akinesis.[29,30] Overall, echocardiography has a low sensitivity to diagnose acute pulmonary embolism, but its sensitivity for massive pulmonary embolism is much higher.[29]

Ultrasound to assess fluid responsiveness is described in greater detail in Chapter 8. Subcostal imaging of the inferior vena cava (IVC) comprises one of the most useful modalities in the evaluation of fluid responsiveness. In general, a small diameter IVC with marked respiratory variability in diameter indicates likely fluid responsiveness, while a large

diameter IVC with lack of respiratory variability indicates unlikely fluid responsiveness. The IVC can be located by rotating the probe in a counterclockwise fashion, while keeping the right atrium in sight from the subcostal view. Because of this, an IVC evaluation is sometimes done as an extension of the FAST exam. In critically ill patients, IVC findings often do not completely explain the clinical picture, and other studies may be needed to fully assess volume status and cardiovascular function.[31]

Limitations of the FAST Examination

While the FAST examination can provide rapid diagnosis of free fluid and expedite care, it has limitations and pitfalls. First, there is a chance of a false negative study. This may be due to sonographer error or insufficient time after injury for enough fluid to accumulate in order to be imaged.[2,9] Free fluid in the abdomen can usually be discovered when as little as 200 ml is present.[9] If an initial FAST examination is negative, repeat exams over the course of the patient's care, particularly if there are significant clinical changes or high suspicion, may eventually reveal free fluid in the abdomen.[2,20] False negative results can also be influenced by other severe injuries. Studies have shown that in patients with minor solid organ injuries, those with comorbid severe head injuries had increased rates of false negative results on FAST examination.[6,32] False negative results can lead to poor patient outcomes, as the undetected pathology may lead to continued deterioration and a missed opportunity for early intervention.

False positive findings can arise from many factors and can lead to unnecessary procedures and testing. Physiologic fluid collections may be misinterpreted as traumatic free fluid. These situations arise due to ovarian cyst rupture, ventriculoperitoneal (VP) shunts, peritoneal dialysis, and preexisting ascites.[3] It can be difficult to discern between new intra-abdominal bleeding and ascites, as they appear similar on ultrasound.[20] Pericardial fat pad or preexisting pericardial effusion may be described as new free fluid and may lead to unnecessary pericardiocentesis and potential patient harm.[3]

Technical difficulty can lead to poor imaging and inability to accurately assess free fluid. This can be secondary to patient body habitus, as morbid obesity can make it difficult to obtain adequate visualization. Traumatic injury itself can make ultrasonography difficult, due to subcutaneous emphysema, patient position, slow rate of bleeding, bowel gas, and intra-abdominal adhesions.[3] Retroperitoneal hematoma and hemorrhage are very difficult to assess with ultrasonography as well.[1,3,9] The FAST exam is also very poor in determining hollow viscus or solid organ injury that is not associated with free fluid in the abdomen, such as early bowel injury or pancreatic insults.[9,33]

Abdominal Aortic Ultrasound

Ultrasound to evaluate the aorta in patients with undifferentiated hypotension can be a useful tool to assess for possible aneurysmal disease as a causative factor.[20] Abdominal ultrasonography has a high sensitivity and specificity for detecting abdominal aortic aneurysms (AAA).[1] It can also be used to assess for possible aortic dissection in cases where the patient presents with symptoms of limb ischemia and/or acute severe abdominal pain.[34] Since it is critical that these diagnoses are made rapidly, the portability and speed of ultrasound makes it an optimal initial exam.

The abdominal aortic ultrasound scanning technique is similar to that used for the FAST examination. The curvilinear probe is best suited for this study, as the aorta is a deep lying structure within the abdomen. With the patient in the supine position, the probe is initially placed in the midepigastrium of the subcostal area in a transverse plane.[20] Firm pressure should be applied to the probe in order to displace any bowel gas that may overlie the abdominal aorta, which is seen just to the left of the lumbar spine.[20] The aorta can then be scanned from the epigastrium down to the bifurcation, at approximately the level of the umbilicus. The takeoffs of the celiac, superior mesenteric, and sometimes inferior mesenteric arteries can be visualized and assessed during this portion of the exam. The transducer should then be turned clockwise 90 degrees to view the aorta in a longitudinal plane, as it is often easier to appreciate the extent of an aortic aneurysm when viewed in this plane.

Once the aorta is identified, care should be taken not only to follow it through its entire course through the abdomen but also to get accurate measurement of its diameter and determine the possible presence of an aneurysm. The normal diameter of the abdominal aorta is less than 3 cm.[20] There are two methods for

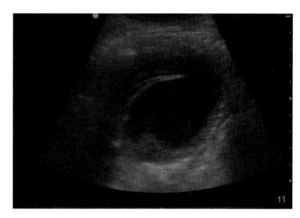

Figure 9.4 Abdominal aortic aneurysm: this patient presented to the emergency department with abdominal pain and hypotension. The transverse view of the aorta was obtained just cephalad to the umbilicus. The abdominal aortic aneurysm is greater than 5 cm in diameter.

measuring the diameter of the aorta: from inner wall to inner wall (ITI) and outer wall to outer wall (OTO).[35,36] The ITI measurement has greater interobserver reliability than the OTO measurement.[35] The anteroposterior diameter is more accurate and reproducible than the transverse diameter in the measurement of abdominal aortic aneurysm.[35,37] If mural hematoma is noted, then OTO measurements should be utilized.[20] Measurements greater than 5.5 cm are concerning in a hypotensive patient, as the risk for rupture is high.[20] If an aneurysm is found, consultation with a vascular surgeon is prudent and further evaluation with a CT scan is often needed for surgical planning (Figure 9.4).

Ultrasound can also be utilized to detect aortic dissection. These patients may present with symptoms of obstruction of the branch arteries from the aorta, including mesenteric ischemia, limb ischemia, and paraplegia.[34] Ultrasound findings that correlate with aortic dissection include visualization of an intimal flap and intramural thrombus.[34] The intimal flap can sometimes originate in the thoracic aorta and extend into the abdominal aorta, affecting the branch arteries, including the celiac, superior mesenteric, and inferior mesenteric. Rapid recognition of this pathology can lead to quick surgical intervention and better patient outcomes. Abdominal aortic ultrasound decreases the time to initial identification of aortic dissection.[34,38] Further evaluation by CT imaging, however, is usually needed for definitive treatment planning.

Gallbladder Ultrasound

Disease of the biliary system is a problem that critical care physicians commonly encounter, and ultrasound is the primary modality for assessment of infectious processes and obstruction.[1,2,28] Signs of gallbladder disease include distention, wall thickening, pericholecystic fluid, biliary sludge, and sonographic Murphy's sign.

The gallbladder examination is performed by placing the ultrasound probe just inferior to the xiphoid process with the probe indicator directed cephalad, directing the ultrasound beam into the liver parenchyma. The probe is then moved toward the right side of the patient's body until the anechoic gallbladder is located.[22] This examination can also be performed during the FAST exam of the RUQ.

Interrogation of the common bile duct should be performed when assessing for possible obstructive disease, particularly if stones are discovered. The common bile duct can be differentiated from vessels of the portal system with the aid of color Doppler. An anechoic structure leaving the gallbladder with no flow will positively identify this structure.[22] Common bile duct measurements greater than 4 cm are suspicious for obstructive disease.

Several errors may occur when performing ultrasound assessment of the biliary system. False positives may instigate further unnecessary testing and interventions. Generalized edema, pre-eclampsia, cardiac failure, and renal failure often are associated with gallbladder wall thickening and may be mistaken for pathologic changes suggestive of cholecystitis.[28] Care should be taken to reduce these errors, but ultimately expert consultation and CT or magnetic resonance cholangiopancreatography may be necessary for definitive diagnosis.

Detection of Pneumoperitoneum

Perforation of hollow viscus in the abdominal cavity can cause critical illness and rapid clinical deterioration. Quick identification of this abnormality in a patient with clinical signs consistent with pneumoperitoneum allows for swift and appropriate medical and surgical intervention to reduce patient morbidity. Free air in the abdomen has a few distinctive features that sonographers must be aware of. Key findings are enhancement of the peritoneal stripe and reverberation artifact from the peritoneum.[1,22] Other findings such as enhanced echogenic free fluid in the abdomen due to spillage of enteric contents can also be appreciated.[22]

Identification of free air is typically discovered incidentally during other ultrasound examinations, such as the FAST examination or ultrasound imaging of the aorta or gallbladder.[22] Air collections from pneumoperitoneum are typically superficial and can be detected by any transducer that can image a depth greater than the thickness of the abdominal wall. The key to recognizing air on an abdominal ultrasound study is that it appears as A-lines, a repeating pattern of horizontal lines generated by reverberation artifact, the same as it appears on thoracic ultrasound (see Chapter 7, "Point-of-Care Ultrasound of the Lung"). Visualization of free air between the liver and abdominal wall reduces the chance of a false positive.[22]

FAST exam key points		
Views	**Main components**	**Notes**
Right Upper Quadrant (perihepatic)	R subphrenic Hepato-renal (Morrison's pouch) Inferior pole kidney	Easiest to perform most sensitive to detect fluid
Left Upper Quadrant (perisplenic)	Spleno-renal L subphrenic L parecolic gutter	Most difficult to perform
Pelvic	Bladder Rectovesical piuch Rectouterine space (Douglas's pouch)	Avoid mistaking normal findings for pathology
Subcostal	Cardiac activity Pericardial effusion	Covered in more detail in other chapters

Conclusions

Abdominal ultrasonography is a powerful tool in the armamentarium of anesthesiologists, critical care physicians, and emergency room physicians. Use of ultrasound to evaluate for possible abdominal pathology following trauma and abdominal surgical procedures in unstable patients can provide useful information to diagnose potential life-threatening conditions. Alone, it can guide rapid medical and interventional treatments and improve patient outcomes. It may also reduce the need for other imaging studies (e.g., CT scan) and possibly prevent unnecessary procedures (e.g., diagnostic peritoneal lavage).

References

1. Kameda T, Taniguchi N. Overview of point-of-care abdominal ultrasound in emergency and critical care. *J Intensive Care* 2016;**4**:53.

2. Pace J, Arntfield R. Focused assessment with sonography in trauma: a review of concepts and considerations for anesthesiology. *Can J Anaesth* 2018;**65**:360–70.

3. American Institute of Ultrasound in Medicine. AIUM practice guideline for the performance of the focused assessment with sonography for trauma (FAST) examination. *J Ultrasound Med* 2014;**33**:2047–56.

4. McGahan JP, Rose J, Coates TL, Wisner DH, Newberry P. Use of ultrasonography in the patient with acute abdominal trauma. *J Ultrasound Med* 1997;**12**:653–62.

5. Laing F, Federle M, Jeffery B, Brown TW. Ultrasonic evaluation of patients with acute right upper quadrant pain. *Radiology* 1981;**140**:449.

6. Savatmongkorngul S, Wongwaisayawan S, Kaewlai R. Focused assessment with sonography for trauma: current perspectives. *Open Access Emergency Medicine* 2017;**9**:57–62.

7. Elbaih AH, Abu-Elela ST. Predictive value of focused assessment with sonography for trauma (FAST) for laparotomy in unstable polytrauma Egyptian patients. *Chin J of Traumatol* 2017;**20**:323–28.

8. Sheng AY, Dalziel P, Liteplo AS, Fagenholz P, Noble VE. Focused assessment with sonography in trauma and abdominal computed tomography utilization in adult trauma patients: trends over the last decade. *Emerg Med Int* 2013;2013:678380.

9. Montoya J, Stawicki SP, Evans DC, et al. From FAST to E-FAST: an overview of the evolution of ultrasound-based traumatic injury assessment. *Eur J Trauma Surg* 2016;**42**:119–26.

10. Ollerton JE, Sugrue M, Balogh Z, et al. Prospective study to evaluate the influence of FAST on trauma patient management. *J Trauma* 2006;**60**:785–91.

11. Jehle D, Guarino J, Karamanoukian H. Emergency department ultrasound in the evaluation of blunt abdominal trauma. *Am J Emerg Med* 1993;**11**(4):342–6.

12. Moore CL, Copel JA. Point-of-care ultrasonography. *N Engl J Med.* 2011;**364**:749–57.

13. Noble VE. Think ultrasound when evaluating for pneumothorax. *J Ultrasound Med* 2012;**31**(3):501–4.

14. Dammers D, El Moumni M, Hoogland II, Veeger N, Ter Avest E. Should we perform a FAST exam in haemodynamically stable patients presenting after blunt abdominal injury: a retrospective cohort study. *Scand J Trauma Resusc Emerg Med* 2017;**25**:1.

15. Melniker LA, Leibner E, McKenney MG, et al. Randomized controlled clinical trial of point-of-care, limited ultrasonography for trauma in the emergency department: the first sonography outcomes assessment program trial. *Ann Emerg Med* 2006;**48**:227–35.

16. Boulanger BR, McLellan BA, Brenneman FD, Ochoa J, Kirkpatrick AW. Prospective evidence of the superiority of a sonography-based algorithm in the assessment of blunt abdominal injury. *J Trauma* 1999;**47**:632–7.

17. Arrillaga A, Graham R, York JW, Miller RS. Increased efficiency and cost-effectiveness in the evaluation of the blunt abdominal trauma patient with the use of ultrasound. *Am Surg* 1999;**65**:31–5.

18. Rozycki GS, Newman PG. Surgeon-performed ultrasound for the assessment of abdominal injuries. *Adv Surg* 1999;**33**:243–59.

19. Rozycki GS, Ballard RB, Feliciano DV, Schmidt JA, Pennington SD. Surgeon-performed ultrasound for the assessment of truncal injuries: lessons learned from 1540 patients. *Ann Surg* 1998;**228**:557–67.

20. Jehle D, Stiller G, Wagner D. Sensitivity in detecting free intraperitoneal fluid with the pelvic views of the FAST exam. *Am J Emerg Med* 2003;**21**:476–8.

21. O'Brien KM, Stolz LA, Amini R, et al. Focused assessment with sonography for trauma examination: re-examining the importance of the left upper quadrant view. *J Ultrasound Med* 2015;**34**:1429–34.

22. Boniface KS, Calabrese KY. Intensive care ultrasound: IV. *Abdominal Ultrasound in Critical Care. Ann Am Thorac Soc* 2013;**10**:713–24.

23. Lobo V, Hunter-Behrend M, Cullnan E, et al. Caudal edge of the liver in the right upper quadrant (RUQ) view is the most sensitive area for free fluid on the FAST exam. *West J Emerg Med* 2017;**18**:270–80.

24. Abrams BJ, Sukumvanich P, Seibel R, Moscati R, Jehle D. Ultrasound for the detection of intraperitoneal fluid: the role of Trendelenberg positioning. *Am J Emerg Med* 1999;**17**:117–20.

25. Ma OJ, Kefer MP, Mateer JR, Thoma B. Evaluation of hemoperitoneum using a single-view vs multiple-view ultrasonographic examination. *Acad Emerg Med* 1995;**2**:581–6.

26. Rozycki G, Ochsner M, Feliciano D, et al. Early detection of hemoperitoneum by ultrasound examination of the right upper quadrant: a multicenter study. *J Trauma* 1998;**45**:878–83.

27. Blackbourne LH, Soffer D, McKenney M, et al. Secondary ultrasound examination increases the sensitivity of the FAST exam in blunt trauma. *J Trauma* 2004;**57**:934–8.

28. Blanco P, Volpicelli G. Common pitfalls in point-of-care ultrasound: a practical guide for emergency and critical care physicians. *Crit Ultrasound J* 2016;**8**:15.

29. Sosland RP, Gupta K. McConnell's sign. *Circulation* 2008;**118**:e517–e518.

30. McConnell MV, Solomon SD, Rayan ME, et al. Regional right ventricular dysfunction detected by echocardiography in acute pulmonary embolism. *Am J Cardiol* 1996;**78**:469–73.

31. Airapetian N, Maizel J, Alyamani O, et al. Does inferior vena cava respiratory variability predict fluid responsiveness in spontaneously breathing patients? *Crit Care* 2015;**19**:400.

32. Tayal VS, Nielsen A, Jones AE, et al. Accuracy of trauma ultrasound in major pelvic injury. *J Trauma* 2006;**61**:1453–57.

33. Gaarder C, Kroepelien CF, Loekke R, et al. Ultrasound performed by radiologists-confirming the truth about FAST in trauma. *J Trauma* 2009;**67**:323–27.

34. Chenkin J. Diagnosis of aortic dissection presenting as ST-elevation myocardial infarction using point-of-care ultrasound. *J Emerg Med* 2017;**53**:880–4.

35. Hartshorne TC, McCollum CN, Earnshaw JJ, Morris J, Nasim A. Ultrasound measurement of aortic diameter in a national screening programme. *Eur J Vasc Endovasc Surg* 2011;**42**:195–9.

36. Thapar A, Cheal D, Hopkins T, et al. Internal or external wall diameter for abdominal aortic aneurysm screening? *Ann R Coll Surg Engl* 2010;**92**(6):503–5.

37. Ellis M, Powell JT, Greenhalgh RM. Limitations of ultrasonography in surveillance of small abdominal aortic aneurysms. *Br J Surg* 1991;**78** (5):614–6.

38. Pare JR, Liu R, Moore CL, et al. Emergency physician focused cardiac ultrasound improves diagnosis of ascending aortic dissection. *Am J Emerg Med* 2016;**34**:486–92.

Noninvasive Measurement of Cardiac Output

Samuel Gilliland, Robert H. Thiele, and Karsten Bartels

Introduction

Adolf Eugen Fick (1829–1901) described the relationship between cardiac output (CO), oxygen uptake (VO_2), and the difference between arterial and venous blood oxygen content (CaO_2–CvO_2) as follows:[1]

$$CO = VO_2/(CaO_2–CvO_2)$$

The "Fick method" involves measurement of mixed venous oxygen content and arterial oxygen content, with oxygen uptake measured using a Douglas bag. The equation is then solved for cardiac output. While the Fick technique is too cumbersome to be used clinically, it has allowed researchers to develop and validate other more practical means of measuring cardiac output.

The principle upon which the Fick technique is based (conservation of mass and energy) is also used in applications where an indicator (e.g., cold fluid) is injected upstream and then measured downstream, as in thermodilution. The advent of the Swan–Ganz catheter in the 1970s, combining thermodilution with the balloon-tipped pulmonary artery catheter (PAC), allowed for the measurement and optimization of cardiac output to become a clinical reality.[2–4] Unfortunately, multiple large prospective randomized-controlled trials failed to show improvement of mortality in critically ill patients with its use.[5–7] These failures were attributed, in part, to the counterbalancing adverse effects of such an invasive monitor, frequent misinterpretation of the data, and perhaps ineffective or harmful treatment based on the data. In response, cardiac output monitoring and "optimization" were not abandoned, but instead less invasive monitoring strategies have been pursued.[8]

As the PAC was the clinical reference standard at the time of these monitors' initial development, many have erroneously interpreted it as the experimental reference standard as well. Additional reference standards include electromagnetic and transit time flow meters, as well as measurement of CO obtained via the Fick method. Cardiac output monitoring modalities described here are assessed comparatively to these standards.

Thermodilution

Injection of an indicator with subsequent measurement on a time-concentration curve form the basis for Stewart's "indicator-dilution" method of determining cardiac output.[9] Flow is calculated with a derivation of the Conservation of Indicator Principle, the "Stewart–Hamilton equation."

$$m = Q \int_0^\infty c(t)dt$$

In this equation, m is the mass of the indicator injected, Q is flow, and c(t) the change in concentration over time.[10] Using temperature as the indicator, Fegler adapted this technique.[4] Additional factors must be considered to apply this to the Swan thermodilution measurements, and thus CO is calculated as

$$CO = V_I (T_B - T_I) K_I * K_2 / \int_0^\infty \Delta T_B(t)dt$$

In this equation V_I is injectate volume, T_B blood temperature, T_I injectate temperature, K_I density factor defined as specific heat multiplied by specific gravity of the injectate divided by the product of the specific heat and gravity of blood, and K_2 is a computation constant taking into account the dead space of the catheter, head exchange in transit, and injection rate. This is then divided by the change in blood temperature over time ($\int_0^\infty \Delta T_B(t)dt$).[11]

Assumptions made by these calculations are important to note, as they may affect interpretation of data or result in inaccurate measurements in particular clinical scenarios. These assumptions are as follows: (1) that the injectate temperature will return to baseline in a finite period of time (as opposed to infinity), (2) that the injectate and the bloodstream are perfectly mixed, and (3) that the measurement of temperature difference is accurate. Clinical scenarios that may invalidate these assumptions include tricuspid regurgitation,[12] frequent repeated measurements,[13] low flow states,[14] and rapid temperature changes following cardiopulmonary bypass.[15,16] Additionally, as PAC thermodilution relies on measurements taken at the right atrium and pulmonary artery, this measurement is of right-sided cardiac output and ignores intracardiac shunting.

The PAC cardiac output, as validated in a large number and variety of experimental models, is accurate and precise, with an error of only 13% for triplicate readings.[17] This, along with its "first to market" position,[2] led to its adoption as the clinical reference standard. Continuous thermodilution catheters, which use a heating element as opposed to injectate, seem to offer similar clinical accuracy, though they do lag behind real-time measurements by up to 5 minutes.[18–20] The additional benefit of the catheter is the ability to measure pulmonary artery pressures (PAP) and pulmonary artery occlusion pressures (PAOP), though the ability of clinicians to reliably interpret this information has been questioned.[21]

Ultrasound-Based Techniques

By relating the frequency of a returning ultrasound beam (Δf) with the frequency of the initial beam (f_0), the speed of sound in tissue (c), and the angle of incidence to a moving reflector (θ), the Doppler equation can calculate the velocity of that reflector (v), or in the case of ultrasound-based techniques of CO monitoring, blood velocity. To calculate CO, that velocity is integrated over time (velocity time integral, or VTI) and then multiplied by a cross-sectional area. This assumes that the measured velocity is equal at all points in the vessel being studied, and that cross-sectional change of the vessel is a negligible source of error.[22]

$$v = c\Delta f / (2f_0 cos(\theta))$$

Validation of Doppler-based devices has been performed both in ex vivo models and animal and human experimental reference standards, similar to the PAC. The accuracy of Doppler compared to thermodilution-derived cardiac output is slightly reduced, though this difference may not be clinically relevant

and may be outweighed by the noninvasive nature of these devices.

An advantage of Doppler-based devices such as the CardioQ (Deltex Medical, Chichester, West Sussex, UK) is ease of use without the requirement for advanced ultrasound skills. The esophageal Doppler probe resembles a gastric tube in size and shape, with a small dedicated probe at the end. It may be inserted orally or nasally and is positioned to image the descending thoracic aorta. Because of this positioning, it fails to capture the 30% of the cardiac output that is diverted proximally and so also fails to directly measure CO. However, assessment of CO by esophageal Doppler as compared to Fick methods reveals only a slightly lower correlation than that of the PAC.[23–25] Of note, the algorithm developed to calculate stroke volume from esophageal Doppler devices is derived from a Doppler/thermodilution database and thus cannot be more accurate than thermodilution itself.[26]

Additional information provided by esophageal Doppler may include stroke volume variation and corrected flow time (FT_c), the latter being time spent in systole corrected for heart rate. Both have been used as a measure of fluid responsiveness and incorporated into goal-directed fluid management strategies.

Arterial Waveform Devices

Arterial waveform analysis is available commercially in two classes of devices, generally split into those requiring calibration and those that do not (i.e., uncalibrated). The underlying principle of both classes is the same and based on Windkessel's model of blood flow.[27] This assumes the volume of blood entering a vessel of infinite length must equal the volume of blood leaving a vessel over the period of cardiac contraction. It also assumes that the vessel will expand during systole and contract during diastole. In this model, the arterioles serve as resistors, while the aorta is a capacitor.[28] Impedance, or resistance to pulsatile flow, is calculated using a variety of techniques, including those based on physical models (e.g., the characteristic impedance [cZ] technique) and models that are empirically derived (e.g., FloTrac/Vigileo).[29] All of these estimates are imperfect, therefore devices utilizing calibration might have some advantage.

Pulse contour devices, similar to esophageal Doppler devices, additionally calculate stroke volume (SV) variation and pulse pressure variation. In some devices, ventricular contractility assessment (rate of left ventricular pressure rise early in systole, or dP/dt$_{max}$), extravascular lung water, and other derived variables may also be determined. Caution must be taken, however, in those patients with a pathology that alters the arterial waveform (e.g., aortic insufficiency).

Calibrated Arterial Waveform Devices

Transpulmonary Thermodilution (PiCCO)

By analyzing the arterial waveform distal to the dicrotic notch, the PiCCO system (Maquet, Rastatt, Germany) treats compliance as a dynamic variable dependent on pressure (C(p)) and incorporates instantaneous pressure changes (dP/dt) into its stroke volume estimate. This is meant to better account for the ventricular output fraction that is stored in capacitance vessels. Furthermore, to account for changes in impedance that occur over time, the PiCCO utilizes intermittent cardiac output calibration with a proprietary temperature-sensing central venous catheter used to perform transpulmonary thermodilution:

$$SV = k_{end\text{-}diastole}\int^{end\text{-}systole} [P(t)/SVR + C(p) \times dP/dt]dt$$

where SVR = systemic vascular resistance.

Transpulmonary thermodilution has been shown to be non-inferior to conventional thermodilution both by experimental reference standards and in multiple animal models.[30–38]

Lithium Dilution (LiDCO Plus)

The PulseCO algorithm is used by LiDCO (LiDCO Ltd, Lake Villa, IL, USA) monitors to estimate aortic blood volume by using a transfer function to determine characteristic impedance.[39] The LiDCO Plus can be calibrated using a lithium dilution curve (LiDCO); alternatively it may be used as an uncalibrated device.

Cardiac output measurements using lithium injected centrally then sampled via a femoral catheter are more accurate than conventional thermodilution according to data from experimental studies conducted in animals; if the lithium is injected peripherally, however, accuracy is reduced.[40–42] Although comparison studies are limited, the available evidence indicates that this calibrated device is reasonably accurate compared to conventional thermodilution.[43–45]

Uncalibrated Arterial Waveform Devices

Empiric Approach (FloTrac)

The FloTrac's (Edwards Lifesciences, Irvine, CA) use of an empirically derived mathematical model, as opposed to a physical model, is a significant departure in arterial waveform analysis.[46] As the device is uncalibrated, accuracy is reduced.[47–55]

Pressure Recording Analytical Method

The Pressure Recording Analytical Method (PRAM) (Hewlett Packard, Andover, MA, USA) operates on the principle that volumetric changes in blood vessels are based on the interplay between arterial compliance, left ventricular ejection force, impedance, and peripheral resistance to flow secondary to wave reflection from vessel bifurcations as well as changing diameter.[56] It also relies on the assumption that these changes occur in the radial direction. Though the PRAM method compares favorably against Doppler-based devices in animal models,[57] experimental reference standards,[56] and conventional thermodilution,[58,59] further validation is needed as the majority of these data come from a single investigatory group.

Calibrated versus Uncalibrated Arterial Waveform Devices

In a study comparing LiDCO, PiCCO, and FloTRAC monitors to intermittent thermodilution, the calibrated devices (LiDCO, PiCCO) had narrower limits of agreement as compared to the uncalibrated device (FloTRAC).[60] These results have been replicated in later studies. Though the benefits of calibration have not been demonstrated universally,[61] the majority of data favor calibrated devices over uncalibrated devices for accuracy and precision.[62–64] Additionally, the accuracy of PulseCO, PiCCO, and FloTrac measurements appears to decrease during periods of hemodynamic instability, making them potentially less useful in acute situations.

Photoplethysmography

The photoplethysmography (PPG) waveform resembles that of an invasively derived waveform in a number of ways. They have both systolic-forward and diastolic-backward components,[65,66] and they are affected by both changes in vascular tone and aortic elasticity.[65,67–69] Thus, the plethysmographic waveform may be similar to an arterial line waveform used to noninvasively characterize cardiac output.

Changes in PPG baseline have been found to be correlated with arterial systolic pulse pressure variation in multiple human studies and may have a similar role in determining fluid responsiveness, especially in mechanically ventilated patients.[70,71] Similar results have been demonstrated in patients undergoing general anesthesia.[72]

By more closely examining the PPG waveform itself with devices such as a reflection mode infrared finger probe (ADInstruments, Sydney, Australia), additional information may be gleaned. Left ventricular ejection time (LVET) is the time between the start of systolic upstroke and the dicrotic notch.[73] LVET measured by Doppler flow of the aorta correlates with that measured by PPG and decreases proportionally to hypovolemia.[74] By examining the pre-ejection period (i.e., the interval between the ECG R wave and the radial artery pulse pressure upstroke), a clinician may be able to determine fluid responsiveness.[75] A prolonged pre-ejection period positively correlates with improvement in cardiac index after fluid challenge.[76]

Left ventricular outflow impedance is affected by vascular tone and pulse wave velocity.[65] With vasoconstriction, the faster pulse wave returns to the left ventricle earlier, which then increases outflow impedance.[77] This is reflected qualitatively by the PPG contour,[78] and quantitatively by the PPG amplitude, reflective index (RI), and PPG-derived stiffness index. A decrease in systemic vascular resistance not only increases the amplitude of the PPG waveform but also shortens the width.[78–84] The dicrotic notch moves leftward with vasoconstriction.[85,86] The RI is determined by the ratio of the amplitudes of the backward and forward waves, which is indirectly related to vascular impedance.[87] A stiffness index depends on the presence of the dicrotic notch (not always readily apparent in the waveform) and is related to the elasticity of the vascular system.[87,88]

As noted in other methodologies discussed here, these measurable variables may be incorporated into algorithms extrapolating cardiac output and may be useful in the future as a real-time, noninvasive CO monitor.

Bioimpedance and Bioreactance

The relationship between intrathoracic blood volume and thoracic electrical resistance is the basis for thoracic electrical bioimpedance (TEB). The maximum impedance change over time is assumed to be related to peak aortic flow rate. Using EKG tracings to determine ventricular ejection time, the peak aortic flow rate is averaged over this period to approximate mean aortic flow rate. It is also assumed that any change in thoracic electrical resistance is solely attributed to a change in intrathoracic blood volume. Given these assumptions, CO measurement with TEB may be significantly altered by pulmonary edema, electrode positioning, and electrical noise. Comparisons to other cardiac output monitors, as well as animal and human experimental reference standards, suggest that it is less accurate than thermodilution and Doppler-based devices. This lack of accuracy is exacerbated by the potential for electrical interference in the operating room, specifically electrocautery.

Electrical velocimetry attempts to improve the accuracy of these older devices and operates under the assumption that aortic blood flow velocity, not thoracic blood volume, is related to thoracic conductivity. Comparison data against thermodilution and Doppler-based estimates of CO are limited.

Bioreactance focuses on the electrical capacitance and induction properties of intrathoracic blood in order to limit error related to electrode positioning, humidity, body size, and temperature. These properties relate stroke volume to phase shift between applied and received voltage.[89] The NICOM (Cheetah Medical, Vancouver, WA) measures CO using this technique and has been compared to both thermodilution[47,89,90] and Doppler-based methods.[91] Few studies have been conducted using this new device, precluding a meaningful assessment – more investigation is needed.

Conclusions

Several methods of cardiac output determination have been devised to obtain similar data to reference standards such as the Fick method. Their relative features are outlined in Table 10.1. Doppler-based techniques have similar accuracy as PACs with the advantage of being less invasive. Calibrated pulse contour devices are more accurate than their uncalibrated counterparts but require intermittent operator intervention to retain that accuracy. Photoplethysmography is

Table 10.1 Cardiac output monitoring modalities characterized qualitatively.

Characteristic	Thermodilution	Doppler	Calibrated Pulse Contour	Uncalibrated Pulse Contour	Photoplethys mography	Bioimpedance	Bioreactance	Partial Rebreathing
Accuracy	+++	++	++	+	+	+	+	+
Response Time	++	+++	+++	+++	+++	+++	+++	+
Convenience	+	++	++	+++	+++	+++	+++	++

Note: + = below average, ++ = average, +++ = better than average.

Source: Thiele RH, Bartels K, Gan TJ. Cardiac output monitoring: a contemporary assessment and review. Crit Care Med 2015;43(1):177–85.

a developing and potentially promising modality but requires further refinement and investigation before being ready for widespread clinical use. Bioimpedance devices do not correlate as well as either thermodilution or Doppler, and bioreactance devices require further study in order to make meaningful comparisons.

References

1. Geerts BF, Aarts LP, Jansen JR. Methods in pharmacology: measurement of cardiac output. *Br J Clin Pharmacol* 2011;**71**(3):316–30.

2. Ganz W, Donoso R, Marcus HS, Forrester JS, Swan HJ. A new technique for measurement of cardiac output by thermodilution in man. *Am J Cardiol* 1971;**27**(4):392–6.

3. Swan HJ, Ganz W, Forrester J, et al. Catheterization of the heart in man with use of a flow-directed balloon-tipped catheter. *N Engl J Med* 1970;**283**(9):447–51.

4. Fegler G. Measurement of cardiac output in anaesthetized animals by a thermodilution method. *Q J Exp Physiol Cogn Med Sci* 1954;**39**(3):153–64.

5. Sandham JD, Hull RD, Brant RF, et al. A randomized, controlled trial of the use of pulmonary-artery catheters in high-risk surgical patients. *N Engl J Med* 2003;**348**(1):5–14.

6. Richard C, Warszawski J, Anguel N, et al. Early use of the pulmonary artery catheter and outcomes in patients with shock and acute respiratory distress syndrome: a randomized controlled trial. *JAMA* 2003;**290**(20):2713–20.

7. Harvey S, Harrison DA, Singer M, et al. Assessment of the clinical effectiveness of pulmonary artery catheters in management of patients in intensive care (PAC-Man): a randomised controlled trial. *Lancet* 2005;**366**(9484):472–7.

8. Porhomayon J, El-Solh A, Papadakos P, Nader ND. Cardiac output monitoring devices: an analytic review. *Intern Emerg Med* 2012;**7**(2):163–71.

9. Stewart G. The output of the heart in dogs. *Am J Physiol* 1921;**57**:27–50.

10. Profant M VK, Eckhardt U. The Stewart-Hamilton equations and the indicator dilution method. *SIAM J Appl Math* 1978;**34**:666–75.

11. Nishikawa T, Dohi S. Errors in the measurement of cardiac output by thermodilution. *Can J Anaesth* 1993;**40**(2):142–53.

12. Cigarroa RG, Lange RA, Williams RH, Bedotto JB, Hillis LD. Underestimation of cardiac output by thermodilution in patients with tricuspid regurgitation. *Am J Med* 1989;**86**(4):417–20.

13. Maruschak GF, Potter AM, Schauble JF, Rogers MC. Overestimation of pediatric cardiac output by thermal indicator loss. *Circulation* 1982;**65**(2):380–3.

14. van Grondelle A, Ditchey RV, Groves BM, Wagner WW Jr, Reeves JT. Thermodilution method overestimates low cardiac output in humans. *Am J Physiol* 1983;**245**(4):H690–2.

15. Bazaral MG, Petre J, Novoa R. Errors in thermodilution cardiac output measurements caused by rapid pulmonary artery temperature decreases after cardiopulmonary bypass. *Anesthesiology* 1992;**77**(1):31–7.

16. Latson TW, Whitten CW, O'Flaherty D. Ventilation, thermal noise, and errors in cardiac output measurements after cardiopulmonary bypass. *Anesthesiology* 1993;**79**(6):1233–43.

17. Yang XX, Critchley LA, Joynt GM. Determination of the precision error of the pulmonary artery thermodilution catheter using an in vitro continuous flow test rig. *Anesth Analg* 2011;**112**(1):70–7.

18. Philip JH, Long MC, Quinn MD, Newbower RS. Continuous thermal measurement of cardiac output. *IEEE Trans Biomed Eng* 1984;**31**(5):393–400.

19. Aranda M, Mihm FG, Garrett S, Mihm MN, Pearl RG. Continuous cardiac output catheters: delay in in vitro response time after controlled flow changes. *Anesthesiology* 1998;**89**(6):1592–5.

20. Goldstein LJ. Response time of the Opti-Q continuous cardiac output pulmonary artery catheter in the urgent mode to a step change in cardiac output. *J Clin Monit Comput* 1999;**15**(7–8):435–9.

21. Iberti TJ, Fischer EP, Leibowitz AB, et al. A multicenter study of physicians' knowledge of the pulmonary artery catheter. *Pulmonary Artery Catheter Study Group*. *JAMA* 1990;**264**(22):2928–32.

22. Schuster AH, Nanda NC. Doppler echocardiographic measurement of cardiac output: comparison with a non-golden standard. *Am J Cardiol*. 1984;**53**(1):257–9.

23. Smith HJ, Grottum P, Simonsen S. Doppler flowmetry in the lower thoracic aorta. An indirect estimation of cardiac output. *Acta Radiol Diagn (Stockh)* 1985;**26**(3):257–63.

24. Davies JN, Allen DR, Chant AD. Non-invasive Doppler-derived cardiac output: a validation study comparing this technique with thermodilution and Fick methods. *Eur J Vasc Surg*. 1991;**5**(5):497–500.

25. Valtier B, Cholley BP, Belot JP, et al. Noninvasive monitoring of cardiac output in critically ill patients using transesophageal Doppler. *Am J Respir Crit Care Med* 1998;**158**(1):77–83.

26. Lowe GC, BM; Philpot, EJ, et al. Oesophageal Doppler Monitor (ODM) guided individualised goal directed fluid management (iGDFM) in surgery – a technical review. Deltex Medical Technical Review; 2010.

27. Kouchoukos NT, Sheppard LC, McDonald DA. Estimation of stroke volume in the dog by a pulse contour method. *Circ Res* 1970;**26**(5):611–23.

28. Essler S, Schroeder MJ, Phaniraj V, et al. Fast estimation of arterial vascular parameters for transient and steady beats with application to hemodynamic state under variant gravitational conditions. *Ann Biomed Eng* 1999;**27**(4):486–97.

29. Wesseling K, de Witt B, Weber A. A simple device for the continuous measurement of cardiac output. *Adv Cardiovasc Phys* 1983;**5**:16–52.

30. Bajorat J, Hofmockel R, Vagts DA, et al. Comparison of invasive and less-invasive techniques of cardiac output measurement under different haemodynamic conditions in a pig model. *Eur J Anaesthesiol* 2006;**23**(1):23–30.

31. Marx G, Schuerholz T, Sumpelmann R, Simon T, Leuwer M. Comparison of cardiac output measurements by arterial trans-cardiopulmonary and pulmonary arterial thermodilution with direct Fick in septic shock. *Eur J Anaesthesiol* 2005;**22**(2):129–34.

32. Pauli C, Fakler U, Genz T, et al. Cardiac output determination in children: equivalence of the transpulmonary thermodilution method to the direct Fick principle. *Intensive Care Med* 2002;**28**(7):947–52.

33. Goedje O, Hoeke K, Lichtwarck-Aschoff M, et al. Continuous cardiac output by femoral arterial thermodilution calibrated pulse contour analysis: comparison with pulmonary arterial thermodilution. *Crit Care Med* 1999;**27**(11):2407–12.

34. Sakka SG, Kozieras J, Thuemer O, van Hout N. Measurement of cardiac output: a comparison between transpulmonary thermodilution and uncalibrated pulse contour analysis. *Br J Anaesth* 2007;**99**(3):337–42.

35. Della Rocca G, Costa MG, Pompei L, Coccia C, Pietropaoli P. Continuous and intermittent cardiac output measurement: pulmonary artery catheter versus aortic transpulmonary technique. *Br J Anaesth* 2002;**88**(3):350–6.

36. Hamzaoui O, Monnet X, Richard C, et al. Effects of changes in vascular tone on the agreement between pulse contour and transpulmonary thermodilution cardiac output measurements within an up to 6-hour calibration-free period. *Crit Care Med* 2008;**36**(2):434–40.

37. Buhre W, Weyland A, Kazmaier S, et al. Comparison of cardiac output assessed by pulse-contour analysis and thermodilution in patients undergoing minimally invasive direct coronary artery bypass grafting. *J Cardiothorac Vasc Anesth* 1999;**13**(4):437–40.

38. Gust R, Gottschalk A, Bauer H, et al. Cardiac output measurement by transpulmonary versus conventional thermodilution technique in intensive care patients after coronary artery bypass grafting. *J Cardiothorac Vasc Anesth* 1998;**12**(5):519–22.

39. Linton NW, Linton RA. Estimation of changes in cardiac output from the arterial blood pressure waveform in the upper limb. *Br J Anaesth* 2001;**86**(4):486–96.

40. Linton RA, Young LE, Marlin DJ, et al. Cardiac output measured by lithium dilution, thermodilution, and transesophageal Doppler echocardiography in anesthetized horses. *Am J Vet Res* 2000;**61**(7):731–7.

41. Kurita T, Morita K, Kato S, et al. Lithium dilution cardiac output measurements using a peripheral injection site comparison with central injection technique and thermodilution. *J Clin Monit Comput* 1999;**15**(5):279–85.

42. Kurita T, Morita K, Kato S, et al. Comparison of the accuracy of the lithium dilution technique with the thermodilution technique for measurement of cardiac output. *Br J Anaesth* 1997;**79**(6):770–5.

43. Linton RA, Band DM, Haire KM. A new method of measuring cardiac output in man using lithium dilution. *Br J Anaesth* 1993;**71**(2):262–6.

44. Costa MG, Della Rocca G, Chiarandini P, et al. Continuous and intermittent cardiac output measurement in hyperdynamic conditions: pulmonary artery catheter vs. lithium dilution technique. *Intensive Care Med* 2008;**34**(2):257–63.

45. Mora B, Ince I, Birkenberg B, et al. Validation of cardiac output measurement with the LiDCO pulse contour system in patients with impaired left ventricular function after cardiac surgery. *Anaesthesia* 2011;**66**(8):675–81.

46. Pratt B, Roteliuk L, Hatib F, Frazier J, Wallen RD. Calculating arterial pressure-based cardiac output using a novel measurement and analysis method. *Biomed Instrum Technol* 2007;**41**(5):403–11.

47. Marque S, Cariou A, Chiche JD, Squara P. Comparison between Flotrac-Vigileo and Bioreactance, a totally noninvasive method for cardiac output monitoring. *Crit Care* 2009;**13**(3):R73.

48. Opdam HI, Wan L, Bellomo R. A pilot assessment of the FloTrac cardiac output monitoring system. *Intensive Care Med* 2007;**33**(2):344–9.

49. Cannesson M, Attof Y, Rosamel P, et al. Comparison of FloTrac cardiac output monitoring system in patients undergoing coronary artery bypass grafting with pulmonary artery cardiac output measurements. *Eur J Anaesthesiol* 2007;**24**(10):832–9.

50. Breukers RM, Sepehrkhouy S, Spiegelenberg SR, Groeneveld AB. Cardiac output measured by a new arterial pressure waveform analysis method without calibration compared with thermodilution after cardiac surgery. *J Cardiothorac Vasc Anesth* 2007;**21**(5):632–5.

51. Biais M, Nouette-Gaulain K, Cottenceau V, et al. Cardiac output measurement in patients undergoing liver transplantation: pulmonary artery catheter versus uncalibrated arterial pressure waveform analysis. *Anesth Analg* 2008;**106**(5):1480–6.

52. Biancofiore G, Critchley LA, Lee A, et al. Evaluation of a new software version of the FloTrac/Vigileo (version 3.02) and a comparison with previous data in cirrhotic patients undergoing liver transplant surgery. *Anesth Analg* 2011;**113**(3):515–22.

53. Saraceni E, Rossi S, Persona P, et al. Comparison of two methods for cardiac output measurement in critically ill patients. *Br J Anaesth* 2011;**106**(5):690–4.

54. Eleftheriadis S, Galatoudis Z, Didilis V, et al. Variations in arterial blood pressure are associated with parallel changes in FlowTrac/Vigileo-derived cardiac output measurements: a prospective comparison study. *Crit Care* 2009;**13**(6):R179.

55. Sander M, Spies CD, Grubitzsch H, et al. Comparison of uncalibrated arterial waveform analysis in cardiac surgery patients with thermodilution cardiac output measurements. *Crit Care* 2006;**10**(6):R164.

56. Romano SM, Pistolesi M. Assessment of cardiac output from systemic arterial pressure in humans. *Crit Care Med* 2002;**30**(8):1834–41.

57. Romagnoli S, Romano SM, Bevilacqua S, et al. Cardiac output by arterial pulse contour: reliability under hemodynamic derangements. *Interact Cardiovasc Thorac Surg* 2009;**8**(6):642–6.

58. Franchi F, Silvestri R, Cubattoli L, et al. Comparison between an uncalibrated pulse contour method and thermodilution technique for cardiac output estimation in septic patients. *Br J Anaesth* 2011;**107**(2):202–8.

59. Scolletta S, Franchi F, Taccone FS, et al. An uncalibrated pulse contour method to measure cardiac output during aortic counterpulsation. *Anesth Analg* 2011;**113**(6):1389–95.

60. Hadian M, Kim HK, Severyn DA, Pinsky MR. Cross-comparison of cardiac output trending accuracy of LiDCO, PiCCO, FloTrac and pulmonary artery catheters. *Crit Care* 2010;**14**(6):R212.

61. Krejci V, Vannucci A, Abbas A, Chapman W, Kangrga IM. Comparison of calibrated and uncalibrated arterial pressure-based cardiac output monitors during orthotopic liver transplantation. *Liver Transpl* 2010;**16**(6):773–82.

62. Johansson A, Chew M. Reliability of continuous pulse contour cardiac output measurement during hemodynamic instability. *J Clin Monit Comput* 2007;**21**(4):237–42.

63. Bein B, Meybohm P, Cavus E, et al. The reliability of pulse contour-derived cardiac output during hemorrhage and after vasopressor administration. *Anesth Analg* 2007;**105**(1):107–13.

64. Zollner C, Haller M, Weis M, et al. Beat-to-beat measurement of cardiac output by intravascular pulse contour analysis: a prospective criterion standard study in patients after cardiac surgery. *J Cardiothorac Vasc Anesth* 2000;**14**(2):125–9.

65. O'Rourke MF, Yaginuma T, Avolio AP. Physiological and pathophysiological implications of ventricular/vascular coupling. *Ann Biomed Eng* 1984;**12**(2):119–34.

66. O'Rourke MF. Pressure and flow waves in systemic arteries and the anatomical design of the arterial system. *J Appl Physiol* 1967;**23**(2):139–49.

67. Wisely NA, Cook LB. Arterial flow waveforms from pulse oximetry compared with measured Doppler flow waveforms apparatus. *Anaesthesia* 2001;**56**(6):556–61.

68. Millasseau SC, Guigui FG, Kelly RP, et al. Noninvasive assessment of the digital volume pulse: comparison with the peripheral pressure pulse. *Hypertension* 2000;**36**(6):952–6.

69. Almond NE, Jones DP, Cooke ED. Noninvasive measurement of the human peripheral circulation: relationship between laser Doppler flowmeter and photoplethysmograph signals from the finger. *Angiology* 1988;**39**(9):819–29.

70. Natalini G, Rosano A, Taranto M, et al. Arterial versus plethysmographic dynamic indices to test responsiveness for testing fluid administration in hypotensive patients: a clinical trial. *Anesth Analg* 2006;**103**(6):1478–84.

71. Cannesson M, Besnard C, Durand PG, Bohe J, Jacques D. Relation between respiratory variations in pulse oximetry plethysmographic waveform amplitude and arterial pulse pressure in ventilated patients. *Crit Care* 2005;**9**(5):R562–8.

72. Cannesson M, Attof Y, Rosamel P, et al. Respiratory variations in pulse oximetry plethysmographic waveform amplitude to predict fluid responsiveness in the operating room. *Anesthesiology* 2007;**106**(6):1105–11.

73. Chan GS, Middleton PM, Celler BG, Wang L, Lovell NH. Automatic detection of left ventricular ejection time from a finger photoplethysmographic pulse oximetry waveform: comparison with Doppler aortic measurement. *Physiol Meas* 2007;**28**(4):439–52.

74. Geeraerts T, Albaladejo P, Declere AD, et al. Decrease in left ventricular ejection time on digital arterial

waveform during simulated hypovolemia in normal humans. *J Trauma* 2004;**56**(4):845–9.

75. Bendjelid K, Suter PM, Romand JA. The respiratory change in preejection period: a new method to predict fluid responsiveness. *J Appl Physiol (1985)* 2004;**96**(1):337–42.

76. Feissel M, Badie J, Merlani PG, Faller JP, Bendjelid K. Pre-ejection period variations predict the fluid responsiveness of septic ventilated patients. *Crit Care Med* 2005;**33**(11):2534–9.

77. Chowienczyk PJ, Kelly RP, MacCallum H, et al. Photoplethysmographic assessment of pulse wave reflection: blunted response to endothelium-dependent beta2-adrenergic vasodilation in type II diabetes mellitus. *J Am Coll Cardiol* 1999;**34**(7):2007–14.

78. Murray WB, Foster PA. The peripheral pulse wave: information overlooked. *J Clin Monit* 1996;**12**(5):365–77.

79. Lund F. Digital pulse plethysmography (DPG) in studies of the hemodynamic response to nitrates–a survey of recording methods and principles of analysis. *Acta Pharmacol Toxicol (Copenh)* 1986;**59** Suppl 6:79–96.

80. Ezri T, Steinmetz A, Geva D, Szmuk P. Skin vasomotor reflex as a measure of depth of anesthesia. *Anesthesiology* 1998;**89**(5):1281–2.

81. Zhang XY, Zhang YT. The effect of local mild cold exposure on pulse transit time. *Physiol Meas* 2006;**27**(7):649–60.

82. Awad AA, Ghobashy MA, Ouda W, et al. Different responses of ear and finger pulse oximeter wave form to cold pressor test. *Anesth Analg* 2001;**92**(6):1483–6.

83. Awad AA, Haddadin AS, Tantawy H, et al. The relationship between the photoplethysmographic waveform and systemic vascular resistance. *J Clin Monit Comput* 2007;**21**(6):365–72.

84. Lee QY, Chan GS, Redmond SJ, et al. Multivariate classification of systemic vascular resistance using photoplethysmography. *Physiol Meas* 2011;**32**(8):1117–32.

85. Lax H, Feinberg AW, Cohen BM. Studies of the arterial pulse wave: I. The normal pulse wave and its modification in the presence of human arteriosclerosis. *J Chronic Dis* 1956;**3**(6):618–31.

86. Dawber TR, Thomas HE, Jr., McNamara PM. Characteristics of the dicrotic notch of the arterial pulse wave in coronary heart disease. *Angiology* 1973;**24**(4):244–55.

87. Millasseau SC, Kelly RP, Ritter JM, Chowienczyk PJ. Determination of age-related increases in large artery stiffness by digital pulse contour analysis. *Clin Sci (Lond)* 2002;**103**(4):371–7.

88. Arnett DK, Evans GW, Riley WA. Arterial stiffness: a new cardiovascular risk factor? *Am J Epidemiol* 1994;**140**(8):669–82.

89. Keren H, Burkhoff D, Squara P. Evaluation of a noninvasive continuous cardiac output monitoring system based on thoracic bioreactance. *Am J Physiol Heart Circ Physiol* 2007;**293**(1):H583–9.

90. Raval NY, Squara P, Cleman M, et al. Multicenter evaluation of noninvasive cardiac output measurement by bioreactance technique. *J Clin Monit Comput* 2008;**22**(2):113–9.

91. Weisz DE, Jain A, McNamara PJ, A EL-K. Non-invasive cardiac output monitoring in neonates using bioreactance: a comparison with echocardiography. *Neonatology* 2012;**102**(1):61–7.

92. Thiele RH, Bartels K, Gan TJ. Cardiac output monitoring: a contemporary assessment and review. *Crit Care Med* 2015;**43**(1):177–85.

Assessing Intravascular Volume Status and Fluid Responsiveness: A Non-Ultrasound Approach

David S. Beebe

Introduction

One of the clinical decisions that anesthesiologists routinely face is "when" and "how much" fluid to give patients in the perioperative period in order to maintain or restore circulating blood volume and pressure. Intravascular volume is commonly affected in the perioperative period by multiple factors, including dehydration due to preoperative medical instruction (i.e., fasting), preoperative bowel preparation, possible vomiting and diarrhea, diuretic administration, third-spacing (i.e., movement of fluid from the intravascular space to the interstitial space), and intraoperative blood loss. Further, cardiac depression and systemic vasodilation due to anesthesia often cause hypotension, which is frequently and erroneously assumed to be due to hypovolemia.

Traditionally, anesthesiologists have relied on standard fluid replacement strategies based upon patient weight, length of time the patient was fasting, blood loss, and type of surgery, in conjunction with heart rate, blood pressure, urine output measurement, and personal "expertise." This approach may be adequate in most circumstances, but given that hypovolemia and hypervolemia are both associated with increased morbidity and mortality, more definitive and objective assessment of intravascular volume would be beneficial.

Accurate assessment of intravascular volume is especially important in certain high-risk patient groups that either do not respond to or may be harmed by fluid administration. Patients with severe sepsis and hypotension are routinely resuscitated by administration of a fluid challenge (e.g., 10–30 ml/kg of crystalloid) to increase preload, cardiac output, and blood pressure. Heart rate, blood pressure, and urine output are measured as surrogate markers of the cardiac output response. Only 50% of these patients, however,

have a positive response to fluid administration. Furthermore, patients with right or left ventricular heart failure may be harmed by fluid administration that does not result in hemodynamic improvement, as fluid overload has been linked to delirium, congestive heart failure, cardiac conduction abnormalities, non-cardiogenic pulmonary edema, hepatic congestion, ileus, acute kidney injury, peripheral edema, wound dehiscence, decubitus ulcers, deep vein thrombosis, and pulmonary embolism.

A priori identification of patients who are likely to respond to fluid administration with an increase in cardiac output and blood pressure would be the optimal approach to resuscitation. Invasive methods used to guide resuscitation for more than 50 years, including central venous pressure and pulmonary capillary wedge pressure measurement, have repeatedly been shown to not predict fluid responsiveness.

Within the past 15–20 years the focus on predicting fluid responsiveness has shifted to measuring the dynamic changes in arterial blood pressure that occur during positive pressure ventilation. Assessment of these dynamic changes is the most sensitive and specific means of predicting fluid responsiveness and recently has been incorporated into bedside devices. Despite this, determination and utilization of dynamic changes in arterial blood pressure remain inconsistently applied. This chapter (1) reviews the physiological principles underlying the dynamic changes in arterial blood pressure with mechanical ventilation that form the basis for systolic pressure variation, pulse pressure variation, stroke volume variation, and plethysmography monitoring; and (2) provides an overview of monitors that incorporate these principles, including their applications, contraindications, and pitfalls.

Physiological Basis of Dynamic Fluid Responsiveness Monitors

Background

Blood pressure varies over the course of a spontaneous respiratory cycle, decreasing with inspiration and increasing during expiration. In the 1970s Rick and Burke observed that with mechanical positive pressure ventilation, blood pressure temporarily increases with inspiration and decreases during expiration; because this is the opposite of what occurs during spontaneous ventilation, the phenomenon was termed "blood pressure respirator paradox."[1] Rick and Burke also observed that there was a relationship between volume status and the range of blood pressure change over the respiratory cycle, yet the facts that hypovolemic patients have greater variation in blood pressure during the respiratory cycle than normovolemic patients and that fluid administration reduces this variation were not regarded as having clinical significance for more than 20 years.[2]

Blood Pressure and Stroke Volume Variation with Positive Pressure Ventilation

Stroke volume (SV) is the amount of blood pumped by each ventricle with each heartbeat. Arterial blood pressure is directly proportional to the SV. Every single blood pressure waveform may be used to directly determine if a change in SV occurred by comparing it to the waveforms that came immediately before and after. As SV varies over the respiratory cycle, so does the arterial pressure waveform. The most common elements used to infer the SV change from the arterial pressure waveform are (1) the integral of the pressure over time (sometimes simply referred to as the area under the arterial pressure curve), (2) the systolic pressure in isolation, and (3) the pulse pressure (i.e., the difference between the systolic and the diastolic blood pressure).

The area under the arterial pressure curve may be used to calculate the SV and determine its change over time, the stroke volume variation (SVV). Other indicators of SVV are the systolic pressure variation (SPV) and the pulse pressure variation (PPV). The SVV, SPV, and PPV may all be used to predict fluid responsiveness and can be used interchangeably. Of these three variables the SPV is the simplest to measure. The PPV and SVV have slightly greater sensitivity and specificity, but all three indices have an area under the curve (i.e., a sensitivity and specificity) approaching the 0.90 range.

Positive pressure ventilation creates the intrathoracic physiology that results in these measures' utility in the determination of fluid responsiveness. Positive pressure ventilation squeezes blood out of the lungs and into the left heart, resulting in increased left ventricular preload and SV. Simultaneously, as intrathoracic pressure rises, the vena cava is compressed, right atrial pressure increases, and venous return to the heart decreases. After a few heartbeats this reduces the amount of blood returning to the right ventricle and causes a decreased left ventricular preload and SV. Assuming that the compliance of the systemic vasculature does not change over the course of the respiratory cycle, the SPV and PPV may be calculated from systolic pressure (SP) and pulse pressure (PP) measurements over one respiratory cycle, respectively, and expressed as percentages.

SPV% = (Maximum SP–Minimum SP)/Mean SP

PPV% = (Maximum PP–Minimum PP)/Mean PP

The SVV may be determined from the area under the tracing of the arterial pressure waveform used to determine the SV over one respiratory cycle, also expressed as a percentage.

SVV% = (Maximum SV–Minimum SV)/Mean SV

The efficacy of SPV, PPV, and SVV measures in predicting fluid responsiveness has been well investigated. Every study has shown that they are highly predictive of fluid responsiveness to such a degree that they should be incorporated into routine clinical practice as a standard of care. A recent meta-analysis by Yang and Du[3] of 22 studies totaling 807 mechanically ventilated patients, 58% of who responded to a fluid challenge, showed that PPV predicted fluid responsiveness with a pooled sensitivity of 0.88 and specificity of 0.89. The median threshold PPV value to predict fluid responsiveness was 12% (interquartile range 10% to 13%).[3] An earlier systematic review of 29 studies that measured both PPV and SVV in a total of 685 patients, 56% of who responded to a fluid challenge, showed similar threshold values for predicting fluid responsiveness (PPV = 12.5 ± 1.6% and SVV = 11.6 ± 1.9%).[4]

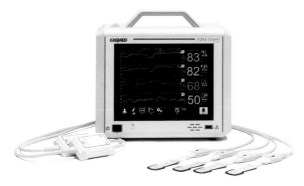

Figure 3.2 CASMED FORESIGHT™ monitor, cables, and oximetry probes. *Printed with permission from the manufacturer.

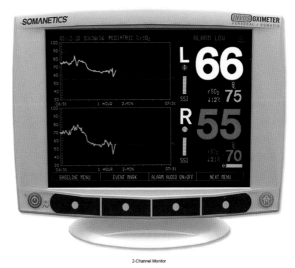

Figure 3.3 Somanetics INVOS™ cerebral oximetry monitor. *Printed with permission from the manufacturer.

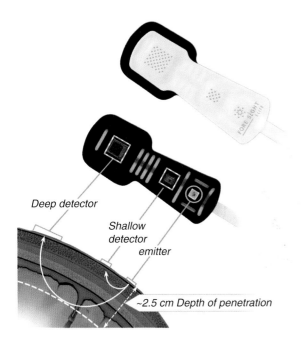

Deep detector

Shallow detector

emitter

~2.5 cm Depth of penetration

Figure 3.4 CASMED FORESIGHT™ oximetry probe and depth of penetration. *Printed with permission from the manufacturer.

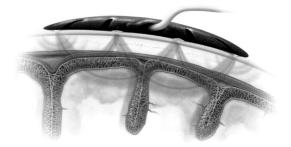

Figure 3.5 Nonin EQUANOX™ cerebral oximetry sensors. *Printed with permission from the manufacturer.

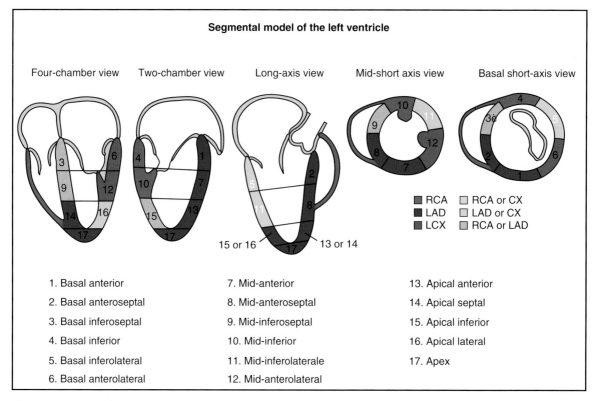

Segmental model of the left ventricle

Four-chamber view   Two-chamber view   Long-axis view   Mid-short axis view   Basal short-axis view

15 or 16   13 or 14

■ RCA   ☐ RCA or CX
■ LAD   ☐ LAD or CX
■ LCX   ☐ RCA or LAD

1. Basal anterior	7. Mid-anterior	13. Apical anterior
2. Basal anteroseptal	8. Mid-anteroseptal	14. Apical septal
3. Basal inferoseptal	9. Mid-inferoseptal	15. Apical inferior
4. Basal inferior	10. Mid-inferior	16. Apical lateral
5. Basal inferolateral	11. Mid-inferolaterale	17. Apex
6. Basal anterolateral	12. Mid-anterolateral	

Figure 5.4 was taken from Badano LP, Picano E. (2015) Standardized Myocardial Segmentation of the Left Ventricle. In: *Stress Echocardiography*. Springer, Cham.

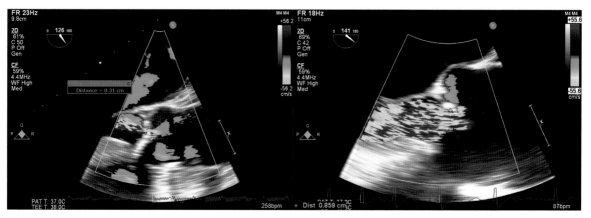

Figure 5.7 Vena contra aortic valve. Mid-esophageal aortic valve long axis. The vena contracta may be used to differentiate among degrees of aortic regurgitation. The image on the left has a narrow vena contracta, which is associated with a mild degree of aortic regurgitation. By contrast, the large vena contracta on the right is associated with a severe degree of aortic regurgitation.

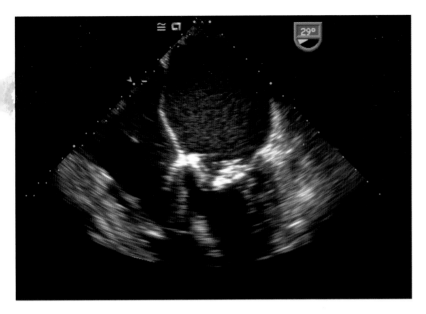

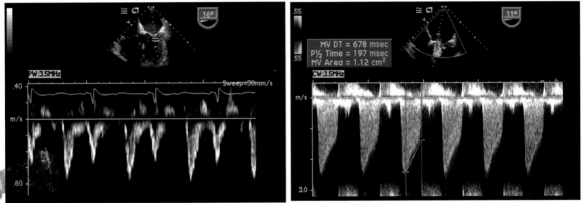

Figure 5.8 Top row: Mid-esophageal four-chamber view. The mitral valve is severely stenotic with severe calcification of the annulus and leaflets. Bottom row: Transmitral Doppler spectrum. The panel on the left is the normal transmitral Doppler flow and the panel on the right is the transmitral flow in the presence of mitral stenosis.

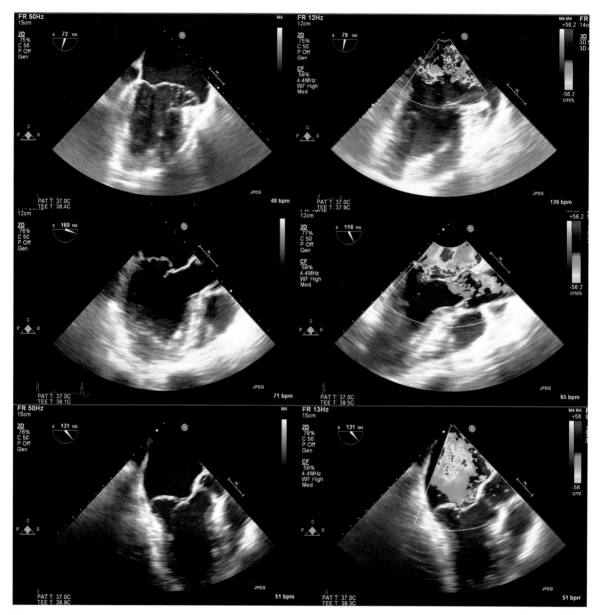

Figure 5.9 Mitral regurgitation. The top row illustrates a Barlow's mitral valve with multiple billowing and prolapsed segments. The second row illustrates a prolapsed posterior leaflet. The posterior leaflet is above the level of the mitral annulus. By contrast, a flail segment is illustrated in the bottom row, with the mitral valve segment pointing toward the atrium.

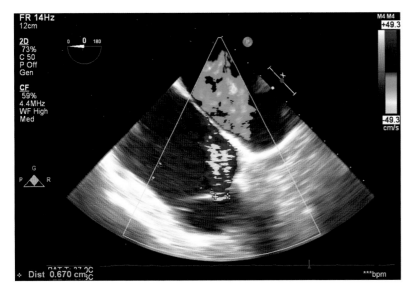

Figure 5.10 Functional tricuspid regurgitation. A mid-esophageal four-chamber view demonstrates a large functional tricuspid regurgitant jet. The vena contracta is measured as the jet emanates from the right ventricle.

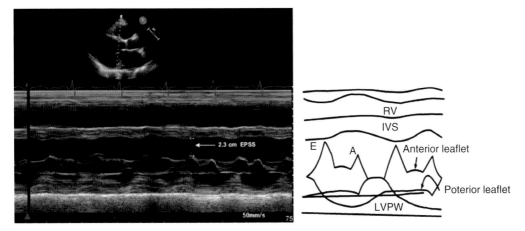

Figure 6.1 E-point septal separation (EPSS) in the parasternal long-axis view of a patient with severe left ventricular systolic dysfunction. EPSS > 8 mm is associated with systolic dysfunction. IVS, interventricular septum; LVPW, left ventricular posterior wall; RV, right ventricle. Reprinted with permission from McKaigney CJ, Krantz MJ, La Rocque CL, et al. E-point septal separation: a bedside tool for emergency physician assessment of left ventricular ejection fraction. *Am J Emerg Med* 2014;32:493–7.

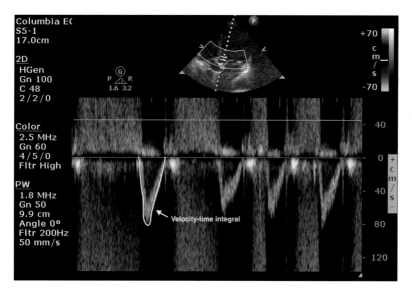

Figure 6.2(b) Apical five-chamber view showing pulsed-wave Doppler (PWD) at the left ventricular outflow tract (LVOT). The velocity-time integral (VTI) function on the ultrasound machine traces the area under the PWD curve, which, when multiplied by the area of the LVOT obtained in the parasternal long-axis view, allows calculation of left ventricular stroke volume. Stroke volume multiplied by heart rate determines cardiac output.

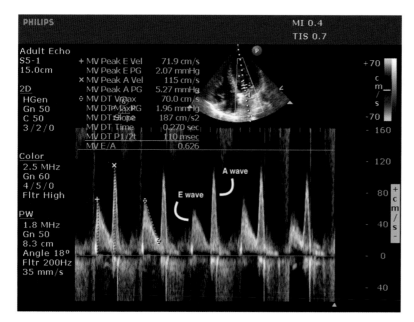

Figure 6.3(a) Apical four-chamber view with pulsed-wave Doppler (PWD) across the mitral valve showing biphasic diastolic flow. The E wave represents early passive filling, whereas the A wave shows atrial contraction during late diastole. Peak E- and A-wave velocities are used to calculate the E/A ratio.

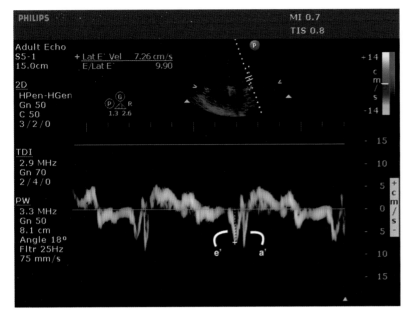

Figure 6.3(b) Apical four-chamber view with tissue Doppler imaging (TDI) of the mitral annulus showing early (e') and late (a') excursion of the mitral annulus during diastole. The E/e' ratio utilizing peak e' velocity is another measure of left ventricular diastolic function.

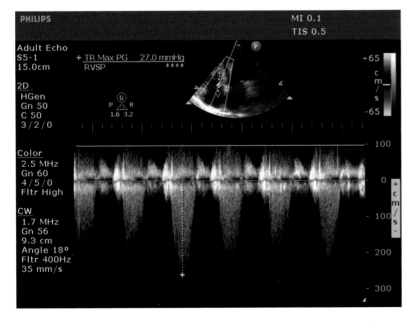

Figure 6.5 Continuous-wave Doppler (CWD) of tricuspid regurgitation (TR) in the apical four-chamber view. Maximal TR jet velocity can be used to calculate right ventricular systolic pressure using the simplified Bernoulli equation and right atrial pressure.

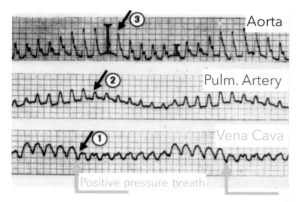

Figure 8.3 Illustration of the heart–lung interaction with positive pressure ventilation in a hypovolemic patient. **(1)** As the pressure increases with the initiation of a mechanical breath, the flow to the RA through the vena cava decreases significantly. **(2)** With a minimal delay the flow in the main pulmonary artery decreases as well, secondary to both an afterload increase and preload decrease. **(3)** The LV SV initially increases as the pulmonary capillaries are drained by the increased intrathoracic pressure and increase the LV preload transiently, however, thereafter preload drops significantly and LV SV drops (red bars).

Source: Michard F. Changes in arterial pressure during mechanical ventilation. *Anesthesiology* 2005; 103(2):419–28.

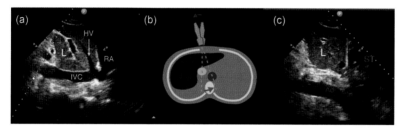

Figure 8.5 Subcostal view required for measurement of the IVC diameter. IVC= inferior vena cava, RA = right atrium, HV = hepatic vein, L = Liver, Ao = aorta, ST = soft tissue layer. **(a)** Subcostal long axis view of the IVC: The IVC is directly attached to the liver parenchyma, receives blood from the hepatic vein (blue arrow) just distal to the diaphragm, and clearly drains into the right atrium; the measurement of the diameter is performed within 3 cm distal to the diaphragm and distal to the HV inlet. **(b)** It is important to differentiate the IVC (blue dot) from the descending aorta (red dot). This is done by tilting the ultrasound beam to the patient's right. **(c)** The resulting view is a subcostal long-axis view of the descending aorta. The aorta is clearly separated from the liver by a soft tissue layer and is not connected to a cardiac chamber at this level.

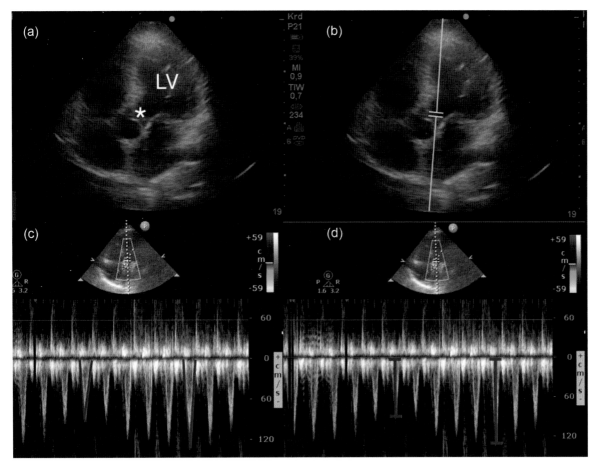

Figure 8.7 Acquisition of the LVOT VTI/ Vmax. **(a)** The apical five-chamber view is obtained with the LVOT (*) positioned in the center of the image. **(b)** The pulsed wave Doppler function is activated and the sample volume (SVol) is placed into the LVOT just above the aortic valve. **(c)** The LVOT is represented by the yellow quadrangle and the aortic valve is highlighted in blue. Once in pulsed wave Doppler mode, the envelopes below the time axis (red dotted line) can be highlighted and the area under the curve can be measured at the point of expiration and inspiration.

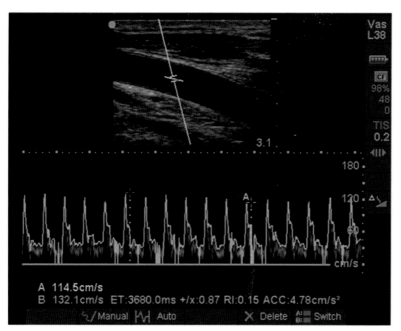

Figure 8.8 Acquisition of the CCA V_{max}. As indicated in the 2D image at the top of the image, the sample volume is placed in the middle of the artery and at an angle less than 60 degrees to the blood flow. Once the Doppler signal has been recorded the maximal and minimal flow velocities are measured, in this case 114,5 cm/s and 132 cm/s[27].

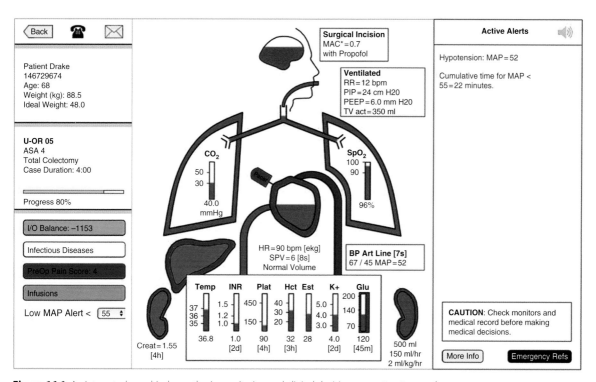

Figure 16.1 An integrated, graphical, anesthesia monitoring and clinical decision support system package.

Source: Kruger GH, Tremper KK. Advanced integrated real-time clinical displays. *Anesthesiol Clin* 2011;29: 487–504.

Kheterpal S, Shanks A, Tremper KK. Impact of a Novel Multiparameter Decision Support System on Intraoperative Processes of Care and Postoperative Outcomes. *Anesthesiology*. 2018; 128:272–282.

For patients without an arterial line, recent advances in pulse oximetry monitoring are promising for predicting fluid responsiveness. An oximetry-derived perfusion index (Pi) reflects the amplitude of the pulse oximetry waveform (PV) calculated from the pulsatile and non-pulsatile infrared signals. Dynamic Pi change, the pleth variability index (PVi), is calculated over the course of a respiratory cycle as:[5]

$$PVi = (Maximum\ PV - Minimum\ PV)/Maximum\ PV$$

Note that in this formula the denominator is the maximum PV value, not the mean value as in the SPV, PPV, and SVV calculations, thus the PVi is not a percentage.

Assessment of Fluid Responsiveness Using SPV, PPV, SVV, and PVi

In patients with normal ventricular contractility, as hypovolemia develops (e.g., due to blood loss, diuresis, inadequate fluid administration), positive pressure ventilation causes an increase in the SPV, PPV, SVV, and PVi, which increase further as hypovolemia becomes more severe. The increase in these indicators is driven by several factors that occur with hypovolemia: (1) the vena cava contains less volume and is more easily compressed or even collapsed during inspiration, resulting in decreased venous return and subsequent decreased left ventricular preload and SV; (2) transmission of the pleural pressure to the right atrium reduces venous return; (3) pulmonary West zone 1 conditions (i.e., pulmonary artery pressure is less than alveolar pressure) predominate as lower pulmonary artery pressures, increased right ventricular afterload, and reduced forward flow to the left ventricle result in a decreased preload and SV.

By contrast, these physiologic changes are not seen in normovolemia when the vena cava and atria are relatively incompressible and West zone 1 conditions are less prominent, so the net effect of a respiratory cycle is minimal change in the SV of both the right and the left ventricles.

The greater the SPV, PPV, SVV, and PVi, the more likely it is that the patient is significantly hypovolemic and that fluid administration will result in a decrease in these indices and an increase in SV and blood pressure. Most of the literature indicates that SPV, PPV, SVV values that are greater than 13% and or a PVi greater than 14 should trigger fluid administration, as the sensitivity is near greater than 0.9. In other words,

fluid administered to the patient has a 90% chance of increasing the SV and blood pressure and only a 10% chance of being ineffective. Conversely, with lower SPV, PPV, SVV, and PVi values, the more likely it is that the patient is not significantly hypovolemic and that fluid administration will not result in a decrease in these indices or an increase in SV and blood pressure. Most of the literature indicates that SPV, PPV, SVV, and PVi values less than 9% should trigger a more cautious approach to fluid administration because the specificity is greater than 0.9; fluid administration has a 90% chance of not increasing the SV and blood pressure, and has only a 10% chance of being effective.

Patients with abnormal ventricular function have unpredictable or no fluid responsiveness, because the ventricle's response to increased preload may be variable or absent.[4,6] The SPV, PPV, SVV, and PVi therefore cannot be used with any degree of certainty in patients with abnormal ventricular function.

Monitors that Display Pulse Pressure Variation, Stroke Volume Variation, and the Pleth Variability Index

Overview

There are now several monitors available for determining some combination or permutation of SPV, PPV, and SVV. However, the SPV and PPV can be determined manually from a hard copy of the arterial tracing or by use of the electronic cursor function built into most monitoring screens. Further, their automatic determination and display have been hard-wired into standard bedside monitoring units to accompany the basic electrocardiogram, automated blood pressure, and pulse oximetry functions. More sophisticated determination of SV, SVV, and other calculated variables requires arterial pressure waveform analysis performed by stand-alone monitors dedicated to this task that also can display SPV and/or PPV. These monitors may require initial and intermittent calibration to a known SV or cardiac output, or rely on proprietary waveform analysis and algorithms without a need to calibrate. There is only one pulse oximeter that has the PVi feature.[5] The utility of these monitors, however, is limited to patients with underlying normal physiologic responses; they are less accurate during intense peripheral vasoconstriction, irregular heart rhythms, aortic regurgitation, and cardiac hypocontractility.

While use of these devices has been slowly increasing, none are currently considered a standard of care, and they are utilized in only a minority of hospitals. Nevertheless, anesthesiologists should have a basic knowledge of them to understand their data and how they might assist in patient management.

Monitors Requiring an Arterial Line and Calibration to a "Known" Cardiac Output

The PiCCO system (MAQUET Holding B.V. & Co., Germany) uses a simple "pulse contour" analysis of the arterial wave form (i.e., integration of the area under the arterial waveform), and intermittent calibration with a transpulmonary thermodilution technique that requires a proprietary thermistor-tipped arterial line and a central line. It continuously monitors the SV, SVV, and PPV. In addition, it has the capability for more sophisticated measurement of global end-diastolic volume, intrathoracic blood volume, and extravascular lung water via mathematical models utilizing physiologic assumptions, although the clinical utility of these parameters is less well established than the SVV.[7]

The original LiDCO system (LiDCO, United Kingdom) also analyzes the arterial waveform to determine the SV, SVV, and PPV. Calibration relies on a lithium dilution technique whereby lithium is injected into a peripheral vein and an ion-selective electrode attached to the arterial line senses the lithium concentration and plots it over time to calculate the SV and cardiac output, which are then used to calibrate the measurement derived from the arterial waveform.[7]

Monitors That Require an Arterial Line and No Calibration

The FloTrac system (Edwards Lifesciences, Irvine, CA) also known as the Vigileo, relies on a special blood flow sensor connected to a standard arterial line. It uses a proprietary algorithm to integrate the sensor data, arterial waveform analysis, and patient demographic data to determine the SV, PPV, and SVV. This algorithm has undergone many variations over the past several years to achieve greater accuracy.[7]

LiDCO has expanded its product line over time and on its most recent website under "Build your hemodynamic monitor" now lists customizable options, including "standard minimally invasive monitoring," "+ add non-invasive monitoring," and "+ add depth of anesthesia module." The LiDCO Rapid[TM] system, like the Flo-Trac, does not require external calibration. Unlike the Flo-Trac, however, any type of arterial catheter at any site can be utilized with this monitor. Long-term trends in the cardiac output, SV, SVV, and PPV are also calculated and displayed. There are several variations of this device that have undergone frequent reinvention and name changes. Most recently, a noninvasive arterial pressure methodology (CNAP[TM]) that utilizes a dual finger cuff to derive beat-to-beat hemodynamic data has been marketed.[8]

Noninvasive Monitors (No Arterial Line Required)

The ClearSight System (Edwards Lifesciences Corporation, Irvine, CA) is a noninvasive monitor of arterial blood pressure that uses a small blood pressure cuff placed on the finger and an infrared light source with a sensor on the other side of the finger to measure the blood volume under the cuff, which changes with pulsation. The device increases and decreases the cuff pressure to keep the measured blood volume constant via a complex algorithm, and calculates the blood pressure as well as the SV and SVV continuously.[9] LiDCO uses a dual finger cuff that appears to net similar information as the ClearSight system, which has been available for a longer period of time.

NICOM[TM] (Cheetah Medical, Vancouver, WA, USA) uses a unique, noninvasive technology termed "bioreactance" that is related to bioimpedance. Bioimpedance, the degree to which the body impedes electric current flow, measures the amplitude of the voltage change that accompanies changes in fluid volume. Bioreactance measures the change in phases of the electrical current via four electrodes applied to the chest in order to detect SV. Studies measuring the cardiac output, SV, and SVV using this device have shown a high level of agreement with data from PiCCO, Flo-Trac, and pulmonary artery catheters.[10] Prior devices utilizing bioimpedance were not widely accepted, and of all the devices relying on electrical current, the NICOM[TM] technology is commercially dominant.

Cardio Q (Deltex Medical Limited, Chichester, UK) is a small Doppler probe placed trans-nasally into the esophagus and positioned facing the adjacent descending aorta. It measures SV and cardiac output and is used to determine the impact of a fluid challenge on these variables; a lack of increase in response to a fluid challenge may help guide the clinician to avoid further fluid administration. Unlike all of the other devices described in this chapter, this device requires training and skill in placing the probe properly in order to obtain adequate signals. In the United Kingdom this device has been subject to several large randomized trials, primarily in the context of bowel surgery, that have demonstrated its impact on decreasing length of stay and postoperative complications. This device has been approved for use by the National Institute for Health Care Excellence.[11]

The Masimo-Radical 7™ pulse oximeter (Masimo Co, Irvine, California) is a unique monitor that calculates the PVi using the plethysmographic waveform. To reiterate, the PVi can be used to determine fluid responsiveness, although it does not determine the SV.[5] As this device is completely noninvasive, it is promising and is undergoing investigation as a means to determine volume responsiveness in children.[12]

Applications

Intraoperative Fluid Management

The main goal of advanced hemodynamic and volumetric monitoring is to objectively guide fluid management. Use of this monitoring is mostly applicable in the intensive care unit but is increasingly used in the perioperative management of high-risk patients, since most of these patients are already on positive pressure ventilation and monitored with an arterial line, and because they have high morbidity and mortality that may be reduced with better fluid management. This monitoring allows for "just in time" fluid administration, initiated when the direct and indirect SV measures indicate significant hypovolemia, but prior to development of hypotension. Fluid management that is guided by advanced hemodynamic and volumetric monitors is associated with better outcomes than standard care based on static variables and intuition, even if there is no difference in the total fluid administered. Furthermore, if the SV indices suggest that a hypotensive patient will not be fluid-responsive, then vasoactive agents should be administered and fluid overload may be avoided.[5,13]

Goal-Directed Therapy: Principles of Fluid Management and Outcomes

Goal-directed therapy protocols were originally developed to treat patients in septic shock[14] but have been applied to other clinical situations, including high-risk patients undergoing major operations. The "goal" is to optimize oxygen delivery, primarily by the administration of fluid, until the SV is maximized. When the stroke volume is on the flat portion of the Starling curve, the SV is maximized, and additional fluid will not increase the cardiac output any further. At this point more fluid will increase the risk of hypervolemia, and the only way to further increase cardiac output is to administer inotropes. While this approach has not been clearly associated with improved outcomes in septic shock patients, it has been incorporated into many enhanced recovery after surgery protocols.[15,16]

Attempts to maximize SV and minimize SPV, PPV, SVV, and PVi, however, may inadvertently result in more fluid administered than necessary. Certain surgeries (e.g., head and neck surgery, pneumonectomy) have better outcomes with mild hypovolemia; administration of more fluid than necessary may be detrimental.[17]

Goal-directed fluid therapy was originally achieved by utilizing some combination of central venous pressure, cardiac output measured from a pulmonary artery catheter, and mixed venous oxygen saturation. More recently, the types of monitors discussed herein have been used in several large studies.[3,5,16] The typical approach is to determine the SPV, PPV, SVV, and/or PVi, and if it is "normal" (i.e., < 9%) only administer maintenance fluid. However, if the index measure is greater than 13%, a fluid challenge would be administered, the response tracked, and the process repeated until the index measure decreases to the normal range. Further volume may be administered if indicated by other determinants (e.g., increased heart rate, decreased end tidal CO_2, decreased urine output) by maintaining a holistic view.

There are two relatively large studies of this approach in patients undergoing major intestinal surgery. The OPTIMISE trial was a multicenter randomized trial of 734 patients age greater than 50 assigned to either standard therapy or a goal-directed fluid therapy protocol utilizing the calibrated LiDCO monitor, intravenous albumin to maximize the stroke volume, and a constant intravenous infusion of dopex-amine (a rarely used inotrope that is not available in the United States). There was no significant difference in primary adverse outcomes (i.e., composite of 30-day moderate or major complications and mortality) or secondary outcomes (e.g., infection, need for ICU admission, length of stay). A meta-analysis of the study data combined with that of 37 other studies of lesser quality, however, showed a significant reduction in complication rates, including infection and length of stay, but no reduction in mortality in the hospital, at 30 days, or at longest follow-up.[15]

The second trial examining goal-directed fluid therapy was the POEMAS study, a multicenter randomized trial that used the NICOM monitor in 142 patients who were randomized to standard therapy or a goal-directed therapy protocol utilizing colloids and inotropic agents to maximize SV. The patients in the treatment group received more colloids, blood, and dobutamine than those receiving standard therapy. There was no difference in complication rates or length of stay between the two groups.[16]

Inevitably, goal-directed therapy will be attempted in a wider range of patient groups and surgical procedures. It is important to note, however, that operative interventions that may impact hemodynamics (e.g., laparoscopy) or require special positioning will result in unpredictable SV measurements and responses. For example, changing from a supine to prone position increases the SVV by as much as 25%. This was considered a normal response in one study, and the trigger for a fluid challenge in the prone position was therefore set to a 20% change from the baseline prone SVV.[18] These are unexpected findings and the approach is very different than in a supine patient.

Historically, goal-directed therapy originated in the context of emergency room treatment of sepsis, based on a well-known publication by Rivers et al.[14] in 2001. More recently, however, three large prospective randomized trials (ProCESS, ARISE, and ProMISe) performed in patients with sepsis found no benefit, and a meta-analysis of patients in these three trials has cast doubt on this approach.[20] Some of the failure to reproduce the Rivers results in the newer trials may be due to a change in resuscitation of the control groups to be more similar to the intervention group in the original Rivers study, as clinicians over time incorporated the initial findings into their everyday management. There is much less evidence supporting goal-directed therapy for conditions other than sepsis. It is sobering that it took almost 15 years to disprove the most widely embraced original indications for goal-directed therapy, and that related approaches are now being incorporated into enhanced surgery protocols with nearly no evidence supporting their use. Also concerning is that once a therapy is incorporated into the mainstream, even when it is shown to be useless or even harmful, removing that therapy is difficult and takes a long period of time.

Pitfalls and Limitations of PPV, SVV, and PVi Monitoring

Two absolute requirements for using PPV, SVV, and PVi measurements are the need for a sinus rhythm and tidal volumes large enough to recreate the necessary physiological challenge. Typically, tidal volumes of 10 ml/kg are required, which are larger than currently recommended in many situations. Successful monitoring may still occur by using smaller tidal volumes chronically, and intermittently use 10 ml/kg for 30–60 seconds to measure these variables.

Additional limitations are very high respiratory rates and abnormal ventricular function. High respiratory rates interfere with complete left ventricle filling and do not allow observation of these phenomena. Abnormal ventricular function interferes with interpretation of these measurements and cannot be detected or quantified by them; therefore, echocardiography may be a better monitoring adjunct in unstable patients with concomitant cardiac disease.[4] In one study, the majority of ICU patients had one or more conditions (e.g., non-sinus rhythm, absolute need for large tidal volumes or high respiratory rates, abnormal right or left ventricular function) that rendered the monitoring useless.[19]

Although discussed previously, it bears repeating that intense peripheral vasoconstriction is an impediment to using these kinds of data and devices, particularly in patients who also have peripheral vascular disease. This limiting factor especially applies to the Clearsight and LiDCO CNAP[TM] monitors which use blood pressure measurements from the finger(s), and the Masimo PVi which is dependent on the plethysmograph and pulse oximetry signal.[5,8,9]

Table 11.1 Summary of nonultrasound monitors to assess intravascular volume status and fluid responsiveness.

Name	Manufacturer	Key Aspects
Calibrated Arterial Waveform Analysis		
PiCCO	MAQUET Holding B.V. & Co., Germany	Requires central line and arterial line Calibrated by thermodilution
LiDCO	LiDCO, London, UK	Requires an arterial line Calibrated by lithium dilution
Uncalibrated Arterial Waveform Analysis		
FloTrac	Edwards Lifesciences, Irvine, California, USA	Requires an arterial line
LIDCO Rapid	LIDCO, London, UK	Requires an arterial line
ClearSight	Edwards Lifesciences, Irvine, California, USA	Non-invasive Finger pressure device
CNAP	LiDCO, London, UK	Non-invasive Finger pressure device
Other Methodologies		
NICOM	Cheetah Medical, Vancouver, WA, USA	Bioreactance
Cardio Q	Deltex Medical Limited, Chichester, UK	Esophageal Doppler
Masimo-Radical 7	Masimo Co, Irvine California, USA	Pulse oximeter-based plethysmography

Intraoperative use of these measurements may not be useful to predict volume responsiveness in patients undergoing thoracotomy or laparoscopy.[21,22] Their use in children in any setting has not been well studied.[23]

Conclusions

Several hemodynamic and volumetric monitoring devices that can predict fluid responsiveness are commercially available (see Table 11.1), but even simple observation of an arterial line tracing may be extremely informative. This approach can improve patient care by helping to objectively answer the perennial "when" and "how much" questions of fluid administration. In theory, these devices should facilitate rapid diagnosis and treatment of hypovolemia, may foster pre-emptive strategies, and assist in avoiding excessive fluid administration. All of the devices described above have undergone numerous iterations over time and are still developing with respect to their underlying data acquisition technology, proprietary algorithms, interface, display, and pricing. In practice, however, there is no convincing evidence that employing these devices for these purposes has any impact on outcome. Nevertheless, as these monitors become less invasive, more sophisticated, and easier to use, they are increasingly utilized in intensive care units and operating rooms.

References

1. Rick J, Burke S. Respirator paradox. *South Med J* 1978;**71**:1376–8.

2. Michard F. Changes in arterial pressure during mechanical ventilation. *Anesthesiology* 2005;**103**:419–28.

3. Yang X, Du B. Does pulse pressure variation predict fluid responsiveness in critically ill patients? A systematic review and meta-analysis. *Crit Care* 2014;**18**:650–63.

4. Marik P, Cavallazzi R, Vasu T, Hirani A. Dynamic changes in arterial waveform derived variables and fluid responsiveness in mechanically ventilated patients: a systematic review of the literature. *Crit Care Med* 2009;**37**:2642–7.

5. Forget P, Lois F, de Kock M. Goal-directed fluid management based on the pulse oximeter-derived pleth variability index reduces lactate levels and improves fluid management. *Anesth Analg* 2010;**111**:910–4.

6. Carsetti A, Cecconi M, Rhodes A. Fluid bolus therapy: monitoring and predicting fluid responsiveness. *Curr Opin Crit Care* 2015;**21**:388–94.

7. Porhomayon J, Zadell G, Congello S, Nader N. Applications of minimally invasive cardiac output monitors. *Intl J Emerg Med* 2012;**5**:18.

8. LiDCO product information retrieved at www.lidco.com on January 24, 2019.

9. Raggi E, Sakai T. Update on finger-application-type noninvasive continuous hemodynamic monitors (CNAP and ccNexfin): physical principles, validation,

and clinical use. *Semin Cardiothorac Vasc Anesth* 2017;**21**:321–9.

10. Waldron N, Miller T, Thacker J, et al. A prospective comparison of a noninvasive cardiac output monitor versus esophageal Doppler monitor for goal-directed fluid therapy in colorectal surgery patients. *Anesth Analg* 2014;**118**:966–75.

11. Conway D, Hussain A, Gall I. A comparison of noninvasive bioreactance with oesophageal Doppler estimation of stroke volume during open abdominal surgery: an observational study. *Eur J Anaesthesiol* 2013;**30**:501–8.

12. Chandler J, Cook E, Petersen C, et al. Pulse oximeter plethysmograph variation and its relationship to the arterial waveform in mechanically ventilated children. *J Clin Monit Comput* 2012;**26**:145–51.

13. Guerin L, Monnet X, Teboul J. Monitoring volume and fluid responsiveness: from static to dynamic indicators. *Best Pract Res Clin Anaesthesiol* 2013;**27**:177–85.

14. Rivers E, Nguyen B, Havstad S, et al. Early goal directed therapy in the treatment of severe sepsis and septic shock. *N Engl J Med* 2001;**345**:1368–77.

15. Pearse R, Harrison D, MacDonald N, et al. Effect of a perioperative, cardiac output-guided hemodynamic therapy algorithm on outcomes following major gastrointestinal surgery: a randomized clinical trial and systematic review. *JAMA* 2014;**311**:2181–90.

16. Pestana D, Espinosa E, Eden A, et al. Perioperative goal-directed hemodynamic optimization using noninvasive cardiac output monitoring in major abdominal surgery: a prospective, randomized, multicenter, pragmatic trial: POEMAS Study (PerOperative goal-directed thErapy in Major Abdominal Surgery). *Anesth Analg* 2014;**119**:579–87.

17. Chau E, Slinger P. Perioperative fluid management for pulmonary resection surgery and esophagectomy. *Semin Cardiothorac Vasc Anesth* 2014;**18**:36–44.

18. Bacchin M, Ceria C, Giannone S, et al. Goal-directed fluid therapy based on stroke volume variation in patients undergoing major spine surgery in the prone position: a cohort study. *Spine* 2016;**41**:E1131–E1137.

19. Mair S, Tschirdewahn J, Gotz S, et al. Applicability of stroke volume variation in patients of a general intensive care unit: a longitudinal observational study. *J Clin Monit Comput* 2017;**31**:1177–87.

20. Rowan K, Angus D, Baily M, et al. Early goal directed therapy for septic shock-a patient level meta-analysis. *N Engl J Med* 2017;**376**:2223–34.

21. Jeong D, Ahn H, Park H, et al. Stroke volume variation and pulse pressure variation are not useful for predicting fluid responsiveness in thoracic surgery. *Anesth Analg* 2017;**125**:1158–65.

22. Liu F, Zhu S, Ji Q, et al. The impact of intra-abdominal pressure on the stroke volume variation and plethysmographic variability index in patients undergoing laparoscopic cholecystectomy. *Biosci Trends* 2015;**9**:129–33.

23. Gan H, Cannesson M, Chandler J, Ansermino J. Predicting fluid responsiveness in children: a systematic review. *Anesth Analg* 2013;**117**:1380–92.

Chapter 12

Assessment of Extravascular Lung Water

Torsten Loop

Introduction

Increased extravascular lung water (EVLW) is caused by abnormal movement of fluid across the pulmonary capillary barrier. It is comprised of all fluids within the extravascular compartment of the lung (i.e., outside of the pulmonary circulation), including intracellular, interstitial, alveolar, lymphatic, and surfactant, but pleural fluid is not considered extravascular lung water. An increase in EVLW may be caused by two primary physiologic derangements: (1) an increased hydrostatic intravascular pressure, as seen in cardiogenic pulmonary edema due to congestive heart failure; and (2) a decrease in the effectiveness of the pulmonary capillary barrier causing an increase in its permeability, as seen in non-cardiogenic pulmonary edema due to acute respiratory distress syndrome (ARDS), septic shock, and other conditions that are associated with less severe or collateral acute lung injuries.[1]

Physiology of Extravascular Lung Water Accumulation

Homeostatic mechanisms prevent appreciable transudation of intravascular fluid into the air-filled alveoli and other extravascular pulmonary tissue. The relationship between fluid flow and hydrostatic pressure (P) is described by the classic Starling equation that describes the balance of hydrostatic and colloidal pressures calculated as (equation 1):[2]

$EVLW = Kf \times [(P_c - P_{ev}) - (\pi c - \pi ev)] - lymphatic$
$flow$

Kf = capillary membrane permeability and filtration coefficient

P_c = hydrostatic pressure in the capillary

P_{ev} = hydrostatic pressure in the extravascular tissue/interstitium

πc = plasma protein oncotic pressure in the capillary

πev = plasma protein oncotic pressure in the extravascular tissue/interstitium

lymphatic flow = the rate of removal of fluid

While the oncotic gradient is primarily determined by protein concentration, the key variable under normal circumstances in the absence of a lung injury is the hydrostatic pressure in the pulmonary capillary microvasculature, which depends on pulmonary blood flow and resistance (equation 2):

$P_c = P_{la} + (PVR \times CO)$

P_c = pulmonary capillary pressure

P_{la} = left atrial pressure

PVR = pulmonary vascular resistance

Under normal circumstances, the small volume of EVLW resulting from the movement of fluid across the capillary membrane is whisked away by the lymphatic system and deposited back into the venous system via the thoracic duct, and hence no accumulation normally occurs. Under pathologic conditions the net movement exceeds the lymphatic system's ability to remove it and EVLW increases.

Very basically, cardiogenic pulmonary edema is caused by increased pressure within the vasculature. Non-cardiogenic pulmonary edema is caused by an increase in the permeability of the membrane separating the extra- and intravascular compartments and perhaps, in very rare cases, by an exceedingly low oncotic pressure. Cardiogenic pulmonary edema is usually ruled out by the absence of heart failure determined by history, echocardiography, or measurement of the left atrial pressure, or its surrogate, the pulmonary capillary wedge pressure.

The tissue and molecular components that control permeability of the membrane separating the extra- and intravascular compartments include the endothelium, the epithelium, an intervening fused basement membrane (i.e., proteoglycan), elastic fibers, and collagen I and III. These structures strongly control the permeability of the pores or channels through which fluid moves.[3]

The lung is resistant to developing an increased EVLW, as the lymphatic drainage is highly effective under normal conditions. The normal value of the EVLW indexed to body weight (EVLWI) is 7.3 ± 2.8 mL/kg, with normal values of EVLWI considered to be less than 10 mL/kg.[4,5] Two recent studies have suggested that EVLW should be indexed to height only, since indexing EVLW to body weight underestimates EVLW in patients who are overweight, as the lungs do not increase in size commensurate with an increase in adipose tissue.[6,7]

Measurement of Extravascular Lung Water

Clinical diagnosis of EVLW is based on patient examination, particularly auscultation focused on the presence or absence of rales, chest radiograph, and most recently, lung ultrasound focused on the presence or absence of B-lines (see Chapter 7).[8] Various experimental imaging methods, such as computer tomography, magnetic resonance imaging, and positron emission tomography, have all been used to quantify EVLW; however, gravimetry as used in experimental investigation of post-morbid specimens is considered to be the gold standard.[9,10] This ex vivo method consists of measuring the difference in the weight of the lungs before and after desiccation, which obviously is not possible in clinical practice.[9] While pulmonary ultrasound to detect B-lines helps assess the presence or absence of increased EVLW, the degree and change of EVLW is not measureable using this technique.[11,12]

One of the first studies to demonstrate the clinical value of measuring EVLW was performed by Sibbald et al. in a broad range of critically ill patients with both acute cardiogenic and non-cardiogenic pulmonary edema using a standard pulmonary artery catheter with a double-indicator thermodilution technique using indocyanine green and temperature change.[13] To quantify the fluid in the pulmonary capillary bed, EVLW was measured by injecting 10 ml of iced saline solution containing 5 mg of indocyanine green dye into the central circulation as a bolus using the central

venous pressure (CVP) port of the pulmonary artery catheter; standard thermodilution cardiac output was measured using the pulmonary artery catheter and indocyanine green concentration was measured via a femoral artery sample collected via an arterial catheter continuously sampling blood. This double-indicator trans-pulmonary thermodilution was reported capable of detecting changes in EVLW of 20% or more and correlated well with gravimetry.[14]

Principles of Transpulmonary Thermodilution

The main advance in the measurement of EVLW has been the ability to utilize a practical single transpulmonary thermodilution (TPTD) technique rather than a cumbersome experimental technique requiring nonstandard processes, including continuous withdrawing of blood via a femoral arterial line, and specialized laboratory equipment to measure the concentration of the green dye. This single injection technique uses one injection of a cold indicator, usually iced saline, into the superior vena cava via a central venous catheter, and detection of temperature change over time via a femoral arterial catheter equipped with a thermistor. This is done by applying a series of assumptions and calculations (see Figure 12.1).[15]

The traditional thermodilution curve used to determine cardiac output is a plot of temperature change on the y axis and time on the x axis. Typically, the curve is asymmetrical, corresponding to the primary dilution and secondly to recirculation. To quantify the specific intrathoracic thermal volume (ITTV) and the pulmonary thermal volume (PTV), the effects of recirculation must be eliminated, and mean transit times must be calculated. The mean transit time (MTt) represents the time when half of the indicator passes the detection in the central artery. It is predominantly determined from the area under the thermodilution curve directly after the drop of the peak. The exponential downslope time (DSt) represents the wash-out function of the indicator. It is calculated from the downslope part of the thermodilution curve. Both mean transit time and exponential downslope time serve as the basis for calculation of the volumes explained in Figure 12.1.

$$ITTV = CO \times MTt$$
$$PTV = CO \times DSt$$
$$GEDV = ITTV - PTV$$
$$ITBV = GEDV \times 1.25$$
$$EVLW = ITTV - ITBV$$

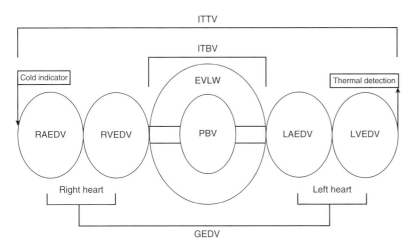

Figure 12.1 Pulmonary thermodilution measurement characteristics. RAEDV = right atrial end-diastolic volume; RVEDV = right ventricular end-diastolic volume; PBV = pulmonary blood volume; EVLW = extravascular lung water; LAEDV = left atrial end-diastolic volume; LVEDV = left ventricular end-diastolic volume; GEDV = cardiac global end-diastolic volume; ITBV = intrathoracic blood volume; ITTV = intrathoracic thermal volume.

ITTV = intrathoracic thermal volume

CO = cardiac output

MTT = mean transit time

PTV = pulmonary thermal volume

EDT = exponential decay time

GEDV = global end-diastolic volume

ITBV = intrathoracic blood volume

EVLW = extravascular lung water

The ITBV calculation assumes that the relationship between GEDV and ITBV is linear.[15] Potential limitations in the accuracy of EVLW measurement include those common to trans-cardiopulmonary thermodilution calculation of cardiac output as well as tricuspid regurgitation, mitral regurgitation, lung resection, obstruction of major pulmonary vessels and large increases in positive end-expiratory pressure.[16]

Clinical Practice

Two commercially available devices that utilize transpulmonary thermodilution, the PiCCO2 (Maquet, Munich, Germany) and the VolumeView/EV 1000® (Edwards Lifesciences, Irvine, CA, USA), may be used to determine EVLW. The estimation of the EVLW and the pulmonary blood volume also allows the calculation of a pulmonary vascular permeability index (PVPI) equal to the ratio of the extravascular lung water index and the pulmonary blood volume. An increased PVPI is consistent with a lung injury, and a lower ratio is more suggestive of a hydrostatic-driven congestive heart failure-type increase in EVLW.[17,18] Calculations of the PVPI and other hemodynamic parameters are based on the Stewart–Hamilton and Newman principles.[19,20] Both devices use the same algorithm and provide comparable measurements.[21,22]

The measurement of EVLWI requires the global end-diastolic volume (GEDV), which is the cardiac volume minus the total pulmonary volume from ITTV (see Figure 12.1). Furthermore, the intrathoracic blood volume (ITBV) is estimated from the GEDV according to the above-mentioned equation ($ITBV = GEDV \times 1.25$).[15] EVLWI is obtained by subtracting ITBV from ITTV. The main drawbacks in measuring EVLW are unreliable data in the case of pulmonary embolism, lung resection, or large pleural effusions.[23] In addition, the EVLW level is indexed to the predicted body weight, not the actual body weight, in order to avoid underestimation of EVLW.[24]

Acute Respiratory Distress Syndrome

From a pathophysiological point of view, measurement of EVLWI or PVPI may be helpful in defining ARDS, by equating the severity of the pathologic increase in pulmonary vascular permeability and alveolar damage with the abnormal increase of EVLWI.[5,25–29] A retrospective analysis of 373 critically ill patients demonstrated that patients with an EVLW greater than 15 mL/kg had a mortality rate of 65%, while patients with an EVLW less than 10 ml/kg had a mortality rate of only 33%.[27] Specifically, the maximum EVLW was significantly higher in non-survivors than in survivors, with a median of 14.3 mL/kg vs. 10.2 mL/kg, respectively. Further, an increase in EVLW may be an indicator of early ARDS and becomes apparent before a large A-a gradient or radiographic change develops.

Septic Shock

In patients with septic shock, EVLW measurements are moderately correlated with markers of acute lung injury such as lung compliance, PaO_2/FiO_2 ratio, radiographic opacification, lung injury score, and outcome.[30,31] EVLWI and permeability indexes were significantly increased in non-survivors at day 3, compared to scores in survivors. Thus, EVLW might be of value as an indicator of prognosis and severity of sepsis-induced acute lung injury.

Goal-Directed Therapy Targeting Extravascular Lung Water

The quantity of EVLW may be a relevant therapeutic target in the fluid management of critically ill patients. Increased positive fluid balance is associated with worse outcomes in acute lung injury (ALI) and ARDS, and by inference EVLW and increased positive fluid balance are linked.[32] The reduction of EVLW via a goal-directed approach is an appealing strategy, with preliminary evidence supporting its potential incorporation into other hemodynamic strategies. In a small clinical study of 16 patients with septic shock requiring mechanical ventilation, measurement of ITBVI and TEDVI was shown to be a more useful indicator of EVLW than standard hemodynamic variables, CVP, and pulmonary wedge pressure.[33] A 1992 randomized, prospective study in critically ill ICU patients with pulmonary edema found that fluid management, primarily by diuresis and fluid restriction, directed by EVLW measurement versus pulmonary artery catheter-directed care, resulted in EVLW decrease and was associated with fewer ventilator days and shorter ICU length of stay.[34] Thus, driving fluid management by EVLW measurements utilizing a bedside monitor might be advantageous.

Cardiac index, PVPI, and EVLWI measured during the postoperative period after single-lung transplantation, demonstrated an EVLWI of 12 mL/kg and a PVPI of 2.3, consistent with hydrostatic pulmonary edema.[35] EVLWI was significantly increased in patients with a lower PaO_2/FiO_2 ratio, 17 mL/kg in the group with PaO_2/FiO_2 less than 150 mmHg versus 12 mL/Kg in the group with PaO_2/FiO_2 greater than 150 mmHg.

Coldermans et al. assessed the prognostic value of an increased EVLWI and the fluid balance in critically ill patients.[36] The best predictor for mortality was an EVLWI of greater than 11 mL/kg, showing a 60% sensitivity and a 57% specificity with a PPV of 61%.

An EVLWI greater than 11 mL/kg was correlated with a higher percentage of ALI (70% versus 34%), higher tidal volumes (8.8 ± 1.9 versus 7.8 ± 1.4 mL/kg), and a trend to higher mortality (61% versus 44%).[36]

EVLW and the associated measurements these devices record have been investigated in a small study of patients with subarachnoid hemorrhage who had surgical clipping, and appeared to lower the incidence of vasospasm and cardiopulmonary complications compared with those managed with standard therapy.[37] Its utility in various cardiac and pulmonary procedures has in some studies shown benefits, but these studies also have been relatively small, had heterogeneous study groups, did not measure the same treatment outcomes, and were inconsistent in their findings.[35,38,39] EVLW reduction by continuous renal replacement therapy has also been demonstrated, but EVLW-guided continuous renal replacement therapy is not a standard.[40]

Application of and Weaning from Mechanical Ventilation

Determination of EVLW seems intuitively helpful in the setting of high levels of mechanical ventilator support and subsequent weaning plans. Several experimental studies performed in animals reveal the protective role of positive end-expiratory pressure application to reduce EVLW.[41,42] Monnet et al. demonstrated that an increase in EVLW during a spontaneous breathing trial was diagnostic of weaning-induced pulmonary edema, with good accuracy and in particular 100% specificity.[43] However, a PubMed search performed on March 5, 2018 using the search words "wean, extravascular, lung, water" identified only 19 publications, none of which used EVLW as a treatment goal or readiness for extubation parameter.

Conclusion

Extravascular lung water is a physiologic variable that can be determined using commercially available devices that utilize a transpulmonary thermodilution technique, and may be subject to targeted therapy including diuresis and treatment of hypotension with vasopressors instead of fluids. The quantity and change in EVLW may be prognostic and can be used in combination with standard vital signs (e.g., blood pressure), pulse pressure variation or stroke volume variation, and cardiac output, to guide therapy in cases where EVLW minimization itself is a reasonable goal, especially in patients with ARDS. However, large or multicenter outcome studies including EVLW into a goal-directed therapeutic strategy are lacking and the approach is not widely practiced.

References

1. Ware LB, Matthay MA. Clinical practice: acute pulmonary edema. *N Engl J Med* 2005;**353**:2788–96.

2. Starling EH. On the absorption of fluids from the connective tissue spaces. *J Physiol* 1896;**19**:312–26.

3. Miserocchi G. Mechanisms controlling the volume of pleural fluid and extravascular lung water. *Eur Respir Rev* 2009;**18**:244–52.

4. Tagami T, Kushimoto S, Yamamoto Y, et al. Validation of extravascular lung water measurement by single transpulmonary thermodilution: human autopsy study. *Crit Care* 2010;**14**:R162.

5. Tagami T, Sawabe M, Kushimoto S, et al. Quantitative diagnosis of diffuse alveolar damage using extravascular lung water. *Crit Care Med* 2013;**41**:2144–50.

6. Huber W, Mair S, Gotz SQ, et al. Extravascular lung water and its association with weight, height, age, and gender: a study in intensive care unit patients. *Intensive Care Med* 2013;**39**:146–50.

7. Phillips CR, Chesnutt MS, Smith SM. Extravascular lung water in sepsis-associated acute respiratory distress syndrome: indexing with predicted body weight improves correlation with severity of illness and survival. *Crit Care Med* 2008;**36**:69–73.

8. Saugel B, Ringmaier S, Holzapfel K, et al. Physical examination, central venous pressure, and chest radiography for the prediction of transpulmonary thermodilution-derived hemodynamic parameters in critically ill patients: a prospective trial. *J Crit Care* 2011;**26**:402–10.

9. Lange NR, Schuster DP. The measurement of lung water. *Crit Care* 1999;**3**:R19–R24.

10. Pearce ML, Yamashita J, Beazell J. Measurement of pulmonary edema. *Circ Res* 1965;**16**:482–8.

11. Volpicelli G, Elbarbary M, Blaivas M, et al. International evidence-based recommendations for point-of-care lung ultrasound. *Intensive Care Med* 2012;**38**:577–91.

12. Enghard P, Rademacher S, Nee J, et al. Simplified lung ultrasound protocol shows excellent prediction of extravascular lung water in ventilated intensive care patients. *Crit Care* 2015;**19**:36.

13. Sibbald WJ, Warshawski FJ, Short AK, et al. Clinical studies of measuring extravascular lung water by the thermal dye technique in critically ill patients. *Chest* 1983;**83**:725–31.

14. Mihm FG, Feeley TW, Jamieson SW. Thermal dye double indicator dilution measurement of lung water in man: comparison with gravimetric measurements. *Thorax* 1987;**42**:72–6.

15. Sakka SG, Ruhl CC, Pfeiffer UJ, et al. Assessment of cardiac preload and extravascular lung water by single transpulmonary thermodilution. *Intensive Care Med* 2000;**26**:180–7.

16. Michard F, Schachtrupp A, Toens C. Factors influencing the estimation of extravascular lung water by transpulmonary thermodilution in critically ill patients. *Crit Care Med* 2005;**33**:1243–7.

17. Kushimoto S, Taira Y, Kitazawa Y, et al. The clinical usefulness of extravascular lung water and pulmonary vascular permeability index to diagnose and characterize pulmonary edema: a prospective multicenter study on the quantitative differential diagnostic definition for acute lung injury/acute respiratory distress syndrome. *Crit Care* 2012;**16**:R232.

18. Monnet X, Anguel N, Osman D, et al. Assessing pulmonary permeability by transpulmonary thermodilution allows differentiation of hydrostatic pulmonary edema from ALI/ARDS. *Intensive Care Med* 2007;**33**:448–53.

19. Jozwiak M, Teboul JL, Monnet X. Extravascular lung water in critical care: recent advances and clinical applications. *Ann Intensive Care* 2015;**5**:38.

20. Brown LM, Liu KD, Matthay MA. Measurement of extravascular lung water using the single indicator method in patients: research and potential clinical value. *Am J Physiol Lung Cell Mol Physiol* 2009;**297**: L547–58.

21. Bendjelid K, Giraud R, Siegenthaler N, Michard F. Validation of a new transpulmonary thermodilution system to assess global end-diastolic volume and extravascular lung water. *Crit Care* 2010;**14**:R209.

22. Kiefer N, Hofer CK, Marx G, et al. Clinical validation of a new thermodilution system for the assessment of cardiac output and volumetric parameters. *Crit Care* 2012;**16**:R98.

23. Monnet X, Teboul JL. Transpulmonary thermodilution: advantages and limits. *Crit Care* 2017;**21**:147.

24. Berkowitz DM, Danai PA, Eaton S, Moss M, Martin GS. Accurate characterization of extravascular lung water in acute respiratory distress syndrome. *Crit Care Med* 2008;**36**:1803–9.

25. LeTourneau JL, Pinney J, Phillips CR. Extravascular lung water predicts progression to acute lung injury in patients with increased risk. *Crit Care Med* 2012;**40**:847–54.

26. Kushimoto S, Endo T, Yamanouchi S, et al; PiCCO pulmonary edema study group. Relationship between extravascular lung water and severity categories of acute respiratory distress syndrome by the Berlin definition. *Crit Care* 2013;**17**:R132.

27. Sakka SG. Extravascular lung water in ARDS patients. *Minerva Anestesiol* 2013;**79**:274–84.

28. Schuster DP. Identifying patients with ARDS: time for a different approach. *Intensive Care Med* 1997;**23**:1197–203.

29. Perel A. Extravascular lung water and the pulmonary vascular permeability index may improve the definition of ARDS. *Crit Care* 2013;**17**:108.

30. Kuzkov VV, Kirov MY, Sovershaev MA, et al. Extravascular lung water determined with single transpulmonary thermodilution correlates with the severity of sepsis-induced acute lung injury. *Crit Care Med* 2006;**34**:1647–53.

31. Wang H, Cui N, Su L, et al. Prognostic value of extravascular lung water and its potential role in guiding fluid therapy in septic shock after initial resuscitation. *J Crit Care* 2016;**33**:106–13.

32. Sakr Y, Vincent JL, Reinhart K, et al. Sepsis occurrence in acutely ill patients investigators: high tidal volume and positive fluid balance are associated with worse outcome in acute lung injury. *Chest* 2005;**128**:3098–108.

33. Boussat S, Jacques T, Levy B, et al. Intravascular volume monitoring and extravascular lung water in septic patients with pulmonary edema. *Intensive Care Med* 2002;**28**:712–8.

34. Mitchell JP, Schuller D, Calandrino FS, Schuster DP. Improved outcome based on fluid management in critically ill patients requiring pulmonary artery catheterization. *Am Rev Respir Dis* 1992;**145**:990–8.

35. Tran-Dinh A, Augustin P, Dufour G, et al. Evaluation of cardiac index and extravascular lung water after single-lung transplantation using the transpulmonary thermodilution technique by the PiCCO2 device. *J Cardiothorac Vasc Anesth* 2018;**32** (4):1731–5.

36. Cordemans C, De Laet I, Van Regenmortel N, et al. Fluid management in critically ill patients: the role of extravascular lung water, abdominal hypertension, capillary leak, and fluid balance. *Ann Intensive Care* 2012;**2**:S1.

37. Mutoh T, Kazumata K, Ishikawa T, Terasaka S. Performance of bedside transpulmonary thermodilution monitoring for goal-directed hemodynamic management after subarachnoid hemorrhage. *Stroke* 2009;**40**:2368–74.

38. Lenkin AI, Kirov MY, Kuzkov VV, et al. Comparison of goal-directed hemodynamic optimization using pulmonary artery catheter and transpulmonary thermodilution in combined valve repair: a randomized clinical trial. *Crit Care Res Pract* 2012;**2012**:821218.

39. Kapoor PM, Magoon R, Rawat RS, et al. Goal-directed therapy improves the outcome of high-risk cardiac patients undergoing off-pump coronary artery bypass. *Ann Card Anaesth* 2017;**20**:83–9.

40. Compton F, Hoffmann C, Zidek W, Schmidt S, Schaefer JH. Volumetric hemodynamic parameters to guide fluid removal on hemodialysis in the intensive care unit. *Hemodial Int* 2007;**11**:231–7.

41. Fernández Mondéjar E, Vazquez Mata G, Cárdnas A, et al. Ventilation with positive end-expiratory pressure reduces extravascular lung water and increases lymphatic flow in hydrostatic pulmonary edema. *Crit Care Med* 1996;**24**:1562–7.

42. Colmenero-Ruiz M, Fernández-Mondéjar E, Fernández-Sacristán MA, Rivera-Fernández R, Vazquez-Mata G. PEEP and low tidal volume ventilation reduce lung water in porcine pulmonary edema. *Am J Respir Crit Care Med* 1997;**155**:964–70.

43. Dres M, Teboul JL, Anguel N, et al. Extravascular lung water, B-type natriuretic peptide, and blood volume contraction enable diagnosis of weaning-induced pulmonary edema. *Crit Care Med* 2014;**42**:1882–9.

Chapter 13

Point-of-Care Hematology

Jacob Raphael, Liza Enriquez, Lindsay Regali, and Linda Shore-Lesserson

Introduction

Perioperative management of hemostasis and coagulopathy is a complex, time-sensitive task for the anesthesiologist caring for patients undergoing surgery. The combination of anticoagulant medications and possible inherent bleeding disorders makes the ability to diagnose potential causes and risks of bleeding and guide therapy critically important.

Point-of-care (POC) testing is an essential tool that has been used in clinical practice for decades and provides rapid results at the bedside. Recent technology has progressed, and several new instruments are commercially available to assist the practitioner in guiding therapy, reducing the administration of unnecessary blood products, and improving patient outcomes.

Monitoring Anticoagulation

The activated clotting time (ACT) is a classic POC test used to guide high-dose heparin therapy in patients undergoing cardiopulmonary bypass (CPB), extracorporeal membrane oxygenation (ECMO), vascular interventions, hemodialysis, and cardiac catheterization. First described by Hattersley in 1966, the ACT uses whole blood and measures clot formation via the intrinsic pathway using surface activators such as celite, kaolin, or glass beads.[1] Devices that easily fit in the palm of hand, use disposable cartridges, and have a test turnaround time of less than 5 minutes have made this test a mainstay of care for more than 25 years. It is, however, influenced by several patient-related and technology-dependent factors other than the effects of heparin, and thus is highly variable and subject to artifact.[2,3] Devices that assess the viscoelastic properties of whole blood are an advance over basic ACT testing, increasing the breadth of hemostatic abnormalities that can be detected and adding a versatility well beyond simply guiding heparinization.

The Sonoclot® (Sonoclot Coagulation & Platelet Function Analyzer, Sienco Inc., Arvada, CO) provides both qualitative and quantitative information on the entire coagulation process, from clot initiation to fibrinolysis.[4] It has been used in obstetric, cardiac, liver, vascular, and trauma surgery to identify platelet dysfunction and predict the risk of bleeding (discussed in more detail later in this chapter). Studies have also shown Sonoclot to be beneficial in managing heparin therapy during cardiac surgery and monitoring for residual heparin after cardiac surgery.[5,6] The test uses a kaolin-based activated clotting time (kACT) to monitor high-dose heparin and a glass bead-activated test (gbACT) to monitor baseline and post-protamine levels (low heparin levels).

The most commonly used viscoelastic POC device is the Thromboelastogram® (TEG).[7] The TEG is used to guide blood product administration and can reduce unnecessary transfusions by using a patient-directed approach to specific transfusion therapy. Thus, it is considered an essential tool to monitor patients who are at high risk for bleeding. In reducing transfusions, TEG has been shown to decrease costs and risks associated with transfusion.[8,9] Its use in goal-directed therapy transfusion algorithms is described in more detail later in this chapter.

TEG has been studied in the monitoring of heparinization during cardiac surgery. It has shown good correlations with the "gold standard" ACT; however, there are not enough data supporting the safety of TEG monitoring as a substitute for ACT monitoring of heparinization during CPB. Current guidelines, therefore, do not make any recommendations for its use in this setting.[10] At present, modifications have been made where the use of heparinase, an enzyme that cleaves heparin, can be used to detect any residual heparin effect after reversal with protamine.

Monitoring Direct Thrombin Inhibitors

Direct thrombin inhibitors (DTIs) are a relatively new class of anticoagulants that act by inhibiting thrombin. They are used primarily as an alternative to heparin for patients with heparin-induced thrombocytopenia (HIT) or acute coronary syndrome, and for stroke prevention in patients with atrial fibrillation.[11] There are currently four parenterally administered DTIs (lepirudin, desirudin, bivalirudin, and argatroban) and one orally administered DTI (dabigatran) available in the United States.[12,13]

Routine plasma-based coagulation testing (i.e., activated partial thromboplastin time) results poorly correlate with DTI anticoagulation and drug concentrations.[14,15] The ecarin clotting time (ECT) is a useful test in measuring thrombin inhibition. Ecarin, a proteolytic activator, cleaves prothrombin to form meizothrombin, a procoagulant that is directly inhibited by DTIs but not by heparin. Thus, the prolongation of the ECT is specific to inhibition by DTIs and has a direct linear relationship with drug levels.[16–19]

A modification of the ECT is the ecarin chromogenic assay (ECA). In this assay meizothrombin breakdown of a chromogenic substrate is measured in the presence of DTIs. This technique has been shown to be more accurate than the standard ECT, but it is not widely clinically available.[20]

A dilute thrombin time assay is available for research purposes to monitor the qualitative effects of dabigatran in plasma. It is currently produced by Hyphen Biomed and marketed in North America by Aniara. Pre-diluted patient plasma is mixed with normal pooled plasma, and purified α-thrombin is added to initiate clotting. Clotting time is recorded and graphed linearly compared to DTI calibrators. The dilute thrombin time assay has been shown to have a direct relationship with dabigatran concentration.[21,22]

Point-of-Care Monitoring of Direct Oral Anticoagulants

Direct oral anticoagulants (DOACs) are increasingly used for antithrombotic prophylaxis in patients with non-valvular atrial fibrillation and at high risk for venous thromboembolism. This new class of medications includes the direct thrombin inhibitor dabigatran and the factor Xa inhibitors rivaroxaban, apixaban, and edoxaban. When compared to vitamin K antagonists (VKA), DOACs have similar thromboprophylaxis efficacy and fewer bleeding complications.[23,24] Perhaps most importantly, DOACs have a more predictable pharmacodynamic profile compared to VKAs, hence routine anticoagulation monitoring is unnecessary. Nevertheless, knowing the exact anticoagulant effect of these medications may be important in patients presenting for emergent or urgent surgical procedures, in posttraumatic hemorrhage, or in anticipation of specific procedures such as neuroaxial anesthesia. Important pharmacokinetic and pharmacodynamic features of these medications are summarized in Table 13.1.[25] Standard laboratory tests do not accurately assess the anticoagulation effect of DOACs,[26] and tests that more specifically assess the factor Xa activity or the thrombin time are needed. However, tests such as a diluted thrombin time or anti-factor Xa activity[27,28] are time-consuming and may not be widely available in the context of emergency clinical conditions. Thus, whole blood POC coagulation tests would be ideal to assess the presence of DOAC-induced anticoagulation.

Dabigatran

Several studies have reported that in the presence of therapeutic plasma levels of dabigatran the ACT is prolonged in a concentration-dependent manner.[19,28,29]

Table 13.1 Pharmacokinetic and pharmacodynamic features of direct oral anticoagulants.

	Dabigatran	Rivaroxaban	Apixaban	Edoxaban
Half Life [a]	12–18 h	5–13 h	12 h	9–11 h
Offset of Action	24–96 h	24–48 h	24–48 h	No Data
Mode of Elimination	Renal: 80% Hepatobiliary: 20%	Hepatobiliary: 66% Renal: 33%	Hepatobiliary: 73% Renal: 27%	Hepatobiliary: 50% Renal: 50%
Elimination by Dialysis	Yes	No	No	No

[a] Assuming normal creatinine clearance

Source: Ruff CT, Giugliano RP, Braunwald E, et al. Comparison of the efficacy and safety of new oral anticoagulants with warfarin in patients with atrial fibrillation: a meta-analysis of randomised trials. *Lancet* 2014;383:955–62.

Using viscoelastic tests, dabigatran-spiked blood (taken from healthy volunteers) exhibits significant prolongation of the reaction (R-time) in both the kaolin-activated TEG* and the RapidTEG* assays.[30–32] Similarly, prolongation of the clotting time (CT) of the INTEM* and EXTEM* assays was reported in dabigatran-treated patients.[33–36] At this time though, no POC test can be used to assess the effect of anti-thrombin inhibitors with the necessary accuracy and reliability required to guide clinical decision-making.

Factor Xa Inhibitors

The ability to detect the effects of factor Xa inhibitors using POC coagulation tests is less predictable than for the direct thrombin inhibitors. Standard TEG* and ROTEM* intrinsic coagulation pathway assays and ACT do not correlate linearly with rivaroxaban concentration[29,30] and in fact may fail to demonstrate a residual anticoagulant effect of rivaroxaban.[37] The effects of rivaroxaban on the extrinsic coagulation pathway assay of ROTEM* (EXTEM) have been studied more extensively, and the results are inconsistent. Eller and colleagues have demonstrated prolongation of EXTEM only with extremely high plasma levels of rivaroxaban,[29] whereas others found prolongation at clinically relevant plasma levels.[38–40] Current evidence suggests that viscoelastic POC tests are also not reliable for detecting the anticoagulation effect of apixaban.[37]

Novel Tests of Global Hemostasis

The Global Thrombosis Test

The global thrombosis test (GTT) (Thromboquest Ltd, London, UK) is a novel POC instrument that assesses platelet function using non-anticoagulated whole blood.[41–44] Platelets are exposed to high shear stress under physiological conditions without the need for different platelet agonists. In this new system, whole blood (WB) flows into a conical test tube in which two ceramic balls are placed (Figure 13.1). The inner surface of the tube has flat segments creating narrow gaps. When WB flows by gravity through the narrow gaps and the upper ball bearing, high shear stress occurs, and platelets are activated. In the space between the ball bearings, platelet aggregation occurs, and thrombin is generated. As clot forms, the gaps are gradually occluded at the level of the lower ball

bearing, reducing and arresting blood flow. The time between two consecutive drops is measured as the occlusion time (OT) or the time to form a thrombus. The machine also measures thrombolysis using a parameter called the clot lysis time (LT).

The GTT has been studied in patients with cardiovascular risk factors,[41] end-stage renal disease,[45] and risk for dabigatran-related bleeding complications,[46,47] but it has not been studied in the perioperative setting.

IMPACT-R™

The original cone and plate(let) analyzer (CPA) is a POC device that uses a cone and plate apparatus and tests platelet function based on the adhesion of platelets to extracellular matrix (ECM) under near physiologic flow conditions.[48] The latest CPA marketed is the IMPACT-R™ (Matis Medical, Beersel, Belgium). This device assesses all aspects of platelet function, from primary hemostasis to ultimate platelet aggregation. Using IMPACT-R, platelet adhesion, activation, and aggregation are measured under arterial flow conditions. Citrated whole blood is placed in a polystyrene well and placed under shear stress by the spinning of a cone on a plate at a speed of 1,800 revolutions/sec. Primary hemostasis causes platelets to adhere to the well, while "platelet-to-platelet" aggregation also occurs. These adherent platelet clumps are then washed, stained, and quantified by an image analyzer. The surface area covered (SC) by the platelets represents platelet adhesion, and the average size (AS) of the platelet groups represents platelet aggregation.[49–51]

IMPACT-R™ has been used to study platelet function in cardiac surgical patients, monitor thrombocytopenic patients, test for congenital and acquired platelet defects, and monitor response to antiplatelet medications.[52–54] The device is available for research only and is not yet commercially available.

Viscoelastic Point-of-Care Coagulation Tests

Conventional laboratory tests have limited value in the perioperative management of patients with coagulopathic bleeding (e.g., CPB-induced coagulopathy, trauma-associated coagulopathy). The prothrombin time (PT, also known as the

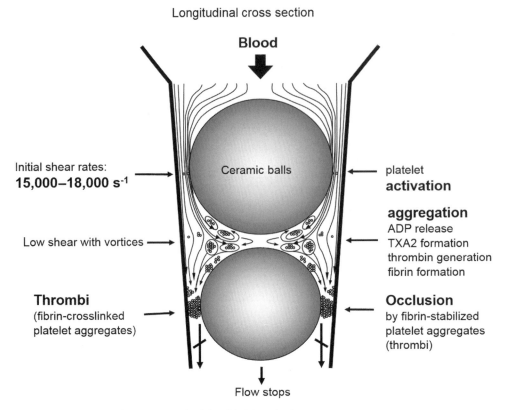

Longitudinal cross section

Blood

Initial shear rates:
15,000–18,000 s⁻¹

Ceramic balls

platelet
activation

aggregation
ADP release
TXA2 formation
thrombin generation
fibrin formation

Low shear with vortices

Thrombi
(fibrin-crosslinked
platelet aggregates)

Occlusion
by fibrin-stabilized
platelet aggregates
(thrombi)

Flow stops

Figure 13.1 Schematic showing principle of the global thrombosis test.

international normalized ratio or INR) and the activated partial thromboplastin time (aPTT) were designed to manage warfarin and heparin anticoagulation, respectively, as well as to evaluate patients with hemophilia and other bleeding disorders. As these tests are performed on plasma and only represent the time to initiation of clot formation, they do not provide data on the platelet–fibrinogen interaction in clot formation and stabilization. Furthermore, these tests are performed in a central laboratory and have a long turnover time (up to 60 minutes), and therefore are not suitable for prediction or management of perioperative hemorrhage.[55,56] Given these limitations, the use of viscoelastic POC coagulation assays to predict excessive bleeding and guide hemostatic therapies in suspected coagulopathic patients has significantly increased over the last two decades and has been incorporated into numerous patient blood management guidelines.[57–61] Several viscoelastic coagulation devices are available for clinical use.

Thromboelastography® (TEG®, Haemonetics, Braintree, MA, USA) and Thromboelastometry (ROTEM®, TEM International GmbH, Munich, Germany)

Both TEG® and ROTEM® are viscoelastic POC whole blood coagulation analyzers that provide global information on the dynamics of clot formation, stabilization, and breakdown, as well as accurately reflect in vivo hemostasis (see Figure 13.2). Results are obtained in less than 30 minutes, making these devices optimal for the perioperative setting. In their early utilization, both systems used a semiautomatic pipette to place citrated whole blood and different activators in a plastic cup. The modern devices are predicated on a similar hemostasis testing principle but utilize a cartridge-based system into which the blood is placed; thus, the test can be run without using a pipette. In TEG® the cup rotates around a pin and a torsion wire translates the resistance to movement into an electrical signal. In ROTEM® the pin rotates while the cup is

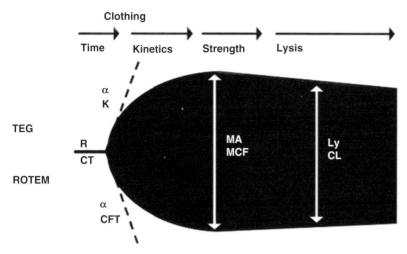

Figure 13.2 Schematic TEG (upper part)/ ROTEM (lower part) trace indicating the commonly reported variables reaction time (R)/ clotting time (CT), clot formation time (CFT), alpha angle (α), maximum amplitude (MA)/ maximal clot firmness (MCF) and lysis (Ly)/clot lysis (CL). Johansson PI, et al. Thromboelastography and thromboelastometry in assessing coagulopathy in trauma. *Scand J Trauma Resusc Emerg Med.* 2009;17:45.

stationary, and the movement of the pin is detected and displayed graphically. As clot develops, the blood becomes more gelatinous and the motion of the cup/ pin is impeded; this is translated graphically as a curve depicting clot kinetics (on the *x* axis), strength (on the *y* axis), and dissolution (combined *x* and *y* axis). The two devices have different names for the tests performed, but both measure the integrity of the intrinsic and extrinsic coagulation pathways, platelet function, fibrinogen function, and fibrinolysis.

After re-calcification, coagulation is initiated by tissue factor to evaluate the extrinsic coagulation pathway, or by a contact activator to evaluate the intrinsic coagulation pathway. Once thrombin is formed, platelets are activated and interact with fibrinogen, causing linkage and development of a dense network of fibrin polymerization. To measure coagulation parameters in anti-coagulated, heparinized patients, lyophilized heparinase can be added to the sample. For evaluation of fibrinogen contribution to clot firmness, a platelet inhibitor may be added to the sample to solely elicit the fibrinogen component of the platelet–fibrinogen interaction. Finally, evaluation of fibrinolysis reveals a very distinctive and easily recognizable pattern. The commercially available TEG® and ROTEM® assays and the normal reference ranges for their analyzed variables are summarized in Tables 13.2 and 13.3, respectively. The latest models TEG® 6s and ROTEM® Sigma have been incorporated into clinical practice. Both devices allow multiple assays using a single cartridge. As these devices are slightly different from the older models, studies are needed to demonstrate the validity of the results obtained by the newer models.

The use of POC-based transfusion algorithms using TEG® or ROTEM® have resulted in significant reduction of allogeneic blood product transfusion in high-risk clinical settings such as cardiovascular surgery,[62–65] trauma,[66–69] and obstetric-related bleeding.[70,71] A large prospective study of more than 7,000 cardiac surgery patients from 17 Canadian centers analyzed transfusion rates and postoperative bleeding endpoints, before and after implementation of the transfusion algorithm using ROTEM® and a platelet POC analyzer (PlateletWorks®). The use of a POC-based transfusion algorithm resulted in a significant decrease in red blood cell (RBC) and platelet transfusions.[72] Furthermore, a prospective study using an algorithm based on ROTEM® and POC platelet analysis (Multiplate® aggregometry) demonstrated reduced RBC and plasma transfusion, compared to a conventional laboratory test-based algorithm. Six-month mortality also was significantly lower in the POC-based group. Many studies that incorporate viscoelastic-based transfusion algorithms and demonstrate reduced transfusion therapy emphasize that *early* use of pro-hemostatic factor concentrates, including fibrinogen concentrates and prothrombin complex concentrates, is key to the intervention.[73–76] The early use of coagulation factor concentrates in bleeding cardiac surgery patients, however, has been questioned,[77,78] and whether this practice improves patient outcomes beyond the reported reduction in transfusion of allogeneic blood products is still debated.[79,80]

In conclusion, POC coagulation analysis using TEG® and ROTEM® transfusion algorithms to guide blood product management has increased

Table 13.2 Commercially available assays for TEG and ROTEM and their clinical indication.

Assay	Activator/Additive	Purpose of Activator/Additive	Clinical relevance
TEG			
	Calcium	Reversal of citrate anticoagulation	Used for samples collected in citrate
KTEG	Kaolin	Intrinsic pathway activation	Evaluation of the intrinsic coagulation pathway
RapidTEG	Tissue Factor + Kaolin	Extrinsic pathway activation	Evaluation of the extrinsic coagulation pathway
HTEG	Heparinase + Kaolin	Neutralize heparin	Diagnose incomplete heparin reversal
Functional Fibrinogen	abciximab	Platelet inhibition	Evaluation of fibrinogen contribution to clot firmness
Platelet Mapping	Activator F (reptilase + factor XIII) + ADP	Platelet activation with and without the contribution of thrombin	Assessment of platelet function
ROTEM			
	Calcium	Reversal of citrate anticoagulation	Used for samples collected in citrate
INTEM	Ellagic acid + Phospholipid	Intrinsic pathway activation	Evaluation of the intrinsic coagulation pathway
EXTEM	Tissue Factor + Phospholipid	Extrinsic pathway activation	Evaluation of the intrinsic coagulation pathway
HEPTEM	Heparinase + Ellagic acid + Phospholipid		Diagnose incomplete heparin reversal
FIBTEM	Cytochalasin D	Platelet inhibition	Evaluation of fibrinogen contribution to clot firmness
APTEM	Aprotinin	Inhibition of fibrinolysis	Diagnosis of hyperfibrinolysis
ROTEM platelet	ADP, Arachidonic acid, TRAP	Platelet activation	Assessment of platelet function

ADP – adenosine diphosphate; TRAP – thrombin receptor activating peptide.

significantly over the last two decades. These coagulation tests are performed on whole blood and more accurately reflect in vivo hemostasis compared to conventional coagulation tests. Furthermore, the results obtained by TEG° and ROTEM° are available much more quickly than conventional laboratory studies. Recent studies with TEG° and ROTEM° have demonstrated early detection and a high positive predictive value for coagulopathic bleeding as well.[81–83]

Sonoclot (Sieno Inc. Arvada, CO, USA)

The mechanism of measurement of the Sonoclot POC device involves the insertion of a plastic probe that is vibrating at an ultrasonic frequency into a sample of whole blood in a glass cuvette. The vibration of the probe is altered as the blood in the sample clots and becomes more gelatinous. Results are provided both graphically (Sonoclot signature) and numerically. The ACT represents the time from activation of the reaction to the beginning of fibrin formation. The kinetics of clot formation and platelet function can also be assessed. Recent studies have demonstrated that Sonoclot parameters are predictive for post-CPB bleeding in adults[5] and children[84] undergoing cardiac surgery.

Another novel use for the Sonoclot analyzer has been reported in heparin-induced thrombocytopenia (HIT) antibody detection. When HIT monoclonal antibody was added to the Sonoclot sample, the anticoagulant activity of heparin was reduced

Table 13.3 Nomenclature of analyzed clot variables and normal reference values in TEG and ROTEM.

	TEG	ROTEM
Clotting time (period to 2 mm amplitude)	R (reaction time) WB: 4–8 min Kaolin: 3–8 min	CT (clotting time) INTEM: 122–208 sec EXTEM: 43–80 sec
Clot kinetics (period from 2 mm-20 mm amplitude)	K (kinetics) WB: 1–4 min Kaolin: 1-3 min	CFT (clot formation time) INTEM: 45–110 sec EXTEM 48–127 sec
Clot strengthening (α angle)	α (slope between R and K) WB: 47°–74° Kaolin: 55°–78°	α (slope of tangent at 2 mm amplitude) INTEM: 70°–12° EXTEM: 65°–80°
Amplitude (at set time points after CT)	A10, A30	A5, A10, A20
Maximal clot strength	MA (maximal amplitude) WB: 55–73 mm Kaolin: 51–69 mm	MCF (maximal clot firmness) INTEM: 51–72 mm EXTEM: 52–70 mm FIBTEM: 9–24 mm
Clot lysis (at set time points)	CL (clot lysis) 30, 60	LY 30, 60
Maximal clot lysis	-	ML (maximal lysis)

WB: whole blood; Kaolin: kaolin-activated re-calcified blood; A5 – amplitude at 5 min; A10 – amplitude at 10 min; A20 – amplitude at 20 min; A30 – amplitude at 30 min.

in a dose-dependent manner, much like in the in vivo disease.[85] Though intriguing, this test has not yet been tested in HIT patients and is not in clinical use.

Quantra Hemostasis Analyzer (HemoSonics LLC, Charlottesville, VA, USA)

The Quantra Hemostasis Analyzer is a novel viscoelastic POC analyzer that uses Sonic Estimation of Elasticity via Resonance (SEER) Sonorheometry, an ultrasound-based technology that uses high-frequency ultrasound pulses to quantify the stiffness of a blood sample during the process of coagulation ex vivo.[86] Several components of hemostasis can be analyzed, including clot time, heparinase clot time, clot stiffness, and platelet and fibrinogen contribution to clot stiffness.[87] Recent studies have shown good correlation between results obtained by the Quantra Hemostasis Analyzer and ROTEM* in cardiac and high-risk spine surgery patients;[88,89] however, discrepancies have been reported when comparing the Quantra Hemostasis Analyzer to TEG*.[90] The clinical experience with this device is very limited; it has been recently approved in the European Union for clinical use but its approval in the United States by the Food and Drug Administration is pending.

Point-of-Care Platelet Function Tests

Platelets play crucial roles in hemostasis and pathological thromboembolic conditions.[91,92] Dual anti-platelet therapy (DAPT) with aspirin and a $P2Y_{12}$ receptor inhibitor has become the main anti-thrombotic treatment in patients with cardiovascular pathological conditions. DAPT is used to treat acute coronary syndrome (ACS), myocardial infarction, stroke, and peripheral arterial disease, and it is prescribed after percutaneous coronary interventions (PCI), coronary artery bypass surgery, and other interventional vascular procedures.

Variability in response to antiplatelet medications makes it essential that the response to antiplatelet drug therapy should be monitored. Drug resistance, manifest as normal platelet reactivity (HPR) despite administration of anti-platelet medication, has been associated with thrombosis and increased incidence of major adverse cardiac events (MACE) after PCI[93,94] and raised the importance of platelet function testing. Additionally, decreased platelet activity exists after CPB and severe trauma and is one of the most important contributing factors to perioperative non-surgical micro-vascular bleeding,[95–98] emphasizing the importance of platelet function testing in surgical patients with excessive bleeding. Platelets are not only crucial for primary hemostasis, but they also augment thrombin generation and promote fibrin polymerization via GPIIb/IIIa receptors. Therefore, decreased platelet function may also result in decreased fibrin polymerization and reduced thrombin generation, further exacerbating coagulopathy and bleeding.[99,100]

In patients treated with antiplatelet therapy, preoperative assessment of platelet function has been shown to predict bleeding complications in cardiac surgery.[101–103] Thus, platelet function testing may be used to individualize and optimize timing of surgery in ACS patients treated with DAPT. The use of platelet function analyses, in combination with viscoelastic coagulation tests as part of goal-directed transfusion management, contributes to decreased perioperative bleeding and reduced transfusion requirements after cardiac surgery[9,65,74,104–106] and trauma.[66,69,107,108]

Light transmission aggregometry (LTA) using platelet-rich plasma is the gold standard for platelet function testing, against which many POC monitors are compared. This in vitro technique is technically cumbersome, time-consuming, and performed under non-physiological conditions,[109] thus it is not widely utilized in the perioperative setting. Several whole blood POC methods for platelet function testing are commercially available (see Table 13.4). Each device has different features, including sample processing, type and potency of platelet agonists, and platform for detecting platelet activity.

VerifyNow System (Accriva Diagnostics, San Diego, CA, USA)

VerifyNow (formerly Ultegra, Accumetrics) is a fully automated whole blood optical-based analyzer that uses agglutination and light transmission to measure $P2Y_{12}$ platelet reactivity units (PRUs). Citrated blood is mixed with fibrinogen-coated polystyrene beads and activated by arachidonic acid (aspirin cartridge), ADP and prostaglandin E_1 ($P2Y_{12}$ cartridge), or thrombin receptor activating peptide (GPIIb/IIIa cartridge). Agglutination between activated platelets and the fibrinogen-coated beads causes the beads to fall out of suspension, thereby resulting in an increase in light transmission through the sample. This increase in light transmittance is converted to a value (i.e., PRU) that is related to the ability of the platelets to be activated or to agglutinate. As the degree of platelet inhibition increases, agglutination decreases, as do PRUs. The normal PRU range is 180–376, and a therapeutic response to $P2Y_{12}$ inhibition is defined as PRU less than 180. HPR in clopidogrel-treated patients is defined as PRU greater than 208.[110] It is important to note that low hematocrit values spuriously increase PRU readings,[111] probably because of a confounding influence on light transmittance. In a retrospective cohort of CABG patients, clopidogrel-treated patients with low agglutination and low PRU were more likely to bleed postoperatively and require transfusion of pro-hemostatic factors.[112] However, in a small group of low-risk CABG patients, neither the VerifyNow nor any other platelet POC test correlated well with blood loss, as assessed by postoperative chest tube output or reduction in hematocrit value.[113] Further research is needed to establish the role of this platelet function assay in predicting peri-procedural bleeding.

Innovance® Platelet Function Analyzer (PFA-100/200, Siemens Healthineers)

The PFA-100 original device was a cartridge-based assay that mimics the bleeding time in an ex vivo test. A small volume of blood is aspirated through an aperture in a membrane coated with platelet agonists until the aperture is completely occluded by a platelet plug. The time to complete occlusion is reported as "closure time." A result greater than 175 seconds is considered abnormal. The newer device, Innovance* PFA-200, has added a P2Y assay to the preexisting cartridges of the earlier model. The Innovance* P2Y cartridge was developed in view of the relative insensitivity of previous cartridges to $P2Y_{12}$ receptor antagonists. This global test of platelet function is easy to use, rapid, requires a small volume of blood (0.8 mL per cartridge), and does not require substantial training. Yet as this is a global platelet adhesion assay, the closure time may be influenced by platelet count, von Willebrand factor levels, and hematocrit. Results need to be carefully interpreted in patients with a platelet count less than 50,000/μL and anemic patients with hematocrit below 25%.[114] It has been reported that patients with blood type O have longer closure times compared to non-O blood groups.[115] A normal closure time may be useful in ruling out a significant platelet defect (high negative predictive value); however, the positive predictive value of closure

Table 13.4 POC platelet function monitoring devices.

Device	Principle	Available Assays	Advantages	Limitations
PFA-100/ 200	Mimics bleeding time Measures time clot time related to high-shear platelet adhesion and aggregation	Col/ADP (CADP) Col/EPI (CEPI) Innovance P2Y assay	Whole blood test Quick Requires small sampling volume	Dependent on platelet count, hematocrit level and von Willebrand factor levels Weak predictive value for periprocedural bleeding[116]
Multiplate	Measures changes in impedance caused by platelet aggregation after exposure to agonists	ADP Arachidonic acid Thrombin receptor activating protein (TRAP)	Whole blood test Run multi channels simultaneously Widely used Good predictive value for bleeding in cardiac surgery	Dependent on platelet count and hematocrit values
VerifyNow	Agglutination between activated platelets and fibrin-coated beads Light transmission through sample is measured	PRU (P2Y$_{12}$ receptor inhibition) aspirin test GPIIb/IIIa test	Whole blood test Simple to use Three antiplatelet medication assays exist	Dependent on hematocrit values Low predictive value in postoperative bleeding
TEG Platelet mapping	Use of kaolin-activated thromboelastography to estimate platelet function	Platelet activation by arachidonic acid (TEG PM$_{AA}$) Platelet activation by ADP (TEG PM$_{ADP}$)	Whole blood test Good correlation with optically monitored platelet aggregation[129] Can be combined with viscoelastic clot assessment	Incomplete inhibition of thrombin-mediated platelet activation may result in underestimation of ADP or AA inhibition Results may be affected by fibrinogen and hematocrit levels
ROTEM Platelet	Impedance aggregometry	ADP-TEM ARA-TEM TRAP-TEM	Whole blood test Can be combined with viscoelastic clot assessment	Significantly different results when compared with multiplatelet aggregometry[132] Limited publications regarding clinical use

AA – arachidonic acid; ADP adenosine diphosphate; GPIIb/IIIa – glycoprotein IIb/IIIa; PRU – P2Y$_{12}$ reaction units; TEG – thromboelastography.

time and peri-procedural bleeding endpoints has been relatively weak.[116,117]

Multiple Electrode Aggregometry (The Multiplate® System, Roche Diagnostics, Rotkreuz, Switzerland)

This assay is based on whole blood impedance aggregometry. It is widely used in DAPT-treated patients to assess platelet function before surgical interventions. Whole blood is collected in a hirudin-containing tube. Each sample is inserted into a test well containing two independent sensor units (electrode wires) and mixed with normal saline and a platelet agonist. Electrical impedance changes are monitored and recorded over six minutes, while activated platelets adhere to the electrodes.[118] Significant agreement with light transmittance aggregometry (LTA) results has been reported.[119] ADP is used as an agonist for detection of P2Y$_{12}$ receptor inhibition (by clopidogrel or other thienopyridines), and thrombin receptor-activating peptide (TRAP) is used for assessment of GPIIb/IIIa inhibition.[120] Results are reported as area under the aggregation curve, and for each reagent there is a different normal range. For example, the normal ADP response is 57–113 aggregation units, and values less than 57 aggregation units represent impaired platelet function.

Several studies have attempted to identify a cutoff level of ADP-initiated platelet aggregation in order to predict major bleeding complications in DAPT-treated patients who require surgical interventions. It has been suggested that for ADP-initiated aggregation a cutoff of greater than 22 aggregation units represents an acceptable bleeding risk in clopidogrel-treated cardiac surgery patients[103] and ticagrelor-treated cardiac surgery patients.[101] It is important to consider that several factors such as age, presence of diabetes,[121] hematocrit level, platelet count, and the delay between blood sample collection and platelet function testing are all known to influence whole blood platelet aggregometry values.[122–124] Despite this fact, whole blood aggregometry has served as an important guide for platelet transfusions in many goal-directed transfusion algorithms.[74,125]

PlateletWorks® (Helena Laboratories, Beaumont, TX, USA)

This device uses the principle of the platelet count ratio to assess platelet reactivity. The platelet count is measured in a standard EDTA tube and tubes into which a platelet agonist (e.g., ADP) has been added. In patients with normal platelet function, the presence of an agonist significantly reduces the platelet count, due to their aggregation into clumps, thus rendering them "unmeasured as platelets." In contrast, the platelet count in the control sample, without an agonist, remains unchanged. In patients with platelet dysfunction, platelets will be refractory to the agonist and will not aggregate, thus reducing the difference between the activated platelet count and the control condition. The ratio of the activated platelet count to the non-activated (control) platelet count is inversely related to platelet reactivity and reflective of platelet function. Although a study that examined the correlation between preoperative platelet dysfunction (as assessed by PlateletWorks®) and postoperative bleeding risk[126] showed no relationship, this analyzer is still valued for its use at the POC during cardiac surgery, and many have successfully incorporated PlateletWorks® into their POC-based transfusion algorithms.[72,105,127] Further research with this device is needed to validate its predictive power for hemmorrhage, determine if it can be used to define a safe level of platelet activity to proceed with interventions despite being on therapy, and determine its cost-effectiveness in transfusion algorithms.

Platelet Testing Using TEG and ROTEM

Both TEG˚ and ROTEM˚ have platforms for POC platelet function analysis. The TEG platelet mapping platform uses thromboelastography to assess platelet function and monitor platelet inhibition by aspirin or P2Y$_{12}$ inhibitors. The standard kaolin TEG is used as a reference for thrombin-mediated platelet activation, which is considered maximal activation. In the platelet mapping assay, heparinized whole blood is mixed with Activator F (reptilase and activated FXIII), which induces fibrin polymerization independent of platelet activation. In another sample, ADP is added, which causes platelet activation if platelets are responsive to ADP. ADP-stimulated maximum amplitude (MA$_{ADP}$) and fibrin-specific MA (MA$_{Fib}$) are used to calculate platelet inhibition in reference to thrombin-mediated MA (MA$_{Thrombin}$) using the following formula:

$$\% \ Platelet \ inhibition = 100 - [(MA_{ADP} - MA_{Fib}) \div (MA_{Thrombin} - MA_{Fib}) \times 100]$$

Alternatively, the area under the curve of ADP-stimulated TEG tracing at 15 minutes (AUC$_{15}$) can be used for quicker results (short TEG). HPR under clopidogrel treatment is defined as less than 30% reduction in the AUC$_{15}$ in the ADP-activated TEG compared to the kaolin TEG.[128]

Comparison of results obtained by TEG˚ platelet mapping with optically monitored platelet aggregation demonstrated good correlation,[129] although incomplete thrombin inhibition by heparin may lead to thrombin-mediated platelet activation and hence underestimation of the degree of platelet inhibition.[130]

ROTEM˚ has a platelet function analyzer that is based on impedance aggregometry. In the ROTEM˚ Delta analyzer two channels are available for whole blood platelet analysis, in addition to the standard four channels that are used for viscoelastic clot analysis. The results are presented by three different parameters: (1) the amplitude at 6 minutes in Ohm (A6), (2) maximum slope (MS) of the aggregation graph in Ohm/min, and (3) area under the curve (AUC) in Ohm x min. Using three types of reagents the effect of different platelet inhibitors can be evaluated: ADP-TEM for detection of P2Y$_{12}$ inhibitors, ARA-TEM (arachidonic acid-TEM) for detection of aspirin and other cyclooxygenase inhibitors, and TRAP-TEM (thrombin receptor agonist peptide-TEM) for measuring platelet inhibition mediated by GPIIb/IIIa antagonists. There are very limited data regarding incorporation of this analyzer into perioperative POC-based transfusion algorithms for patients with excessive bleeding.[67,131]

Conclusion

The perioperative management of patients receiving anticoagulant medication or developing intraoperative coagulopathy relies heavily on the ability to rapidly and accurately detect hemostasis abnormalities and guide therapy. Point-of-care devices aimed at coagulation testing have progressed, and there are several commercially available devices that allow for detection of a wide variety of specific defects. With increased utilization of these tests and the implementation of goal-directed blood management protocols, blood product administration will be precise and rational, and total product administration should decrease.

References

1. Hattersley PG. Activated coagulation time of whole blood. *JAMA* 1966;**196**:436–40.

2. Garvin S, FitzGerald DC, Despotis G, Shekar P, Body SC. Heparin concentration-based anticoagulation for cardiac surgery fails to reliably predict heparin bolus dose requirements. *Anesth Analg* 2010;**111**:849–55.

3. Gravlee GP, Arora S, Lavender SW, et al. Predictive value of blood clotting tests in cardiac surgical patients. *Ann Thorac Surg* 1994;**58**:216–21.

4. Hett DA, Walker D, Pilkington SN, Smith DC. Sonoclot analysis. *Br J Anaesth* 1995;**75**:771–6.

5. Bischof DB, Ganter MT, Shore-Lesserson L, et al. Viscoelastic blood coagulation measurement with Sonoclot predicts postoperative bleeding in cardiac surgery after heparin reversal. *J Cardiothorac Vasc Anesth* 2015;**29**:715–22.

6. Dzemali O, Ganter MT, Zientara A, et al. Evaluation of a new Sonoclot device for heparin management in cardiac surgery. *Clin Appl Thromb Hemost* 2017;**23**:20–6.

7. Luddington RJ. Thromboelastography/thromboelastometry. *Clin Lab Haematol* 2005;**27**:81–90.

8. Ak K, Isbir CS, Tetik S, et al. Thromboelastography-based transfusion algorithm reduces blood product use after elective CABG: a prospective randomized study. *J Card Surg* 2009;**24**:404–10.

9. Shore-Lesserson L, Manspeizer HE, DePerio M, Francis S, Vela-Cantos F, Ergin MA. Thromboelastography-guided transfusion algorithm reduces transfusions in complex cardiac surgery. *Anesth Analg* 1999;**88**:312–9.

10. Shore-Lesserson L, Baker RA, Ferraris VA, et al. The Society of Thoracic Surgeons, The Society of Cardiovascular Anesthesiologists, and The American Society of ExtraCorporeal Technology: Clinical Practice Guidelines-Anticoagulation During Cardiopulmonary Bypass. *Ann Thorac Surg* 2018;**105**:650–62.

11. Di Nisio M, Middeldorp S, Buller HR. Direct thrombin inhibitors. *N Engl J Med* 2005;**353**:1028–40.

12. Stangier J, Rathgen K, Stahle H, Gansser D, Roth W. The pharmacokinetics, pharmacodynamics and tolerability of dabigatran etexilate, a new oral direct thrombin inhibitor, in healthy male subjects. *Br J Clin Pharmacol* 2007;**64**:292–303.

13. Stangier J, Stahle H, Rathgen K, Fuhr R. Pharmacokinetics and pharmacodynamics of the direct oral thrombin inhibitor dabigatran in healthy elderly subjects. *Clin Pharmacokinet* 2008;**47**:47–59.

14. Nielsen VG, Steenwyk BL, Gurley WQ, Pereira SJ, Lell WA, Kirklin JK. Argatroban, bivalirudin, and lepirudin do not decrease clot propagation and strength as effectively as heparin-activated antithrombin in vitro. *J Heart Lung Transplant* 2006;**25**:653–63.

15. Samama MM, Guinet C. Laboratory assessment of new anticoagulants. *Clin Chem Lab Med* 2011;**49**:761–72.

16. Nowak G. The ecarin clotting time, a universal method to quantify direct thrombin inhibitors. *Pathophysiol Haemost Thromb* 2003;**33**:173–83.

17. Siegmund R, Boer K, Poeschel K, Wolf G, Deufel T, Kiehntopf M. Comparison of the ecarin chromogenic assay and different aPTT assays for the measurement of argatroban concentrations in plasma from healthy individuals and from coagulation factor deficient patients. *Thromb Res* 2008;**123**:159–65.

18. Vaishnava P, Eagle KA. Coronary stents and risk for noncardiac surgery: much ado about something, nothing, or DAPT? *J Am Coll Cardiol* 2016;**67**:1050–2.

19. van Ryn J, Stangier J, Haertter S, et al. Dabigatran etexilate–a novel, reversible, oral direct thrombin inhibitor: interpretation of coagulation assays and reversal of anticoagulant activity. *Thromb Haemost* 2010;**103**:1116–27.

20. Lange U, Nowak G, Bucha E. Ecarin chromogenic assay–a new method for quantitative determination of direct thrombin inhibitors like hirudin. *Pathophysiol Haemost Thromb* 2003;**33**:184–91.

21. Avecilla ST, Ferrell C, Chandler WL, Reyes M. Plasma-diluted thrombin time to measure dabigatran concentrations during dabigatran etexilate therapy. *Am J Clin Pathol* 2012;**137**:572–4.

22. Love JE, Ferrell C, Chandler WL. Monitoring direct thrombin inhibitors with a plasma diluted thrombin time. *Thromb Haemost* 2007;**98**:234–42.

23. Ufer M. Comparative efficacy and safety of the novel oral anticoagulants dabigatran, rivaroxaban and apixaban in preclinical and clinical development. *Thromb Haemost* 2010;**103**:572–85.

24. Ruff CT, Giugliano RP, Braunwald E, et al. Comparison of the efficacy and safety of new oral anticoagulants with warfarin in patients with atrial fibrillation: a meta-analysis of randomised trials. *Lancet* 2014;**383**:955–62.

25. Levy JH, Spyropoulos AC, Samama CM, Douketis J. Direct oral anticoagulants: new drugs and new concepts. *JACC Cardiovasc Interv* 2014;**7**:1333–51.

26. Favaloro EJ, Lippi G. Laboratory testing in the era of direct or non-vitamin K antagonist oral anticoagulants: a practical guide to measuring their activity and avoiding diagnostic errors. *Semin Thromb Hemost* 2015;**41**:208–27.

27. Douxfils J, Mullier F, Robert S, et al. Impact of dabigatran on a large panel of routine or specific coagulation assays. Laboratory recommendations for monitoring of dabigatran etexilate. *Thromb Haemost* 2012;**107**:985–97.

28. Douxfils J, Tamigniau A, Chatelain B, et al. Measurement of non-VKA oral anticoagulants versus classic ones: the appropriate use of hemostasis assays. *Thromb J* 2014;**12**:24.

29. Eller T, Busse J, Dittrich M, et al. Dabigatran, rivaroxaban, apixaban, argatroban and fondaparinux and their effects on coagulation POC and platelet function tests. *Clin Chem Lab Med* 2014;**52**:835–44.

30. Dias JD, Norem K, Doorneweerd DD, et al. Use of thromboelastography (TEG) for detection of new oral anticoagulants. *Arch Pathol Lab Med* 2015;**139**:665–73.

31. Solbeck S, Meyer MA, Johansson PI, et al. Monitoring of dabigatran anticoagulation and its reversal in vitro by thromboelastography. *Int J Cardiol* 2014;**176**: 794–9.

32. Solbeck S, Ostrowski SR, Stensballe J, Johansson PI. Thromboelastography detects dabigatran at therapeutic concentrations in vitro to the same extent as gold-standard tests. *Int J Cardiol* 2016;**208**:14–8.

33. Cotton BA, McCarthy JJ, Holcomb JB. Acutely injured patients on dabigatran. *N Engl J Med* 2011;**365**:2039–40.

34. Davis PK, Musunuru H, Walsh M, et al. The ex vivo reversibility of dabigatran-induced whole-blood coagulopathy as monitored by thromboelastography: mechanistic implications for clinical medicine. *Thromb Haemost* 2012;**108**:586–8.

35. Herrmann R, Thom J, Wood A, et al. Thrombin generation using the calibrated automated thrombinoscope to assess reversibility of dabigatran and rivaroxaban. *Thromb Haemost* 2014;**111**:989–95.

36. Stein P, Bosshart M, Brand B, et al. Dabigatran anticoagulation and Stanford type A aortic dissection: lethal coincidence: case report with literature review. *Acta Anaesthesiol Scand* 2014;**58**:630–7.

37. Iapichino GE, Bianchi P, Ranucci M, Baryshnikova E. Point-of-care coagulation tests monitoring of direct oral anticoagulants and their reversal therapy: state of the art. *Semin Thromb Hemost* 2017;**43**:423–32.

38. Escolar G, Arellano-Rodrigo E, Lopez-Vilchez I, et al. Reversal of rivaroxaban-induced alterations on hemostasis by different coagulation factor concentrates – in vitro studies with steady and circulating human blood. *Circ J* 2015;**79**:331–8.

39. Korber MK, Langer E, Ziemer S, et al. Measurement and reversal of prophylactic and therapeutic peak levels of rivaroxaban: an in vitro study. *Clin Appl Thromb Hemost* 2014;**20**:735–40.

40. Perzborn E, Heitmeier S, Laux V, Buchmuller A. Reversal of rivaroxaban-induced anticoagulation with prothrombin complex concentrate, activated prothrombin complex concentrate and recombinant activated factor VII in vitro. *Thromb Res* 2014;**133**:671–81.

41. Saraf S, Christopoulos C, Salha IB, Stott DJ, Gorog DA. Impaired endogenous thrombolysis in acute coronary syndrome patients predicts cardiovascular death and nonfatal myocardial infarction. *J Am Coll Cardiol* 2010;**55**:2107–15.

42. Saraf S, Wellsted D, Sharma S, Gorog DA. Shear-induced global thrombosis test of native blood: pivotal role of ADP allows monitoring of P2Y12 antagonist therapy. *Thromb Res* 2009;**124**:447–51.

43. Yamamoto J, Inoue N, Otsui K, Ishii H, Gorog DA. Global Thrombosis Test (GTT) can detect major determinants of haemostasis including platelet reactivity, endogenous fibrinolytic and thrombin generating potential. *Thromb Res* 2014;**133**:919–26.

44. Yamamoto J, Yamashita T, Ikarugi H, et al. Gorog thrombosis test: a global in-vitro test of platelet function and thrombolysis. *Blood Coagul Fibrinolysis* 2003;**14**:31–9.

45. Sharma S, Farrington K, Kozarski R, et al. Impaired thrombolysis: a novel cardiovascular risk factor in end-stage renal disease. *Eur Heart J* 2013;**34**:354–63.

46. Otsui K, Gorog DA, Yamamoto J, et al. Global thrombosis test – a possible monitoring system for the effects and safety of dabigatran. *Thromb J* 2015;**13**:39.

47. Rosser G, Tricoci P, Morrow D, et al. PAR-1 antagonist vorapaxar favorably improves global thrombotic status in patients with coronary disease. *J Thromb Thrombolysis* 2014;**38**:423–9.

48. Kenet G, Lubetsky A, Shenkman B, et al. Cone and platelet analyser (CPA): a new test for the prediction of bleeding among thrombocytopenic patients. *Br J Haematol* 1998;**101**:255–9.

49. Gerrah R, Snir E, Brill A, Varon D. Platelet function changes as monitored by cone and plate(let) analyzer

during beating heart surgery. *Heart Surg Forum* 2004;7:E191–5.

50. Spectre G, Brill A, Gural A, et al. A new point-of-care method for monitoring anti-platelet therapy: application of the cone and plate(let) analyzer. *Platelets* 2005;**16**:293–9.

51. Varon D, Lashevski I, Brenner B, et al. Cone and plate (let) analyzer: monitoring glycoprotein IIb/IIIa antagonists and von Willebrand disease replacement therapy by testing platelet deposition under flow conditions. *Am Heart J* 1998;**135**:S187–93.

52. Gerrah R, Brill A, Tshori S, et al. Using cone and plate (let) analyzer to predict bleeding in cardiac surgery. *Asian Cardiovasc Thorac Ann* 2006;**14**:310–5.

53. Shenkman B, Schneiderman J, Tamarin I, et al. Testing the effect of GPIIb-IIIa antagonist in patients undergoing carotid stenting: correlation between standard aggregometry, flow cytometry and the cone and plate(let) analyzer (CPA) methods. *Thromb Res* 2001;**102**:311–7.

54. Shenkman B, Matetzky S, Fefer P, et al. Variable responsiveness to clopidogrel and aspirin among patients with acute coronary syndrome as assessed by platelet function tests. *Thromb Res* 2008;**122**:336–45.

55. Toulon P, Ozier Y, Ankri A, et al. Point-of-care versus central laboratory coagulation testing during haemorrhagic surgery. A multicenter study. *Thromb Haemost* 2009;**101**:394–401.

56. Haas T, Fries D, Tanaka KA, et al. Usefulness of standard plasma coagulation tests in the management of perioperative coagulopathic bleeding: is there any evidence? *Br J Anaesth* 2015;**114**:217–24.

57. Society of Thoracic Surgeons Blood Conservation Guideline Task F, Ferraris VA, Brown JR, et al. 2011 update to the Society of Thoracic Surgeons and the Society of Cardiovascular Anesthesiologists blood conservation clinical practice guidelines. *Ann Thorac Surg* 2011;**91**:944–82.

58. Task Force on Patient Blood Management for Adult Cardiac Surgery of the European Association for Cardio-Thoracic S, the European Association of Cardiothoracic Anaesthesiology (EACTA), Boer C, Meesters MI, et al. 2017 EACTS/EACTA Guidelines on patient blood management for adult cardiac surgery. *J Cardiothorac Vasc Anesth* 2018;32(1):88–120.

59. Carson JL, Guyatt G, Heddle NM, et al. Clinical practice guidelines from the AABB: red blood cell transfusion thresholds and storage. *JAMA* 2016;**316**:2025–35.

60. Rossaint R, Bouillon B, Cerny V, et al. The European guideline on management of major bleeding and coagulopathy following trauma: fourth edition. *Crit Care* 2016;**20**:100.

61. Shaylor R, Weiniger CF, Austin N, et al. National and international guidelines for patient blood management in obstetrics: a qualitative review. *Anesth Analg* 2017;**124**:216–32.

62. Shore-Lesserson L, Manspeizer HE, DePerio M, et al. Thromboelastography-guided transfusion algorithm reduces transfusions in complex cardiac surgery. *Anesth Analg* 1999;**88**:312–9.

63. Rahe-Meyer N, Solomon C, Winterhalter M, et al. Thromboelastometry-guided administration of fibrinogen concentrate for the treatment of excessive intraoperative bleeding in thoracoabdominal aortic aneurysm surgery. *J Thorac Cardiovasc Surg* 2009;**138**:694–702.

64. Ranucci M, Baryshnikova E, Ranucci M, Silvetti S, Surgical and Clinical Outcome Research (SCORE) Group. Fibrinogen levels compensation of thrombocytopenia-induced bleeding following cardiac surgery. *Int J Cardiol* 2017;**249**:96–100.

65. Weber CF, Gorlinger K, Meininger D, et al. Point-of-care testing: a prospective, randomized clinical trial of efficacy in coagulopathic cardiac surgery patients. *Anesthesiology* 2012;**117**:531–47.

66. Spahn DR. TEG(R)- or ROTEM(R)-based individualized goal-directed coagulation algorithms: don't wait–act now! *Crit Care* 2014;**18**:637.

67. Stein P, Kaserer A, Spahn GH, Spahn DR. Point-of-care coagulation monitoring in trauma patients. *Semin Thromb Hemost* 2017;**43**:367–74.

68. Schochl H, Nienaber U, Maegele M, et al. Transfusion in trauma: thromboelastometry-guided coagulation factor concentrate-based therapy versus standard fresh frozen plasma-based therapy. *Crit Care* 2011;**15**:R83.

69. Gonzalez E, Moore EE, Moore HB, et al. Goal-directed hemostatic resuscitation of trauma-induced coagulopathy: a pragmatic randomized clinical trial comparing a viscoelastic assay to conventional coagulation assays. *Ann Surg* 2016;**263**:1051–9.

70. Snegovskikh D, Souza D, Walton Z, et al. Point-of-care viscoelastic testing improves the outcome of pregnancies complicated by severe postpartum hemorrhage. *J Clin Anesth* 2018;**44**:50–6.

71. Butwick AJ, Goodnough LT. Transfusion and coagulation management in major obstetric hemorrhage. *Curr Opin Anaesthesiol* 2015;**28**:275–84.

72. Karkouti K, Callum J, Wijeysundera DN, et al. Point-of-care hemostatic testing in cardiac surgery: a stepped-wedge clustered randomized controlled trial. *Circulation* 2016;**134**:1152–62.

73. Ranucci M, Baryshnikova E, Crapelli GB, et al. Randomized, double-blinded, placebo-controlled trial of fibrinogen concentrate supplementation after

complex cardiac surgery. *J Am Heart Assoc* 2015;**4**: e002066.

74. Gorlinger K, Dirkmann D, Hanke AA, et al. First-line therapy with coagulation factor concentrates combined with point-of-care coagulation testing is associated with decreased allogeneic blood transfusion in cardiovascular surgery: a retrospective, single-center cohort study. *Anesthesiology* 2011;**115**:1179–91.

75. Tanaka KA, Esper S, Bolliger D. Perioperative factor concentrate therapy. *Br J Anaesth* 2013;**111** Suppl 1: i35-49.

76. Da Luz LT, Nascimento B, Shankarakutty AK, Rizoli S, Adhikari NK. Effect of thromboelastography (TEG(R)) and rotational thromboelastometry (ROTEM(R)) on diagnosis of coagulopathy, transfusion guidance and mortality in trauma: descriptive systematic review. *Crit Care* 2014;**18**:518.

77. Rahe-Meyer N, Levy JH, Mazer CD, et al. Randomized evaluation of fibrinogen vs placebo in complex cardiovascular surgery (REPLACE): a double-blind phase III study of haemostatic therapy. *Br J Anaesth* 2016;**117**:41–51.

78. Bilecen S, de Groot JA, Kalkman CJ, et al. Effect of fibrinogen concentrate on intraoperative blood loss among patients with intraoperative bleeding during high-risk cardiac surgery: a randomized clinical trial. *JAMA* 2017;**317**:738–47.

79. Afshari A, Wikkelso A, Brok J, Moller AM, Wetterslev J. Thromboelastography (TEG) or thromboelastometry (ROTEM) to monitor haemotherapy versus usual care in patients with massive transfusion. *Cochrane Database Syst Rev* 2011:CD007871.

80. Deppe AC, Weber C, Zimmermann J, et al. Point-of-care thromboelastography/thromboelastometry-based coagulation management in cardiac surgery: a meta-analysis of 8332 patients. *J Surg Res* 2016;**203**:424–33.

81. Laursen TH, Meyer MAS, Meyer ASP, et al. Thromboelastography early amplitudes in bleeding and coagulopathic trauma patients: results from a multicenter study. *J Trauma Acute Care Surg* 2018;**84**:334–41.

82. Dirkmann D, Gorlinger K, Dusse F, Kottenberg E, Peters J. Early thromboelastometric variables reliably predict maximum clot firmness in patients undergoing cardiac surgery: a step towards earlier decision making. *Acta Anaesthesiol Scand* 2013;**57**:594–603.

83. Song JG, Jeong SM, Jun IG, Lee HM, Hwang GS. Five-minute parameter of thromboelastometry is sufficient to detect thrombocytopenia and hypofibrinogenaemia in patients undergoing liver transplantation. *Br J Anaesth* 2014;**112**:290–7.

84. Rajkumar V, Kumar B, Dutta V, Mishra AK, Puri GD. Utility of Sonoclot in prediction of postoperative

bleeding in pediatric patients undergoing cardiac surgery for congenital cyanotic heart disease: a prospective observational study. *J Cardiothorac Vasc Anesth* 2017;**31**:901–8.

85. Wanaka K, Asada R, Miyashita K, et al. Novel HIT antibody detection method using sonoclot(R) coagulation analyzer. *Thromb Res* 2015;**135**:127–9.

86. Corey FS, Walker WF. Sonic estimation of elasticity via resonance: a new method of assessing hemostasis. *Ann Biomed Eng* 2016;**44**:1405–24.

87. Ferrante EA, Blasier KR, Givens TB, et al. A novel device for the evaluation of hemostatic function in critical care settings. *Anesth Analg* 2016;**123**:1372–9.

88. Huffmyer JL, Fernandez LG, Haghighian C, Terkawi AS, Groves DS. Comparison of SEER sonorheometry with rotational thromboelastometry and laboratory parameters in cardiac surgery. *Anesth Analg* 2016;**123**:1390–9.

89. Naik BI, Durieux ME, Knisely A, et al. SEER sonorheometry versus rotational thromboelastometry in large volume blood loss spine surgery. *Anesth Analg* 2016;**123**:1380–9.

90. Reynolds PS, Middleton P, McCarthy H, Spiess BD. A comparison of a new ultrasound-based whole blood viscoelastic test (SEER Sonorheometry) versus thromboelastography in cardiac surgery. *Anesth Analg* 2016;**123**:1400–7.

91. Bhatt DL. Role of antiplatelet therapy across the spectrum of patients with coronary artery disease. *Am J Cardiol* 2009;**103**:11A–9A.

92. Jennings LK. Role of platelets in atherothrombosis. *Am J Cardiol* 2009;**103**:4A–10A.

93. Breet NJ, van Werkum JW, Bouman HJ, et al. High on-aspirin platelet reactivity as measured with aggregation-based, cyclooxygenase-1 inhibition sensitive platelet function tests is associated with the occurrence of atherothrombotic events. *J Thromb Haemost* 2010;**8**:2140–8.

94. Breet NJ, van Werkum JW, Bouman HJ, Ten Berg JM, Hackeng CM. Platelet function tests for the monitoring of P2Y12 inhibitors. *Expert Opin Med Diagn* 2010;**4**:251–65.

95. Orlov D, McCluskey SA, Selby R, et al. Platelet dysfunction as measured by a point-of-care monitor is an independent predictor of high blood loss in cardiac surgery. *Anesth Analg* 2014;**118**:257–63.

96. Zaffar N, Joseph A, Mazer CD, et al. The rationale for platelet transfusion during cardiopulmonary bypass: an observational study. *Can J Anaesth* 2013;**60**:345–54.

97. Wohlauer MV, Moore EE, Thomas S, et al. Early platelet dysfunction: an unrecognized role in the acute coagulopathy of trauma. *J Am Coll Surg* 2012;**214**:739–46.

98. Nekludov M, Bellander BM, Blomback M, Wallen HN. Platelet dysfunction in patients with severe traumatic brain injury. *J Neurotrauma* 2007;**24**:1699–706.

99. Bolliger D, Tanaka KA. Point-of-care coagulation testing in cardiac surgery. *Semin Thromb Hemost* 2017;**43**:386–96.

100. Tanaka KA, Bolliger D, Guzzetta NA. Clinical and practical aspects of restoring thrombin generation in acute coagulopathic bleeding. *Anesth Analg* 2017;**124**:701.

101. Malm CJ, Hansson EC, Akesson J, et al. Preoperative platelet function predicts perioperative bleeding complications in ticagrelor-treated cardiac surgery patients: a prospective observational study. *Br J Anaesth* 2016;**117**:309–15.

102. Mahla E, Prueller F, Farzi S, et al. Does platelet reactivity predict bleeding in patients needing urgent coronary artery bypass grafting during dual antiplatelet therapy? *Ann Thorac Surg* 2016;**102**:2010–7.

103. Ranucci M, Colella D, Baryshnikova E, Di Dedda U, Surgical, Clinical Outcome Research Group. Effect of preoperative P2Y12 and thrombin platelet receptor inhibition on bleeding after cardiac surgery. *Br J Anaesth* 2014;**113**:970–6.

104. Kane LC, Woodward CS, Husain SA, Frei-Jones MJ. Thromboelastography–does it impact blood component transfusion in pediatric heart surgery? *J Surg Res* 2016;**200**:21–7.

105. Karkouti K, McCluskey SA, Callum J, et al. Evaluation of a novel transfusion algorithm employing point-of-care coagulation assays in cardiac surgery: a retrospective cohort study with interrupted time-series analysis. *Anesthesiology* 2015;**122**:560–70.

106. Ranucci M, Baryshnikova E, Pistuddi V, et al. The effectiveness of 10 years of interventions to control postoperative bleeding in adult cardiac surgery. *Interact Cardiovasc Thorac Surg* 2017;**24**:196–202.

107. Schochl H, Nienaber U, Hofer G, et al. Goal-directed coagulation management of major trauma patients using thromboelastometry (ROTEM)-guided administration of fibrinogen concentrate and prothrombin complex concentrate. *Crit Care* 2010;**14**:R55.

108. Theusinger OM, Stein P, Levy JH. Point of care and factor concentrate-based coagulation algorithms. *Transfus Med Hemother* 2015;**42**:115–21.

109. Born GV, Cross MJ. Effect of adenosine diphosphate on the concentration of platelets in circulating blood. *Nature* 1963;**197**:974–6.

110. Nishi T, Ariyoshi N, Nakayama T, et al. Increased platelet inhibition after switching from maintenance clopidogrel to prasugrel in Japanese patients with stable coronary artery disease. *Circ J* 2015;**79**:2439–44.

111. Kakouros N, Kickler TS, Laws KM, Rade JJ. Hematocrit alters VerifyNow P2Y12 assay results independently of intrinsic platelet reactivity and clopidogrel responsiveness. *J Thromb Haemost* 2013;**11**:1814–22.

112. Rosengart TK, Romeiser JL, White LJ, et al. Platelet activity measured by a rapid turnaround assay identifies coronary artery bypass grafting patients at increased risk for bleeding and transfusion complications after clopidogrel administration. *J Thorac Cardiovasc Surg* 2013;**146**:1259–66, 66 e1; discussion 66.

113. Berger PB, Kirchner HL, Wagner ES, et al. Does preoperative platelet function predict bleeding in patients undergoing off pump coronary artery bypass surgery? *J Interv Cardiol* 2015;**28**:223–32.

114. Carcao MD, Blanchette VS, Stephens D, et al. Assessment of thrombocytopenic disorders using the platelet function analyzer (PFA-100). *Br J Haematol* 2002;**117**:961–4.

115. Cho YU, Jang S, Park CJ, Chi HS. Variables that affect platelet function analyzer-100 (PFA-100) closure times and establishment of reference intervals in Korean adults. *Ann Clin Lab Sci* 2008;**38**:247–53.

116. Fattorutto M, Pradier O, Schmartz D, Ickx B, Barvais L. Does the platelet function analyser (PFA-100) predict blood loss after cardiopulmonary bypass? *Br J Anaesth* 2003;**90**:692–3.

117. Ng KF, Lawmin JC, Tsang SF, Tang WM, Chiu KY. Value of a single preoperative PFA-100 measurement in assessing the risk of bleeding in patients taking cyclooxygenase inhibitors and undergoing total knee replacement. *Br J Anaesth* 2009;**102**:779–84.

118. Bolliger D, Seeberger MD, Tanaka KA, et al. Pre-analytical effects of pneumatic tube transport on impedance platelet aggregometry. *Platelets* 2009;**20**:458–65.

119. Paniccia R, Antonucci E, Maggini N, et al. Assessment of platelet function on whole blood by multiple electrode aggregometry in high-risk patients with coronary artery disease receiving antiplatelet therapy. *Am J Clin Pathol* 2009;**131**:834–42.

120. Mazzeffi MA, Lee K, Taylor B, Tanaka KA. Perioperative management and monitoring of antiplatelet agents: a focused review on aspirin and P2Y12 inhibitors. *Korean J Anesthesiol* 2017;**70**:379–89.

121. Bolliger D, Filipovic M, Matt P, et al. Reduced aspirin responsiveness as assessed by impedance aggregometry is not associated with adverse outcome

after cardiac surgery in a small low-risk cohort. *Platelets* 2016;**27**:254–61.

122. Kaiser AF, Neubauer H, Franken CC, et al. Which is the best anticoagulant for whole blood aggregometry platelet function testing? Comparison of six anticoagulants and diverse storage conditions. *Platelets* 2012;**23**:359–67.

123. Rubak P, Villadsen K, Hvas AM. Reference intervals for platelet aggregation assessed by multiple electrode platelet aggregometry. *Thromb Res* 2012;**130**:420–3.

124. Stissing T, Dridi NP, Ostrowski SR, Bochsen L, Johansson PI. The influence of low platelet count on whole blood aggregometry assessed by multiplate. *Clin Appl Thromb Hemost* 2011;**17**:E211–7.

125. Rahe-Meyer N, Winterhalter M, Boden A, et al. Platelet concentrates transfusion in cardiac surgery and platelet function assessment by multiple electrode aggregometry. *Acta Anaesthesiol Scand* 2009;**53**:168–75.

126. Carroll RC, Chavez JJ, Snider CC, Meyer DS, Muenchen RA. Correlation of perioperative platelet function and coagulation tests with bleeding after cardiopulmonary bypass surgery. *J Lab Clin Med* 2006;**147**:197–204.

127. Dalen M, van der Linden J, Lindvall G, Ivert T. Correlation between point-of-care platelet function testing and bleeding after coronary artery surgery. *Scand Cardiovasc J* 2012;**46**:32–8.

128. Sambu N, Hobson A, Curzen N. "Short" thromboelastography as a test of platelet reactivity in response to antiplatelet therapy: validation and reproducibility. *Platelets* 2011;**22**:210–6.

129. Craft RM, Chavez JJ, Snider CC, Muenchen RA, Carroll RC. Comparison of modified thrombelastograph and plateletworks whole blood assays to optical platelet aggregation for monitoring reversal of clopidogrel inhibition in elective surgery patients. *J Lab Clin Med* 2005;**145**:309–15.

130. Tantry US, Bliden KP, Gurbel PA. Overestimation of platelet aspirin resistance detection by thrombelastograph platelet mapping and validation by conventional aggregometry using arachidonic acid stimulation. *J Am Coll Cardiol* 2005;**46**:1705–9.

131. Fabbro M, 2nd, Winkler AM, Levy JH. Technology: is there sufficient evidence to change practice in point-of-care management of coagulopathy? *J Cardiothorac Vasc Anesth* 2017;**31**:1849–56.

132. Ranucci M, Baryshnikova E, Crapelli GB, et al. Electric impedance platelet aggregometry in cardiac surgery patients: a comparative study of two technologies. *Platelets* 2016;**27**:185–90.

Assessment of Intraoperative Blood Loss

Kyle James Riley and Daniel Katz

Overview

Accurate intraoperative estimation of blood loss is important to guide fluid administration, assess the need to transfuse packed red blood cells and other blood products, and anticipate the severity of post-operative anemia. Avoidance of transfusion is a general goal as blood products are expensive, there is a limited and sometimes inadequate supply, and blood transfusion is associated with increased risk for a variety of postoperative complications.[1–6] Despite the need to accurately quantify surgical blood loss for these purposes, surprisingly there is no gold standard. A variety of methods exist, each with its own advantages and disadvantages.

Monitoring Standard and Practice Guidelines

American Society of Anesthesiologists Standards and Guidelines

The American Society of Anesthesiologists (ASA) Standards for Basic Anesthetic Monitoring sets the most basic standards of anesthetic monitoring. These standards set the requirement for continual ("repeated regularly and frequently in steady rapid succession") monitoring of oxygenation, ventilation, circulation, and temperature.[7] ASA practice guidelines for perioperative blood management have been developed to assist in decisions regarding perioperative blood transfusions and adjuvant therapies.[8] They include recommendations to optimize conditions to reduce potential blood loss, and advocate the use of transfusion algorithms, specialized testing, and restrictive strategies. With regard to determining the extent of blood loss, however, the guidelines simply state the following:[8]

- The literature is inadequate to evaluate the efficacy of measuring blood loss through observation of

surgical sponges, clot size and shape, and suction canister volumes or visual assessment of the blood in the surgical field

- The use of more accurate volumetric and gravimetric measurement techniques may reduce the risk of underestimating blood loss

In the survey of consultant expert and ASA member opinions, both groups strongly agreed that there is a need to:[8]

- Assess the presence of bleeding by a periodic visual assessment of the surgical field
- Perform quantitative measurement of blood loss, including evaluation of surgical sponges and surgical drains, using standard methods

AABB Guidelines

The AABB, formerly known as the "American Association of Blood Banks," is an international, not-for-profit association of individuals and institutions involved in the fields of cellular therapies and transfusion medicine.[9,10] The AABB clinical guidelines for red blood cell (RBC) transfusion thresholds, based on a review of randomized clinical trials, made recommendations for appropriate use of a restrictive transfusion strategy, but provided no recommendations on how to estimate blood loss and only weakly recommended using hemoglobin concentration (Hb) to guide transfusion decision-making.[11–14]

Blood Loss Assessment Methods

Visual Assessment (Subjective Measurement)

In the latest ASA Practice Guidelines survey,[8] 91.6% of the consultant group and 92.7% of the ASA membership responded as agreeing or strongly agreeing with the need to "periodically perform a visual assessment of the surgical field with the surgeon to assess the presence of excessive microvascular (i.e., coagulopathy) or surgical bleeding." Because of its convenience and efficiency, or because other methods may not be available or practical, a visual assessment of blood loss by the anesthesiologist and/or surgeon is commonly used and often referred to as "subjective assessment."[15,16] The literature, however, is replete with studies that demonstrate the inaccuracies of visual blood loss assessment.[1,17–20] There is a tendency to overestimate blood loss volume when blood loss is low and underestimate blood loss volume when blood loss is high,[19] and the degree of inaccuracy of blood loss estimation increases as blood loss itself increases.[20]

It was demonstrated that a brief didactic training course can significantly improve the visual blood loss assessment.[19,21] The improvement after training, however, was transient, as there was a significant decay in estimation accuracy by 9 months after training was completed. The median error in blood loss estimation was −47.8% pre-training, improved to −13.5% immediately following training, but worsened to −34.6% at the 9-month follow-up.[21]

Assay Method

The assay method, also called "photometric analysis," is a set of reliable techniques for measuring blood loss.[16] It is often used in studies as the reference standard against which other blood loss determination methods are compared. The basic procedure is as follows, with all Hb values always expressed in g/dL:[1]

Determine the patient's preoperative Hb (Hb_{preop}). For surgical sponges:

1. Collect all soiled sponges
2. Rinse each sponge with saline solution and compress to remove and collect all rinse liquid; repeat 3–4 times
3. Use a plasma/low Hb photometer or plasma spectrometer to determine rinse Hb (Hb_{Rinse})
4. Determine mass of product rinse liquid (M_{Rinse}) in grams
5. Volume of rinse liquid is:
   $V_{Rinse} = M_{Rinse}/100\ g/dL$, where 100 g/dL is density used for liquids
6. $M_{SpongeHb} = Hb_{Rinse} \times V_{Rinse}$, where $M_{SpongeHb}$ is the mass of Hb loss in grams
7. $V_{SpongeBloodLoss} = M_{SpongeHb}/Hb_{Preop}$, where $V_{SpongeBloodLoss}$ is the volume of sponge blood loss in dL

For blood collected in suction canisters:

1. Gently remix effluent
2. Use a plasma/low Hb analyzer or plasma spectrometer to determine the canister Hb ($Hb_{Canister}$)
3. Determine mass of suction canister liquid ($M_{Canister}$ in grams)
4. Volume of canister liquid is:
   $V_{Canister} = M_{Canister}/(100\ g/dL)$
5. $M_{CanisterHb} = Hb_{Canister} \times V_{Canister}$
6. $V_{CanisterBloodLoss} = M_{CanisterHb}/Hb_{Preop}$

The total volume of blood loss is:

$$V_{Total} = V_{SpongeBloodLoss} + V_{CanisterBloodLoss}$$

Studies may also determine a baseline assay yield rate by applying banked blood of a known quantity to sponges and determining an expected recovery rate for the specific extraction and analysis procedure being used.[1,22] These yield rates (YR) range from 89.5% using manual compression, to 98.99% using a centrifuge to extract the rinse liquid.

Applying a YR, the equation for total volume of blood loss becomes:

$$V_{Total} = (V_{SpongeBloodLoss}/YR) + V_{CanisterBloodLoss}$$

where YR is in decimal % (e.g., 0.895 used for 89.5%).

Gravimetric Blood Loss Determination

Because of issues with visual estimation, the use of the gravimetric method, also called the "quantitative method," is recommended to determine blood loss by national organizations, including the Association of Women's Health, Obstetric and Neonatal Nurses (AWHONN), the California Maternal Quality Care Collaborative (CMQCC), and the Council on Patient Safety in Women's Healthcare.[1]

In a study analyzing the accuracy of different blood loss determination methods during cesarean delivery procedures, Doctorvaladan and colleagues[1] used the following gravimetric procedure and formulas to determine blood loss.

Prior to procedure:

1. Record weights of empty suction canisters
2. Record weights of 3 packs of 5 sponges each and determine average sponge weight (M_{Dry})

During procedure:

1. At uterine incision, record the canister volume using graduated markings ($V_{Canister1}$)
2. After all amniotic fluid is aspirated, record the second measurement of canister volume ($V_{Canister2}$)
3. $V_{Amniotic} = V_{Canister2} - V_{Canister1}$
4. Record total amount of irrigation fluid used ($V_{Irrigation}$)

Post-procedure:

1. Record the weight of each sponge (M_{Wet})
2. Record the weight of each canister effluent ($M_{CanisterEffluent}$)
3. Quantitative blood loss (QBL) is calculated using the following formulas (fluid density is 1.0 g/mL):

$$V_{SpongeQBL} = (M_{Wet} - M_{Dry})/(1.0 \ g/mL)$$

$$V_{CanisterQBL} = M_{CanisterEffluent}/(1.0 \ g/mL)$$

$$V_{TotalQBL} = \Sigma V_{SpongeQBL} + \Sigma V_{CanisterQBL} - V_{Amniotic} - V_{Irrigation}$$

$V_{TotalQBL}$ is the total quantitative blood loss calculated as the sum of all the quantitative blood loss of each sponge, plus the sum of the quantitative blood loss of each canister, minus the volume of amniotic fluid and minus the volume of irrigation fluid used.

Limitations of the gravimetric method include the following:[1,16,22,23]

- It is time-consuming and impractical for real-time intraoperative use
- The presence of non-sanguineous fluids and other substances, including amniotic fluid, ascites, saline, and other tissues, decrease its accuracy
- The assumption that the patient's blood hemoglobin concentration stays constant is incorrect if administered intravenous (IV) fluids which progressively dilute the patient's blood[23]

New technology has been introduced that may help reduce the effort and time associated with the gravimetric blood loss method. The Triton L&D (Gauss Surgical Inc., Los Altos, CA) is a blood loss monitor for labor and delivery that uses a tablet-based application containing a customizable list of blood absorbent items with pre-determined dry weights. A scale, connected to the tablet using Bluetooth, is used to weigh individual or batches of blood-soiled items.

The application then uses the stored dry weights and soiled weights to calculate and track blood loss.[24,25]

Blood Loss Formulas, Hemoglobin Monitoring, and Hematocrit Monitoring

Blood Loss Formula

Studies dating back to 1974[26–29] developed mathematical formulas that use changes in hematocrit (Hct) to calculate an estimated blood loss or an allowable blood loss limit during surgical procedures to determine transfusion triggers. The theoretical dilution equation that models the problem of isovolemic hemodilution is the differential equation:[27]

$$dHct/Hct = dV_{BloodLoss}/V$$

where Hct = hematocrit, dHct is the change in Hct, $dV_{BloodLoss}$ = blood loss (change in blood volume), and V = patient's total blood volume.

Integration over the limits from initial to final yields:

$$V_{BloodLoss} = V \times [ln(Hct_{Initial}) - ln(Hct_{Final})]$$

or

$$V_{BloodLoss} = V \times [ln(Hct_{Initial}/Hct_{Final})]$$

with ln(X) being the natural log of X.

Bourke and Smith[27] replaced the natural log function by an approximation using a Taylor series with the higher-ordered terms dropped:

$$V_{BloodLoss} = V \times (Hct_{Initial} - Hct_{Final}) \times (3 - Hct_{Avg})$$

where $Hct_{Avg} = (Hct_{Initial} + Hct_{Final})/2$

Gross[29] proposed the following simpler equation that more closely approximates the plot of the logarithmic formula:

$$V_{BloodLoss} = V \times ((H_{Initial} - H_{Final})/H_{Avg})$$

where H can be either the Hct or Hb. Hct-based blood loss equations have also been used to evaluate treatments to reduce bleeding. One such study performed by Barrachina and colleagues assessed total blood loss 48 hours after hip replacement surgery with different regimens of tranexamic acid (TXA).[2] This study used the formula proposed by Camarasa et al.[30] to calculate blood loss volumes across the different TXA treatments.

In a comparison of hematocrit-based blood loss equations, Lopez-Picado et al.[31] determined whether applying different blood loss formulas to the data from Barrachina's study[2] would have affected the findings. They compared the four most frequently used formulas of Bourke and Smith,[27] Gross,[29] Mercuriali et al.[32] and Camarasa,[30] as well as their own equation that combined Camarasa's blood loss formula with the International Council for Standardization in Haematology's (ICSH) total blood volume calculation (see Appendix 1 for a further description of the equations). In evaluating the five blood loss equations, Lopez-Picado et al.[31] found that:

- Use of the formulas based on anthropometric and laboratory parameters to calculate patient blood loss would not have affected the clinical conclusions of the Barrachina et al. study
- Use of Gross's equation would negate the significance of some of the Barrachina et al. study findings, probably because it does not take transfusions into account
- There were no significant differences in the total patient blood volumes calculated using the three total blood volume formulas
- There was a very low level of agreement of their chosen reference method and the other formulas

The authors concluded that, in some cases, the differences in the blood loss amounts calculated by the different formulas could affect clinical decisions.

Hemoglobin and Hematocrit Monitoring

Hb and Hct are diagnostic parameters that can be obtained from an automated hematology analyzer in a satellite clinical laboratory or from a point-of-care (POC) device.[33,34] The determination of Hb in a clinical laboratory using an automated analyzer is considered the gold standard for Hb/Hct measurement, the major drawback being the delay in obtaining test results.[35] These machines lyse the RBCs and then use spectrophotometry (CO-oximetry) to determine the concentration of Hb. The wavelengths of light used are not always stated by the manufacturers, but 525 nm is utilized by at least one of them. Once the Hb concentration is determined, the Hct may be

calculated as the number of RBCs per the mean cell volume, or simply as the product of the Hb × 2.941.

Maslow and colleagues[34] compared three POC testing devices to the hospital reference analyzer for cardiac surgery patients. The devices were the GEM 4000 (Instrumentation Laboratory, Bedford, MA), the i-STAT (Abbot Point of Care, Princeton, NJ), and the Radical-7 Pulse CO-Oximeter (Masimo, Irvine, CA).

Device Overview

- The GEM 4000 uses CO-oximetry measurement the absorption of multi-wavelengths of light by the different Hb structures. The Hct value is calculated as the Hb concentration × 3. Cellular reflectors that cause light to scatter may affect the results of CO-oximetry based devices.
- The i-STAT device uses conductivity to measure the Hct based on an electrical current; a higher Hct results in less current passing through the blood. The Hct × 0.34 is used to calculate the Hb concentration. Hemodilution, reduced serum protein levels, and heparinization affect sample conductivity and hence the accuracy of conductivity-calculated Hct.
- The Radical-7 Pulse CO-Oximeter uses a non-invasive percutaneous sensor that measures Hb using multiple wavelengths of light. It provides continuous, real-time monitoring of Hb concentrations. Digital perfusion, sensor position, movement, and external light interference can affect the sensor results.

Device Performance

- The GEM 4000 data correlated with the lab standard ($r = 0.97$), but it had a positive bias (overestimation) that was stable over the phases of surgery and range of Hb/Hct data.
- The i-STAT data correlated with the lab standard ($r = 0.97$) and had the lowest mean bias, but that bias switched from overestimation before cardiopulmonary bypass to underestimation after cardiopulmonary bypass. Also, the bias was positive at higher Hb values and negative at lower Hb values – so higher Hb concentrations were overestimated and lower ones underestimated.
- The Radical-7 Pulse CO-Oximeter data correlated with the lab standard ($r = 0.84$), but not as highly as the other two devices. It consistently overestimated the lab standard, but with a smaller bias prior to surgery that increased during surgery

and peaked after protamine administration. The bias was positive for all Hb values and the positive bias increased as Hb values decreased – so lower Hb concentrations were overestimated to a larger degree than higher Hb concentrations.

Transfusion Decisions

In a small study of 24 consecutive elective adult cardiac surgery patients,[34] if these POC devices had been used in conjunction with a restricted transfusion trigger value of Hb 7 g/dL or Hct 21, then:

- Using the GEM 4000, no patients would have undergone an unnecessary transfusion
- Using the i-STAT, three patients would have undergone an unnecessary transfusion
- Using the Radical-7, no patients would have undergone an unnecessary transfusion

Continuous Real-Time Hemoglobin Monitoring

Two studies looked at the effect on blood transfusions of continuous and noninvasive spectrophotometry hemoglobin (SpHb) monitoring during surgery using the Radical-7 Pulse CO-Oximeter.

Ehrenfeld and colleagues[6] conducted a study in elective orthopedic surgery patients with a moderate overall risk of requiring transfusion, randomized to have continuous intraoperative SpHb monitoring versus standard care without SpHb monitoring; there was no standardized transfusion protocol. In the SpHb group, 0.6% (1 out of 170) of patients received transfusions, while in the standard care group, 4.5% (7 out of 157) of patients received transfusions (risk difference is −0.04; 95% CI: −0.007, −0.004). The groups did not differ with respect to preoperative patient characteristics, outcomes after surgery, or the incidence of postoperative complications at 28 days. The only effect of SpHb monitoring in this study was to reduce the rate of transfusions by 87%, from 4.5% to 0.6%, a 3.9% absolute reduction. But this was a relatively small study in which even the control group transfusion rate was relatively low.

Awada and colleagues[5] evaluated the impact of continuous SpHb monitoring by Radical-7 Pulse CO-Oximeter on blood transfusions in 86 high blood-loss neurosurgery patients in a prospective cohort study. Information recorded included estimated blood loss (EBL), Hb, and SpHb values, units transfused, timing of each blood draw, and the start of each transfusion. The control group did not have

SpHb monitoring and started receiving intermittent blood sampling starting when their EBL reached 15% or more. In both groups, a transfusion was initiated when Hb or SpHb was ≤ 10 g/dL and continued until the EBL was replaced and the Hb was > 10 g/dL. The control and SpHb-monitored groups were similar in surgical procedures and demographics (except that the SpHb group was lower in weight). Preoperatively, the only significant clinical group difference was that the SpHb group had an average baseline Hb about 1 g/dL lower than the control group.

This study found no difference in the percentage of patients transfused; however, in the SpHb group, transfused patients received an average of 1.6 units fewer units ($p < 0.01$), the percent of patients receiving more than 3 RBC units was reduced from 73% to 32% ($p < 0.01$), the post-transfusion Hb values averaged 0.5 g/dL less ($p < 0.01$), and the average delay in time to transfusion was reduced from 50.2 to 9.2 minutes ($p < 0.001$). The study also found that in the SpHb group the Radical-7 Pulse CO-Oximeter values had a very small bias compared to the laboratory Hb values (0.0 ± 0.8 g/dL) and the limits of agreement were −1.6 to 1.5 g/dL.

These studies demonstrated that continuous real-time monitoring of Hb concentrations can affect intraoperative blood transfusion decision-making, reduce decision delay, and decrease the number of patients and total quantity of blood transfused. Everything else being equal, restrictive transfusion strategies require better information about the patient's Hb in addition to blood loss. Continuous monitoring of SpHb concentrations is a promising method that may promote more timely decision-making.

Imaging Analysis

The Triton OR System (Gauss Surgical Inc., Los Altos, CA) uses photo-imaging technology and cloud-based machine-learning (ML) algorithms to determine hemoglobin mass either on sponges or in suction canisters. The images are taken using a tablet computer, encrypted, and transferred to a remote server. For blood-soaked sponges, Gauss Feature Extraction Technology, similar to facial recognition software, processes the photo by identifying relevant areas of the image, makes adjustments for differences in lighting conditions, and filters out the effects of non-sanguineous fluids. Proprietary ML computational models then determine the mass of the Hb from the image and the result is signalled back to the device within seconds.[22–23]

Studies have shown that the Triton OR System data strongly correlate with an R= 0.91 to 0.95 for Hb and estimated blood loss volumes to multiple reference methods.[1,15,22–23,36] It also demonstrated low levels of bias in blood loss estimates by sponge Hb measurement (.01 to 0.7 g Hb per sponge),[22–23] and suction canister content (50 mL).[1] In all of the blood loss determination comparison studies, the Triton OR system performed significantly better than visual and gravimetric estimations of blood loss. It generally had a higher correlation with the studies' reference assay methods, lower biases, and a narrower range of biases.[1,15,22,36]

In a retrospective analysis of cesarean delivery data,[37] clinical outcomes were evaluated for 2,025 patients whose blood loss was visually determined by consensus between obstetrician and anesthesiologist at procedure conclusion (traditional group), and 756 patients whose blood loss was determined by scanning all surgical sponges as the procedure progressed and the surgical canisters, typically at procedure end, using the Triton OR system (device group). All patients were pre-procedurally evaluated for postpartum hemorrhage (PPH) risk as being low, medium or high, and separate analyses of outcome measures were performed for each PPH risk group. Overall, the characteristics of traditional and device groups were similar, with the device group having more multiparous (78.7% versus 67.9%; $p < 0.01$) and slightly older patients (32.2 versus 31.7 years of age, $p < 0.01$). The average measured blood loss, both overall and for the high PPH risk group, was lower in the device group at 555.8 mL and 622.9 mL respectively than in the traditional group at 662.1 mL and 683.2 mL ($p < 0.0001$ for both comparisons). Blood loss greater than 1000 mL was more frequently identified in the device group than the traditional group (14.1% versus 3.5%, $p < 0.0001$). Additionally, the blood loss measurement in the device group demonstrated higher correlation to the PPH risk scores than the traditional group (linear trend difference $p = 0.0024$). The percent of patients receiving transfusions in both groups was not significantly different, but the device group had fewer units transfused (1.83 versus 2.56, $p < 0.038$). The device group patients also had a shorter length of stay (average 4.0 days versus 4.4 days, $p < 0.0006$). The study authors concluded that clinically significant

hemorrhage was identified more frequently by the Triton system than by visual estimation and that, possibly due to earlier recognition and treatment, use of the device reduced blood transfusions.

Conclusion

Table 14.1 summarizes the major advantages and disadvantages of each methodology used to track or quantify blood loss.

While an accurate assessment of Hb/Hct and intraoperative blood loss is critical in optimization of resuscitation and transfusion, their determination in the operating room environment in real time remains challenging. Noninvasive strategies are ideal, but all currently available devices suffer from a variety of practical and statistical problems. A combination of these strategies seems to significantly reduce unnecessary transfusions in select populations, and when used by an educated provider with a support system or decision tree, can affect outcomes.

Appendix I

Source and overview of the five blood loss calculation methods used by Lopez-Picado et al.:[31]

1. Bourke and Smith:[27] this method uses the approximation for natural log with the product of 3 minus the mean hematocrit value. Applied Nadler's formula for total blood volume of the patient.
2. Gross:[29] this method uses the formula simplification that calculates blood loss utilizing the initial hematocrit, final hematocrit, and the mean of these two values. Volumes transfused are not taken into account. Applied Moore's formula for total blood volume of the patient.
3. Mercuriali et al.:[32] this method uses the hematocrit values preoperatively and at 5 days postoperatively and estimates the volume of red cells. Takes into account the total volume of blood transfused. Applied Nadler's formula for total blood volume of the patient.
4. Camarasa et al.:[30] this formula calculates blood loss using the preoperative hematocrit value and the hematocrit at the time of performing the calculation. It takes into consideration transfusions, differentiating between blood from autologous and homologous transfusions, as well as blood recovery systems. Applied a simplified

Table 14.1 Major advantages/disadvantages of different technology to monitor or quantify blood loss.

Methodology	Advantages	Disadvantages
Assay Method	high accuracy	expensive performed only post-procedure involves a laboratory procedure wide adoption is not practical
Visual Estimation	easy perform as needed	low accuracy high variability
Gravimetric	quantitative more practical than assay method	relatively high effort performed only post-procedure
Automated Hematology Analyzer	high accuracy perform as needed	invasive slow turnaround time does not measure losses measures Hb/Hct at one point in time only
Invasive POC Hb/Hct Analyzer (e.g. GEM 4000, i-STAT)	good accuracy perform as needed	invasive accuracy can be situational (bias different at high and low end of spectrum)
Noninvasive Hb analyzer (Radical-7)	good accuracy perform as needed noninvasive real time	accuracy can be situational (bias different at high and low end of spectrum)
Hb/Hct Formulas	moderately easy perform as needed	requires total blood volume estimate no gold standard formula inherits the accuracy and inaccuracy of the required Hb/Hct determination
Imaging Analysis (Triton)	easy near real time highly accurate low bias/variability	small positive bias over the assay method limited to sponges and canisters

version of Moore's formula that uses weight and sex to calculate the total blood volume of the patient.

5. Lopez-Picado et al.:[31] this method uses Camarasa's blood loss calculation but applied the ICSH total blood volume calculation.

All of the formulas include a calculation of the patient's total blood volume based on different variables as follows:[31]

1. Moore: weight (kg), build (values for obese, thin, normal, muscular builds), and sex[29]
2. Nadler: weight (kg), height (cm), and sex
3. ICSH: body surface area and sex

Total Blood Volume and Blood Loss Formulas used in Lopez-Picado et al.[31]

- Estimation of total blood volume of the patient (ETBV)

1. Moore:
   i. Women: $ETBV(ml) = weight \times 65$
   ii. Men: $ETBV(ml) = weight \times 70$

2. Nadler:
   i. Women: $ETBV(ml) = 183 + (0.000356 \times height)^3 + (33 \times weight)$
   ii. Men: $ETBV(ml) = 604 + (0.0003668 \times height)^3 + (32.2 \times weight)$

3. ICSH
   i. Women: $ETBV(ml) = plasma\ volume(ml) + red\ cell\ volume(ml)$
   $= (weight^{0.425} \times height^{0.725}) \times (0.007184 \times 2.217) + (age(years) \times 1.06)$
   ii. Men: $ETBV(ml) = plasma\ volume(ml) + red\ cell\ volume(ml)$
   $= (weight^{0.425} \times height^{0.725}) \times (0.007184 \times 3.064) - 825$

- Estimation of blood loss volume (EBLV)

1. Bourke: $EBLV(ml) = ETBV\ Moore(ml) \times (initial\ hematocrit - final\ hematocrit) \times (3 - mean\ hematocrit)$

2. Gross: $EBLV(ml) = ETBV\ Moore(ml) + (initial\ hematocrit - final\ hematocrit)/ (mean\ hematocrit)$

3. Mercuriali: $EBLV(ml) = ETBV\ Nadler(ml) \times (initial\ hematocrit\ -\ hematocrit\ day5) + transfused\ red\ cell\ volume(ml)$

4. Camarasa:

$EBLV(ml) = ETBV\ Moore \times (initial\ hematocrit\ -\ final\ hematocrit) + transfused\ red\ cell\ volume\ /\ mean\ hematocrit$

1 U packed homologous blood = 170 ml
1 U packed autologous blood = 140 ml

100 ml of recovered blood = 54 ml

5. New formula:

$EBLV(ml) = ETBV\ ICSH \times (initial\ hematocrit\ -\ final\ hematocrit) + transfused\ red\ cell\ volume\ /\ mean\ hematocrit$

1 U packed homologous blood = 450 ml × hematocrit of the blood transfused
1 U packed autologous blood = 450 ml × hematocrit in the pre-surgical anesthesia consult

References

1. Doctorvaladan S, Jelks A, Hsieh E, et al. Accuracy of blood loss measurement during cesarean delivery. *Am J Perinatol Reports* 2017;7:e93–100.

2. Barrachina B, Lopez-Picado A, Remon M, et al. Tranexamic acid compared with placebo for reducing total blood loss in hip replacement surgery. *Anesth Analg* 2016;**122**:986–95.

3. Frank SM, Savage WJ, Rothschild JA, et al. Variability in blood and blood component utilization as assessed by an anesthesia information management system. *Anesthesiology* 2012;**117**:99–106.

4. Guinn NR, Broomer BW, White W, Richardson W, Hill SE. Comparison of visually estimated blood loss with direct hemoglobin measurement in multilevel spine surgery. *Transfusion* 2013;**53**:2790–4.

5. Awada WN, Mohmoued MF, Radwan TM, Hussien GZ, Elkady HW. Continuous and noninvasive hemoglobin monitoring reduces red blood cell transfusion during neurosurgery: a prospective cohort study. *J Clin Monit Comput* 2015;**29**:733–40.

6. Ehrenfeld JM, Henneman JP, Bulka CM, Sandberg WS. Continuous non-invasive hemoglobin monitoring during orthopedic surgery: a randomized trial. *J Blood Disord Transfus* 2014;**5**(237):1–5.

7. Standards for Basic Anesthetic Monitoring – American Society of Anesthesiologists., www.asahq.org/quality-and-practice-management/practice-guidance-resource-documents/standards-for-basic-anesthetic-monitoring accessed: 11/11/2017.

8. Practice Guidelines for Perioperative Blood Management. *Anesthesiology* 2015;**122**:241–75.

9. www.aabb.org/ accessed: 11/12/2017

10. Wiegmann TL, Mintz PD. The growing role of AABB clinical practice guidelines in improving patient care. *Transfusion* 2015;**55**:935–6.

11. Tobian AAR, Heddle NM, Wiegmann TL, Carson JL. Red blood cell transfusion: 2016 clinical practice guidelines from AABB. *Transfusion* 2016;**56**:2627–30.

12. Yazer MH, Triulzi DJ, DI S. AABB red blood cell transfusion guidelines. *JAMA* 2016;**316**:1984–5.

13. Carson JL, Guyatt G, Heddle NM, et al. Clinical practice guidelines from the AABB. *JAMA* 2016;**316**:2025–35.

14. Carson JL, Grossman BJ, Kleinman S, et al. Red blood cell transfusion: a clinical practice guideline from the AABB*. *Ann Intern Med* 2012;**157**:49–58.

15. Sharareh B, Woolwine S, Satish S, Abraham P, Schwarzkopf R. Real time intraoperative monitoring of blood loss with a novel tablet application. *Open Orthop J* 2015;**9**:422–6.

16. Schorn MN. Measurement of blood loss: review of the literature. *J Midwifery Womens Health* 2010;**55**:20–7.

17. Stafford I, Dildy GA, Clark SL, Belfort MA. Visually estimated and calculated blood loss in vaginal and cesarean delivery. *Am J Obstet Gynecol* 2008;**199**:519.e1-7.

18. Bose P, Regan F, Paterson-Brown S. Improving the accuracy of estimated blood loss at obstetric haemorrhage using clinical reconstructions. *BJOG* 2006;**113**:919–24.

19. Dildy GA, Paine AR, George NC, Velasco C. Estimating blood loss: can teaching significantly improve visual estimation? *Obstet Gynecol* 2004;**104**:601–6.

20. Eipe N, Ponniah M. Perioperative blood loss assessment – How accurate? *Indian J Anaesth* 2006;**50**:35–8.

21. Toledo P, Eosakul ST, Goetz K, Wong CA, Grobman WA. Decay in blood loss estimation skills after web-based didactic training. *Simul Healthc* 2012;**7**:18–21.

22. Holmes AA, Konig G, Ting V, et al. Clinical evaluation of a novel system for monitoring surgical hemoglobin loss. *Anesth Analg* 2014;**119**:588–94.

23. Konig G, Holmes AA, Garcia R, et al. In vitro evaluation of a novel system for monitoring surgical hemoglobin loss. *Anesth Analg* 2014;**119**:595–600.

24. Gauss S. Triton L&D – Gauss Surgical, www.gausssurgical.com/tritonld accessed:12/04/2019

25. Gauss S. Gauss Surgical Receives FDA Clearance for Second Generation Triton for Real-Time Monitoring of Surgical Blood Loss – Gauss Surgical., www.gauss surgical.com/news/2017/6/22/gauss-surgical-receives-fda-clearance-for-second-generation-triton-for-real-ti me-monitoring-of-surgical-blood-loss accessed:12/04/2019.

26. Kallos T, Smith TC. Replacement for intraoperative blood loss. *Anesthesiology* 1974;**41**:293–5.

27. Bourke DL, Smith TC. Estimating allowable hemodilution. *Anesthesiology* 1974;**41**:609–11.

28. Ward CF, Meathe EA, Benumof JL, Trousdale F. A computer nomogram for loss replacement. *Anesthesiology* 1980;**53**:S126.

29. Gross JB. Estimating allowable blood loss: corrected for dilution. *Anesthesiology* 1983;**58**:277–80.

30. Camarasa MA, Ollé G, Serra-Prat M, et al. Efficacy of aminocaproic, tranexamic acids in the control of bleeding during total knee replacement: a randomized clinical trial. *Br J Anaesth* 2006;**96**:576–82.

31. Lopez-Picado A, Albinarrate A, Barrachina B. Determination of perioperative blood loss: accuracy or approximation? *Anesth Analg* 2017;**125**:280–6.

32. Mercuriali F, Inghilleri G. Proposal of an algorithm to help the choice of the best transfusion strategy. *Curr Med Res Opin* 1996;**13**:465–78.

33. Vos JJ, Kalmar AF, Struys MM, et al. Accuracy of non-invasive measurement of haemoglobin concentration by pulse co-oximetry during steady-state and dynamic conditions in liver surgery. *Br J Anaesth* 2012;**109**:522–8.

34. Maslow A, Bert A, Singh A, Sweeney J. Point-of-care hemoglobin/hematocrit testing: comparison of methodology and technology. *J Cardiothorac Vasc Anesth* 2016;**30**:352–62.

35. Lamhaut L, Apriotesei R, Combes X, et al. Comparison of the accuracy of noninvasive hemoglobin monitoring by spectrophotometry (SpHb) and HemoCue® with automated laboratory hemoglobin measurement. *Anesthesiology* 2011;**115**:548–54.

36. Konig G, Waters JH, Javidroozi M, et al. Real-time evaluation of an image analysis system for monitoring surgical hemoglobin loss. *J Clin Monit Comput* 2018;**32**:303–10.

37. Rubenstein A, Zamudio S, Al-Khan A, et al. Clinical experience with the implementation of accurate measurement of blood loss during cesarean delivery: influences on hemorrhage recognition and allogeneic transfusion. *Am J Perinatol* 2018;**35**:655–9.

Chapter 15

Respiratory Monitoring in Low-Intensity Settings

Andrew B. Leibowitz and Adel Bassily-Marcus

Introduction

Respiratory failure is a common occurrence in low-intensity hospital settings (i.e., settings other than operating rooms, post-anesthesia care units (PACUs), or intensive care units (ICUs)), and accounts for a large percentage of intra-hospital transfers to ICUs. Traditional monitoring of respiratory function in low-intensity settings is challenging and has limitations. It relies on clinical observations of skin color appearance and counting the respiratory rate, both of which are unreliable, time-consuming, and only performed intermittently.[1] It is difficult to detect cyanosis in dark-skinned individuals and anemic patients. Cyanosis is a very late sign of respiratory insufficiency, usually only developing just prior to a cardiopulmonary arrest when there are limited opportunities for intervening. Additionally, clinical observation cannot determine the depth of respiration or the underlying pathology interfering with effective gas exchange.

Patients with morbid obesity and obstructive sleep apnea (OSA) are especially at risk for respiratory compromise in low-intensity hospital settings. In a meta-analysis of 17 studies involving 7,162 postoperative patients, OSA was associated with an increased risk of respiratory failure (odds ratio 2.42) and cardiac events (odds ratio is 1.63).[2] The prevalence of known OSA in hospitalized patients has increased significantly over the years, yet it remains underdiagnosed despite widespread use of screening tools such as the STOP-BANG Questionnaire, Berlin Questionnaire, and Sleep Apnea Clinical Score. A study of 28,921 nonemergent inpatient surgical patients who were classified as having no OSA, known OSA, or positive screening for OSA (i.e., patients who denied a history of OSA but had a STOP-BANG score greater than 3), found that adverse respiratory events (primarily hypoxemia) were much more common in the two OSA groups.[3] The incidence of postoperative episodes of hypoxemia identified using pulse oximetry oxygen saturation (SpO_2) less than 85% was 27.1% in the no OSA group, 39.5% in the known OSA group, and 39.9% in the positive OSA screening group. Highlighting the risk of undiagnosed OSA, the positive OSA screening group had significantly higher rates of reintubation, ICU admission, prolonged hospitalization, and all-cause 30-day mortality, compared to the other groups.

Another group of patients who are at high risk for respiratory compromise in low-intensity hospital settings are those treated with opioids. An American Society of Anesthesiologists (ASA) Closed Claims database study that reviewed 92 malpractice claims related to postoperative opioid-induced respiratory depression determined that 97% of the events were preventable had there been better monitoring and response.[4] In the PRODIGY (**PR**ediction of **O**pioid-induced respiratory **D**epression **I**n patients monitored by capno**G**raph**Y**) study 1,496 adult patients who were on a general hospital ward and received parenteral opioid therapy for post-surgical and non-surgical pain as the primary analgesic modality were monitored with capnography and pulse oximetry.[5] Impressively, 46% of patients experienced opioid-induced respiratory depression. These data indicate that there is tremendous unmet need for better monitoring of respiratory function in low-intensity settings.

Respiratory function monitors that are commonly used in procedural and ICU settings are designed for use in immobile patients for brief periods of time in areas where the staff-to-patient ratio is high, such as PACUs and ICUs where the ratio is 1:1 or 1:2, or "stepdown" and "intermediate care units" where the ratio usually does not exceed 1:4. While these monitors may be used in low-intensity settings, the required wires and tubes and the potential for motion artifact make their use in low-intensity settings challenging. Patients find the devices uncomfortable to wear, they impede patient mobility, and they are frequently disconnected either intentionally or accidentally. As a result, there is a high frequency of false positive alarms and long periods of time with no monitoring.

Ideally, respiratory monitoring in low-intensity settings would reliably identify patients with respiratory compromise early enough to trigger effective interventions (e.g., naloxone administration, incentive spirometry, pulmonary toilet, continuous positive airway pressure therapy, high flow nasal oxygen) that decrease the need for ICU transfer and tracheal intubation and improve outcomes by reducing mortality. The respiratory function monitoring modalities that are currently utilized in low-intensity hospital settings are continuous pulse oximetry, expired carbon dioxide (CO_2) measurement, photoplethysmography (PPG), bioimpedance-based respiratory minute volume monitoring, and acoustic monitoring, although none are widely used or accepted as a standard of care. This chapter reviews these approaches, their advantages, and their limitations.

Pulse Oximetry

Pulse oximetry (reviewed in Chapter 4) is widely used in emergency rooms, operating rooms, and ICUs to monitor oxygen saturation as an indicator of respiratory function. It is noninvasive, accurate, inexpensive, simple to use, and requires minimal training.

In brief, pulse oximeters use small diodes that emit light in the 660 nm and 940 nm wavelengths aimed through a body part (i.e., fingertip or earlobe). These wavelengths are absorbed in different amounts by oxygenated and deoxygenated blood, and the resultant transmitted light is detected by a sensor on the other side of the body part. An internal processor uses the data to determine the SpO_2. These devices are accurate to within ± 2% of the arterial blood oxygen saturation (SaO_2) determined from an arterial blood sample using a CO-oximeter utilizing spectrophotometry, a much more sophisticated device located in the main laboratory of most hospitals.

Pulse oximeters are commonly used in low-intensity settings, but there are no accepted standards for indications, required staffing ratio of patients assigned to this level of monitoring, alarm settings, or staff alarm notification. New advances have focused on automatic notification systems to pagers, phones, and other devices via a wireless network (e.g., Masimo Patient SafetyNet System), but this approach is not widespread.

Given the availability and low cost of pulse oximetry, it is surprising how little investigation there has been of its use in low-intensity settings. A recent review of four studies comparing pulse oximetry to usual nursing care in surgical patients prescribed opioids in the postoperative period revealed a pooled trend toward decreased ICU transfers of 34% ($p = 0.06$), but the four studies were heterogeneous in both their design and outcomes.[6] A Cochrane review of studies in which 22,992 patients were randomized to usual care versus the addition of pulse oximetry monitoring found that hypoxemia and related events were detected more frequently in the pulse oximetry monitored patients. There was, however, no evidence that use of pulse oximetry significantly affected any outcome variable, including ICU transfers and mortality.[7]

There are multiple limitations that must be taken into consideration when interpreting this literature. There is a need to identify at-risk patients who might benefit from monitoring and as a result have fewer ICU transfers and at least a decrease in interventions ranging from minor (e.g., naloxone administration and non-invasive ventilator support) to major (e.g., tracheal intubation). Alarm settings have not been standardized, and there is no widely accepted lower limit that has an acceptable high positive predictive value and low false alarm rate. Notification systems vary widely in clinical practice and across studies. Differences in method of signaling to hospital staff, such as devices that emit an auditory signal that require staff to be within hearing range versus devices with automatic notification via a pager-type technology, would expectedly yield different results.

One of the greatest limitations of this literature is that many studies have failed to account for supplemental oxygen use. Increasing the FiO_2 to near 0.3 via nasal cannula or face mask oxygen supplementation allows the pCO_2 to rise to 90 mmHg before the SpO_2 would decrease to less than 94%. Further, the PaO_2 may decrease from approximately 600 mmHg (e.g., on high FiO_2 via facemask) to as low as 75 mmHg, a dramatic increase in the alveolar-arterial gradient, before a noticeable decrease in the SpO_2 from 100% to less than 94%. Desaturation noted when the SpO_2 changes from near 100% to less than 94% will then progress rapidly as the steep portion of the oxygen hemoglobin dissociation curve is approached.

Some historical context may help put this into perspective. Pulse oximetry became an operating room standard in 1987, before there was definitive evidence that it impacted outcomes. Even as late as 1991, the lack of evidence was troubling, but as stated in a prescient review, "the 'proof' that a given device is efficacious is often difficult: to define its effectiveness in large populations may be impossible ... it would be foolish to ignore [a monitor's] potential value for lack of 'proof' for such may never be forthcoming."[8] This statement also sums up the current circumstance in low-intensity settings – high-risk patients are experiencing morbidity and mortality, several noninvasive and relatively inexpensive monitors should in theory provide a substantive measure of safety, and it is best to proceed with their deployment for this purpose without the proof.

Expired CO_2 Monitoring

There are three main methods of monitoring expired CO_2. The most commonly employed method uses sensors that measure absorption of infrared light by CO_2. These sensors may be *mainstream,* placed directly into the breathing circuit (e.g., Masimo EMMA™ Mainstream Capnometer, United States), or *sidestream* requiring aspiration of gas through tubing attached to the device containing the sensor (e.g., Philips Respironics LoFLo Side-Stream CO_2 Sensor Module, Netherlands). A second method uses chemical indicators (Medtronic Nellcor™ Easy Cap, United States). These are most commonly used for very short periods of time to confirm tracheal intubation by a change in color of the indicator. The third method by Mass or Raman spectroscopy is an older cumbersome technology that is usually performed in a centralized location, although it is now rarely used.

Capnometry is the measurement of the partial pressure (concentration) of CO_2 in respiratory gases. A capnogram is a graphic display of the partial pressure of expired CO_2 over time, which has a waveform configuration. End-tidal CO_2 ($EtCO_2$) is the CO_2 at the end of an expiratory cycle and is normally 35–45 mmHg. Capnography is an operating room standard to assess the presence and adequacy of ventilation. The detection of expired CO_2 is the "gold standard" to verify tracheal intubation. In many ICUs capnography is routinely used in mechanically ventilated patients and is sometimes used in non-intubated spontaneously breathing patients, most commonly for a period of time immediately after extubation, and on occasion in patients at high risk of respiratory arrest. The expired CO_2 can also be used to assess adequacy of

perfusion, such as during advanced cardiac life support, and could provide insight into the percentage of dead space ventilation and metabolic abnormalities. The absence of expired CO_2 indicates lack of ventilation and/or perfusion; a significant decline in $EtCO_2$ urgently prompts the clinician to reassess ventilation and perfusion.

Trending the $EtCO_2$ and respiratory rate are accurate indicators of respiratory compromise, but their routine use in large groups of patients has not been clearly associated with improved outcomes. In a study of 133 patients monitored with minute-by-minute vital signs, pulse oximetry, and $EtCO_2$, a subset of patients (including those with OSA) benefited from $EtCO_2$ monitoring, but overall, 84% of the alarms triggered by an $EtCO_2$ value less than 20 or greater than 50 mm were false.[9] As discussed in Chapter 18, alarm fatigue is a significant issue and high rates of false alarms inevitably lead to the device's alarms to go unheeded, rendering it useless and possibly even a medical-legal risk.

A review of five studies compared capnography with or without pulse oximetry, to usual nursing care in surgical patients prescribed opioids in the postoperative period.[6] It revealed a trend toward increased recognition of respiratory depression, although none of the studies examined the impact on rescue team activation, ICU transfers, or mortality. This review also commented on capnography's disadvantages, including false alarms and alarm fatigue.

A more recent study of 80 women with a STOP-Bang score greater than 3 who underwent cesarean delivery with intrathecal morphine and were monitored with continuous capnography and pulse oximetry for 24 hours revealed that 53% experienced an apnea event (i.e., no breath for 30–120 seconds).[10] Standard nursing monitoring did not detect a single one of these events, although no clinically relevant events occurred in any patient. Eighty-two percent of the capnography patients reported itchy nose, nausea, interference with nursing, and overall inconvenience. These discomforts and the frequent alerts may limit capnography application after cesarean delivery.

The main limitation of capnography in low-intensity environments is a high false alarm rate. This problem, as noted in every investigation and in clinical practice, is mostly due to patient noncompliance with wearing the device and wiring or tubing. Other common causes of false alarms include mouth breathing rendering nasal cannula sampling useless, clogging of the sampling tubing in sidestream devices, and interference of mainstream sensors by respiratory debris and humidity.

A novel technology related to expired CO_2 monitoring is transcutaneous CO_2 monitoring ($tcCO_2$). This technology may be limited because detection of apnea is not really possible, but $tcCO_2$ will rise with hypoventilation, and in low-intensity settings this detection may be adequate. There is little literature about this method other than confirming its correlation to the arterial blood gas pCO_2.[11]

Photoplethysmography

Photoplethysmography (PPG) is an optical measurement technique used in pulse oximetry that is used to detect blood volume changes in the microvasculature. All pulse oximeters utilize this technology to display the pulsatile signal. As reviewed in Chapter 11, respiration impacts cardiac stroke volume, which in turn affects the blood volume within the microvasculature. Because PPG detects blood volume changes within the microvasculature, it can be used to determine respiratory rate, in combination with the standard pulse oximetry indicators of SpO_2 and heart rate.[12]

As this technology is relatively new, investigation has focused simply on its accuracy and not on its impact. One study compared PPG respiratory rate monitoring using the Medtronic Nellcor™ device to $EtCO_2$ monitoring in 79 healthy subjects and patients in low-intensity settings who had a respiratory rate range of 4–34 breaths per minute.[13] There was excellent correlation and limits of agreement between the two methods, suggesting they could be used interchangeably.

The obvious benefit to PPG respiratory monitoring is that accurate continuous determination of respiratory rate combined with SpO_2 data provides measures of both respiratory rate and efficacy using a noninvasive sensor that is well tolerated. The commercial availability of PPG respiratory rate monitoring is relatively new, and its impact on patient outcomes has not been reported. It seems to have the potential benefits of capnography without the patient acceptance issues, and at very least might allow for automated respiratory rate acquisition in a continuous fashion and eliminate the need for manual counting by staff.

This pulse oximetry functionality may be able to detect respiratory compromise using a quantitative data synthesis of respiratory rate, SpO_2, and heart rate, as well as time-trend analyses of these variables, and an algorithmically calculated risk alert triggering an alarm.

Bioimpedance-Based Respiratory Volume Monitoring

Until recently, the use of bioimpedance for clinical purposes has focused on monitoring cardiac output (e.g., Cheetah NOCOM Bioreactance® Cheetah Medical, MA, USA), and its utility for monitoring respiration was overlooked. Because inspiration and expiration expand and contract the lungs' and chest's volume, impedance to electrical current will change over the respiratory cycle, and this change may be used to detect the rate and depth of respiration. Use of simple bioimpedance measured via EKG leads built into standard bedside monitors (e.g., GE Dash 300, General Electric, United States) to measure only respiratory rate has been a simple feature often taken for granted. Respiratory volume monitoring (RVM) is a new approach that provides an absolute and graphic measurement of respiratory rate, tidal volume, and minute ventilation (Expiron™ 1Xi Respiratory Motion, Inc, United States). Uniquely, the depth of respiration and the respiratory rate may be trended, and alarm settings may reveal very early respiratory compromise (e.g., change of only 20% from baseline), before the patient becomes hypercarbic and long before they may become hypoxemic. Thus, this method has distinct advantages over pulse oximetry, $EtCO_2$, and PPG monitoring.

Bioimpedance-based RVM has been mostly studied in the immediate postoperative period. It is highly dependent on baseline calibration, does not lend itself to use in patients that are fairly mobile, and because it is a very new technology compared to pulse oximetry, $EtCO_2$, and PPG, education and training of staff are critical.

The available data, though limited, are encouraging. Bioimpedance-based RVM was studied in 50 patients who received opioids in a PACU, 18 of whom were classified as high-risk for respiratory depression based on initial minute ventilation measurement being less than 80% of that predicted.[14] The RVM monitoring showed that 13 of the 18 (72%) high-risk patients had a significant decline in the minute ventilation, versus only 1 of the 32 (3%) opioid-receiving patients not at high risk. RVM monitoring also detected apnea, likely of no consequence, in 12 of the 82 patients who received no opioids, a false alarm rate that may be unacceptable. This very exacting protocol that identified at-risk patients as those with a baseline MV less than 80% of the predicted value had a sensitivity of 93% (13 true positives and 1 false negative) and specificity of 86% (31 true negatives and 5 false positives), an encouraging finding.

In another study of 48 healthy volunteers coached to change their respiratory rate, RVM monitoring reached detection of the new steady state more rapidly that the $EtCO_2$ monitoring.[15] This suggests that RVM monitoring can detect respiratory changes early, but evidence of improved outcomes is still lacking.

Acoustic Respiratory Rate Monitoring

Acoustic Respiratory Rate (RRa®) monitoring is essentially detection of respiratory vibrations originating in the walls of the large airways during breathing that are transformed into electrical signals and generate a displayed respiratory rate. As this technology is proprietary to Masimo, it is usually paired with some combination of their pulse oximeter and other technologies.

Early iterations of this technology were plagued by problems with ambient noise and motion artifacts, but these have mostly been eliminated by iterative technologic advances in the sensor and algorithm. The main advantage of RRa is that minimal training is required, the technology is easily understood, it is easy to apply as it is well tolerated, and does not have to be removed and reapplied in ambulating patients.

In a study that included 14 trauma patients that had their respiratory rate monitored with RRa, simple bioimpedance, and $EtCO_2$ as the standard, RRa had a much lower bias and better agreement than simple biopedance.[16] In another study of 62 children ages 2–16, acoustic respiratory rate monitoring was well tolerated 87% of the total monitoring time, and was much more accurate and had fewer false alarms than the simple impedance method.[17]

A much larger investigation performed at Dartmouth-Hitchcock Medical Center entailing 8,712 days of monitoring revealed three main findings. One, there was a high rate (22.7%) of patients that refused the monitoring. Two, with a respiratory rate alarm threshold set to ≤ 6 and ≥ 40 breaths per minute, and a notably low threshold for SpO_2 less than 80%, the majority of alarms (43%) were due to low oxygen saturation, and 21% were due to abnormal

respiratory rate. Three, the number of rescue events, care escalations, ICU transfers, and opioid reversals were not impacted by RRa monitoring. Surprisingly, even in patients with severe oxygen desaturation, respiratory rates were frequently in the normal range.

Conclusion

Currently there is no single respiratory monitoring modality that is widely utilized in low-intensity settings. Furthermore, there is no monitor that has the requisite sensitivity, specificity, and patient acceptance for use in low-intensity settings, though newer monitors are coming closer to this goal. A significant limitation of these technologies is the high rate of false alarms and lack of evidence of improved patient outcomes, particularly with regard to reducing the need to transfer patients to an ICU and reducing mortality. It is highly likely that a monitor will be developed that combines SpO_2 with one or more of these other modalities, utilizes an algorithmic analysis to determine a composite variable that identifies respiratory compromise at an early stage, and does not have a high rate of false alarms that precludes widespread adaptation.

References

1. Lynn LL, Curry JP. Patterns of unexpected in-hospital deaths: a root cause analysis. *Patient Safety in Surgery* 2011; **5**(3):1–24.

2. Hai, F, Porhomayon J, Vermont L, et al. Postoperative complications in patients with obstructive sleep apnea: a meta-analysis. *J Clin Anesth* 2014; **26**(8):591–600.

3. Fernandez-Bustamante A, Bartels K, Clavijo C, et al. Preoperatively screened obstructive sleep apnea is associated with worse postoperative outcomes than previously diagnosed obstructive sleep apnea. *Anesth Analg* 2017;**125**(2):593–602.

4. Lee LA, Caplan RA, Stephens LS, et al. Postoperative opioid-induced respiratory depression: a closed claims analysis. *Anesthesiology* 2015;**122**(3):659–65.

5. Khanna AK, Overdyk FJ, Greening C, Di Stefano P, Buhre WF. Respiratory depression in low acuity hospital settings – seeking answers from the PRODIGY trial. *J Crit Care* 2018;**47**:80–7.

6. Lam T, Nagappa M, Wong J, et al. Continuous pulse oximetry and capnography monitoring for postoperative respiratory depression and adverse events: a systemic review and meta-analysis. *Anesth Analg* 2017;**125**:2019–29.

7. Pedersen T, Nicholson A, Hovhannisyan K, et al. Pulse oximetry for perioperative monitoring. *Cochrane*

Database of Systematic Reviews 2014, Issue 3. Art. No.: CD002013.

8. Duncan PG, Cohen MM. Pulse oximetry and capnography in anaesthetic practice: an epidemiological appraisal. *Can J Anaesth* 1991;**38**(5):619–25.

9. Blankush JM, Freeman R, McIlvaine J, et al. Implementation of a novel postoperative monitoring system using automated Modified Early Warning Scores (MEWS) incorporating end-tidal capnography. *J Clin Monit Comput* 2017;**31**(5):1081–92.

10. Weiniger C, Akdagli S, Turvall E, et al. Prospective observational investigation of capnography and pulse oximetry monitoring after cesarean delivery with intrathecal morphine. *Anesth Analg* 2019;**128**(3):513–22.

11. Chhajed PN, Gehrer S, Pandey KV. Utility of transcutaneous capnography for optimization of non-invasive ventilation pressure. *J Clin Diagn Res* 2016;**10**(9):OC06–OC09.

12. Charlton PH, Bonnici T, Tarassenko L, et al. As assessment of algorithms to estimate respiratory from the electrocardiogram and photoplethysmogram. *Physiol Meas* 2016;**37**(4):610–26.

13. Bergese SD, Mestek ML, Kelley SD, et al. Multicenter study validating accuracy of a continuous respiratory rate measurement derived from pulse oximetry: a comparison with capnography. *Anesth Analg* 2017; **124**(4):1153–9.

14. Voscopoulos C, MacNabb CM, Freeman J, et al. Continuous noninvasive respiratory volume monitoring for the identification of patients at risk for opioid-induced respiration and obstructive breathing patterns. *J Trauma Acute Care Surg.* 2014;**77**:(s208–215).

15. Williams GW II, George CA, Harvey BC, Free JE. A comparison of measurements of changes in respiratory status in spontaneously breathing volunteers by the expiron noninvasive respiratory volume monitor versus the capnostream capnometer. *Anesth Analg* 2017;**124**:120–6.

16. Menner A, Hu P, Stansbury L, et al. Acoustic sensor versus electrocardiographically derived respiratory rate in unstable trauma patients. *J Clin Monit Comput* 2017;**31**:765–72.

17. Patino M, Kalin M, Griffin A, et al. Comparison of postoperative respiratory monitoring by acoustic and transthoracic impedance technologies in pediatric patients at risk or respiratory depression. *Anesth Analg* 2017;**124**(6)1937–42.

18. McGrath SP, Pyke J, Taenzer AH. Assessment of continuous acoustic respiratory rate monitoring as an addition to a pulse oximetry-based patient surveillance system. *J Clin Monit Comput* 2017;**31**(3):561–91.

Chapter 16

The Electronic Health Record as a Monitor for Performance Improvement

David B. Wax

Introduction

The first consistent use of anesthesia records is thought to have been in 1895 when Cushing and Codman kept "ether charts" as part of a wager to see who could most improve their anesthesia skills. Cushing later remarked that "we both became very much more skillful ... particularly due to the detailed attention which we had to put upon the patient by the careful recording of the pulse rate throughout the operation." By 1920, Silk remarked on the "importance of observing the variations in blood pressure of a patient while under an anaesthetic."[1] Thus, there was early recognition that measuring vital signs in order to record them, and then observing trends in those recordings, could lead to improved care. This elevated anesthesia records to the status of patient monitors rather than just banal transcripts.

Nearly a century later, innovation took a wrong turn when an automated anesthesia record-keeping system was reported that simply used a video camera pointed at the anesthesia workstation for the entire case.[2] While this provided a high fidelity record of everything the practitioner saw and did, and might be ideal for a courtroom, there was no way to utilize any of the recorded data other than to replay the footage. Around the same time, however, computerized anesthesia record-keepers were being developed that stored information electronically as discrete data, allowing them to be later retrieved and analyzed for myriad purposes.[3] These systems were initially called AARKS (automated anesthesia record keepers) and then AIMS (anesthesia information management systems), as their scope of use widened beyond just automatically creating a paper intraoperative record.

Some AIMS are homegrown systems, others are standalone commercial products, and still others are modules integrated into a comprehensive EHR/EMR (electronic health/medical record) that encompasses all aspects of care rather than just anesthesia care. The former are highly customized to meet local needs, but they may lack interoperability with other systems. The latter may not fit perfectly into local workflows, but they get closer to the goal of a universal health record.

It is projected that 84% of academic anesthesiology departments (and an unknown number of community practices) in the United States will utilize an AIMS by 2020.[4] These systems create a wealth of data that can be used for clinical, administrative, training, legal, research, compliance, and other purposes. Such "big data" are the fuel for countless research efforts that will eventually lead to improvements in practice.[5] However, the focus of this chapter will be on more immediate uses of AIMS data to inform decisions and improve our practice in real time as other bedside patient monitors do.

Electronic Anesthesia Records

At its most fundamental level, an electronic anesthesia record is simply a digital (and more legible) version of a traditional paper anesthesia record. The primary value of these records is the same now as it was described long ago: measurement and documentation of physiologic data, and observation of their trends, can help practitioners provide better care. As a visual representation of data aggregated from various other patient monitors over time, the AARK itself is a patient monitor that provides unique insight beyond the standalone monitors that feed it.

There was initial concern that moving from a paper record to an electronic record could actually decrease its effectiveness as a clinical tool. The theory was that, with the computer automatically recording vital signs, practitioners could/would be less attentive to the patient's state. There was also fear that monitoring artifacts or non-reassuring data might be permanently recorded in the record and possibly increase malpractice exposure. Some of these fears were allayed in various studies on these matters.

Regarding vigilance, two studies showed that use of an AARK did not decrease practitioner awareness of their patient's state.[6,7] A later study found that where internet surfing was available as a potential distraction on the same workstation as the AARK, practitioners did spend substantial amounts of time looking at something other than the AARK, but this did not adversely impact the incidence of abnormal patient hemodynamics.[8] Other studies showed that paper records were incomplete and inaccurate, while AARK records better reflected reality than the "railroad tracks" of vital signs on paper records.[9–12] Regarding malpractice claims, one study showed that using an AIMS helped result in dismissal, settlement, or successful litigation of cases, and did not hinder the defense.[13] AIMS metadata have also been utilized to discourage attending anesthesiologists from improperly attesting to clinical events that have not yet occurred.[14]

Beyond the basic "ether chart," the AIMS record may include pre-anesthesia notes, procedure notes, post-anesthesia notes, medication and nursing orders, and administrative data. As part of an enterprise EHR, this documentation is potentially viewed by other anesthesia care teams as well as other specialists, administrators, and payers.[15] It can also be viewed remotely when supervising resident/CRNA cases.

As more centers adopt them, concerns about pitfalls of EHRs extend to anesthesia and critical care practices.[16–19] In fact, in a 2013 poll of healthcare leaders, health information technology (HIT) was voted the "safety hazard of the year."[20] The most commonly cited concerns are those of copy/paste functionality and automated note templates which lead to "note bloat" and repetition of irrelevant or erroneous information that can fatigue or mislead subsequent caregivers.[21] Other concerns include excessive time spent on ever-increasing documentation, patient dissatisfaction with practitioner computer use during consultations, alert fatigue, privacy and security risks, potential for documentation in the wrong patient's record, and alienation of senior practitioners not accustomed to computers. Despite these concerns, EHR adoption has accelerated due to regulatory and financial incentives to utilize HIT.[22,23] Anesthesiology EHRs may be less subject to some of these concerns, as the majority of the record is not subject to copy and paste, and patients are generally unaware of the time spent on recordkeeping.

Decision Support Systems

The computers running AIMS no longer just capture, display, and store clinical data for review. Their processing power is now utilized to make use of those data for performance improvement with integrated decision support systems (DSS).[24–27] These algorithms take physiologic data from monitors, clinical information entered by practitioners, laboratory data, and other inputs and algorithmically generate a recommendation that is provided real time or near real time to the practitioner to guide care. The algorithms themselves can be based on standards, guidelines, regulations, checklists, study protocols, corrective actions, or presumed best practices. They need to be designed so as not to trigger inappropriately and cause alert fatigue. In this way, the anesthesia record becomes more than just a "dumb" monitor mirroring patient state – it becomes an accessory brain for the practitioner to interpret the data and act appropriately upon it. This type of assistance becomes increasingly important as more and more research generates more and more predictive algorithms, scoring systems, and evidence-based recommendations that individual practitioners cannot reasonably be expected to know and utilize all of without assistance. The aggregation, synthesis, and dissemination of knowledge by DSS help overcome this barrier to adoption of evidence-based medicine.[28] This is not without controversy, however, as legitimate criticism of evidence-based medicine can decrease acceptance of DSS.[29,30]

There is a multitude of EHR-based DSS. Overall, they appear to have positive or neutral impacts on patient outcomes.[31] There is currently little to no regulatory oversight of these systems as there is for other medical devices, leaving developers and users to ensure the quality and safety of their own systems. It remains to be seen if these systems will become a significant source of adverse events or malpractice litigation.

Most DSS are directed at improving patient care, though some focus on practitioner issues and others focus on administrative issues. Unfortunately, only those DSS that are formally published, anecdotally disclosed, or built into commercial EHRs are known and will be described here. This likely leaves many other systems in use that are known only to their developers and users.

Antibiotic Administration

Some of the earliest AIMS-based interventions were directed at improving on-time administration of antibiotics in an effort to follow guidelines for prevention of surgical site infections.[32–36] These systems utilized some combination of on-screen reminders, real-time alerts (pager/text messaging), and performance reports to ensure pre-incision antibiotic administration and intraoperative re-dosing as needed.

Postoperative Nausea/Vomiting Prophylaxis

Risk factors for postoperative nausea and vomiting (PONV) have been known for some time, but antiemetic prophylaxis is still not always tailored to individual patients. DSS has been utilized to change this.[37,38] The systems work by using data from the preoperative evaluation (e.g., age, gender) and intraoperative record (e.g., opioids, inhaled anesthetics, procedure type) to identify risk factors for PONV and then make real-time recommendations to the practitioner about anti-emetic agents to administer.

Blood Pressure

Since both hypotension and hypertension have been associated with adverse outcomes, some DSS have focused on limiting blood pressure extremes. One DSS monitored for hypotension in the setting of high levels of inhaled anesthetic, as well as hypertension in the setting of vasoconstrictor infusion, and alerted practitioners of the conditions.[39] This system led to changes in practitioner behavior, but patient outcomes were not reported. Another system monitored for a "double low" state of hypotension and low bispectral index and suggested intervention.[40] Unfortunately, this seemed to have little effect on practitioner behavior or short-term outcomes.

Corrective Actions

The root cause analyses and peer review processes that follow near misses or adverse events can identify causative or contributory factors that are amenable to preventive measures based on DSS. One of the earliest reports of this involved liability partly resulting from a gap in vital sign recording (and alleged gap in patient monitoring). DSS was subsequently utilized to alert practitioners when the AIMS vital sign stream is lost so they can intervene promptly.[41–43] Another example is an apnea alert that is triggered if

cardiopulmonary bypass ends and the AIMS does not detect vital signs associated with resumption of ventilation. A "rule of thumb" DSS is exemplified by a "rule of fours" alert that is triggered to raise awareness if the AIMS data indicate over 4 units of blood transfused, 4 liters of fluids, base deficit of 4, and 4 hours of surgery. Abnormal point-of-care lab results have also been used to trigger alerts to the attending anesthesiologist who may be out of the room and otherwise unaware of such results.[44] Retained guidewires have led to electronic checklist items that confirm guidewire removal when a central line is placed. Electronic procedure notes for intrathecal opioid injections or neuraxial/peripheral nerve catheter placements have also been used to trigger notifications to a pain management service to ensure continuity of care.

Chart Review

Self-reporting of adverse events is imperfect due to various human and technical factors. The literature indicates that electronic queries of AIMS records are significantly more reliable than manual reporting of incidents.[45–47] Additionally, the volume of clinical documentation in an EHR often exceeds an amount that can be efficiently or reasonably reviewed manually prior to rendering care. Based on this, a DSS was created that screens old AIMS records for both discrete data and narrative documentation suggestive of critical intraoperative events (e.g., difficult intubation, laryngospasm, bronchospasm, difficult IV access). Cases with such events detected are flagged so that, if the same patient returns for another procedure, the practitioner is forewarned of the potential problem and can anticipate or prevent it from recurring.[48]

Crisis Avoidance

Another exciting area of DSS are those systems that attempt to identify impending crises in advance so that early intervention can be initiated. This is made possible by an enterprise-wide EHR that aggregates physiologic data from various patient areas and automatically screens them using evidence-based criteria of impending clinical deterioration. This process occurs in the background so it does not require the patient's chart to be already accessed/open to trigger the monitoring/screening and alerts. Such systems have been used to identify patients developing SIRS/sepsis, respiratory failure, and acute kidney injury.[49–52] These alerts (and the protocols employed once they are triggered) are in their infancy, with most just deployed in the last 5 years, so the outcome data are preliminary. The "weak link" seems to be provider response and adherence to protocol, perhaps as a result of alert fatigue, false alarms, and the overall embrace of protocols, bundles, care maps, and algorithms that make adherence to any one of these more difficult.

DSS Packages

Just as guidelines are now coming in packages (e.g., ERAS protocols), DSS are also being packaged together to provide optimal care.[53-56] Some of these systems are layered on top of an EHR and aggregate data to present them to the clinician in a more visually/graphically or animated way than the standalone (mostly numeric) monitors they originated from. They also have triggers more complex than the simple low/high limits on most standalone monitors. Decision support in these systems may be implicit (e.g., an image of lungs turning from green to red with hypercarbia) or explicit (alerts

and reminders), and combines best-practice evidence from a variety of areas conveniently in one place (see Figure 16.1).

Risk Reduction

Various other EHR-based systems have been implemented in the anesthesia, pain management, and critical care realms. These include surgical "time outs," anesthesia workstation preparation, beta blocker administration, opioid prescribing, central line-associated bloodstream infection (CLABSI) reduction practices, venous thromboembolism (VTE) prophylaxis, antibiotic stewardship, urinary catheter avoidance, glucose control, ventilator management, blood transfusion restriction, and rational lab and radiology testing.[57-69]

Drug Diversion

Anesthesia practitioners are at risk for substance use disorder, and early detection and intervention can be life-saving. To this end, DSS have been used to

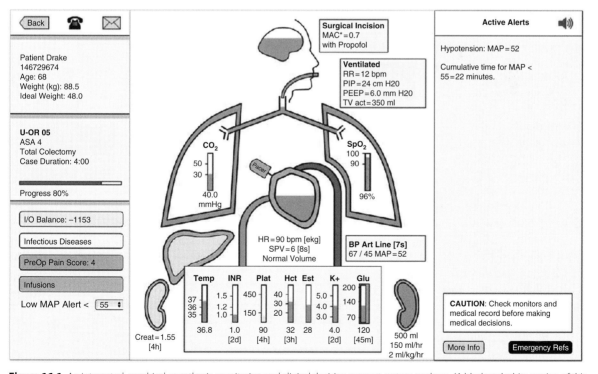

Figure 16.1 An integrated, graphical, anesthesia monitoring and clinical decision support system package. (A black and white version of this figure will appear in some formats. For the color version, please refer to the plate section).

Kheterpal S, Shanks A, Tremper KK. Impact of a Novel Multiparameter Decision Support System on Intraoperative Processes of Care and Postoperative Outcomes. *Anesthesiology*. 2018; 128:272–282.
Source: Kruger GH, Tremper KK. Advanced integrated real-time clinical displays. *Anesthesiol Clin* 2011; 29: 487–504.

monitor AIMS drug administration records and pharmacy records and identify discrepancies and patterns that have been associated with drug diversion.[70,71]

Relief Equity

Inequitable work hours can be a source of job dissatisfaction and burnout in healthcare workers. Two DSS systems have been described that utilize AIMS case information to determine recent departure times for attendings and residents and provide this information to the on-call team (see Figure 16.2).[72,73] This helps balance work hours by prioritizing early relief for those who have recently worked late. This has traditionally been accomplished with maintenance of paper or grease-board "diaries" and "group think," and is prone to human error and explicit and implicit bias.

Resident Monitoring

DSS have also been applied to monitoring of residents for training and evaluation purposes. One area of use is to provide AIMS-based case data for each resident

to clinical coordinators so they can schedule residents as necessary to meet their ACGME minimum case requirements.[74] Another effort to assign residents to cases of appropriate acuity involved using information from the EHR to calculate case risk stratification scores for use during resident scheduling.[75] Another use is facilitating staff evaluations mandated by the ACGME. AIMS-based reminders can identify all the faculty/resident dyads for each clinical day and send reminders to encourage completion of mutual evaluations in a timely fashion.[76,77] An (unsuccessful) effort was even made to use AIMS data about intraoperative blood pressure management by residents to predict their performance on later competency exams.[78]

Cost Containment

Pharmaceutical costs can be a significant component of anesthesia practice expenses. In order to reduce spending, AIMS data have been leveraged to monitor patterns of medication selection by individual practitioners and provide negative feedback to those

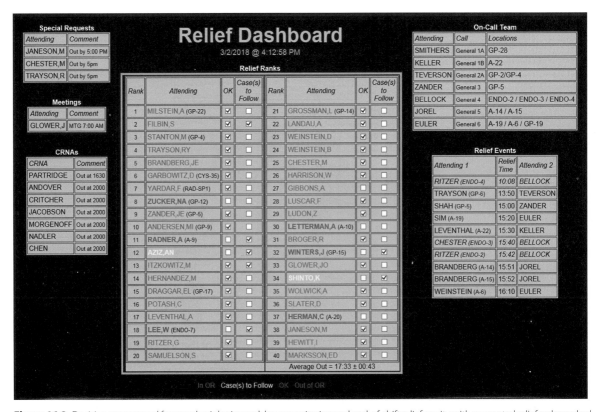

Figure 16.2 Decision support tool for anesthesiologist work hour monitoring and end-of-shift relief equity with suggested relief order ranked by descending average of departure times on prior five weekdays (Mount Sinai Hospital, New York, NY USA).

utilizing more costly agents than their peers.[79] Excessive fresh gas flow when using inhaled anesthetics can also increase costs (and air pollution). Efforts have been made using AIMS data and DSS to monitor fresh gas flow rates and encourage practitioners to reduce them if they exceed norms.[80,81]

Billing

Much of the return-on-investment for EHRs is purported to result from improved revenue collection by monitoring documentation and billing processes to ensure rapid clean bill submission (i.e., minimal charge lag) and maximal payment (i.e., gross collection rate) for services. Early efforts in this regard were aimed at identifying a minimum dataset necessary to have a bill that would be paid without delay or denial due to incomplete items. A background process would screen AIMS cases prior to claim submission and alert practitioners if deficiencies were found so they could be remedied.[82,83] Maximizing reimbursement was the goal of another system that would check the AIMS data for invasive blood pressure data and send an alert if no procedure note was filed for the placement of the arterial catheter (thus precluding billing for it).[84] Other algorithms have been used to avoid lost bills by verifying that every case on the OR schedule on a given day results in a billing entry. Still other efforts have used AIMS data and DSS in monitoring operating room utilization to minimize delays and maximize efficiency.[85,86]

Compensation

Physician compensation can also be driven with AIMS data. A modified fee-for-service system has been described in which productivity pay is allocated among the faculty based on case complexity and duration as documented in the AIMS case records.[87] In complex multisite practices, this may be an effective means of adjudicating relative "value" of individuals' work based on real-time knowledge of the work burden, assuring compensation fairness and encouraging productivity.

Compliance

Various quality measures and regulations (e.g., EHR meaningful use [HITECH-MU], Surgical Care Improvement Project [SCIP], Merit-Based Incentive Payment System [MIPS], Department of Health [DOH] regulations, Joint Commission [JC]

standards) require reporting of data to surveyors, payers, and registries in order to qualify for incentive payments or avoid penalties or citations. Missing data can thus result in sub-maximal revenue or accreditation issues. In order to ensure complete data for reporting, EHRs can be designed with reminders and warnings that prevent practitioners from omitting items that are mandatory for reporting compliance. This can be a simple reminder that a particular mandatory item in a preoperative note is incomplete or a postoperative note is missing, or a more complicated DSS that, for example, alerts the anesthesia team that no patient temperature has been recorded in an ongoing general or neuraxial anesthetic case of greater than one hour.

Conclusions

Electronic anesthesia records and decision support systems have become an integral part of the modern monitoring armamentarium. Together they act as both historian and consultant. These systems are still in their infancy and will continue to grow in both number and complexity for the benefit of patients, practitioners, and systems.

References

1. Zeitlin GL. History of Anesthesia Records. American Society of Anesthesiologists Newsletter. www.woodlibrarymuseum.org/news/pdf/Zeitlin.pdf

2. Piepenbrink JC, Cullen JI Jr, Stafford TJ. The use of video in anesthesia record keeping. *Biomed Instrum Technol* 1990;**24**:19–24.

3. Kenney GNC. Implementation of computerized anaesthetic records. *Baillière's Clinical Anaesthesiology* 1990;**4**:1–6.

4. Stol IS, Ehrenfeld JM, Epstein RH. Technology diffusion of anesthesia information management systems into academic anesthesia departments in the United States. *Anesth Analg* 2014;**118**:644–50.

5. Levin MA, Wanderer JP, Ehrenfeld JM. Data, big data, and metadata in anesthesiology. *Anesth Analg* 2015;**121**:1661–7.

6. Loeb RG. Manual record keeping is not necessary for anesthesia vigilance. *J Clin Monit* 1995;**11**:9–13.

7. Allard J, Dzwonczyk R, Yablok D, Block FE Jr, McDonald JS. Effect of automatic record keeping on vigilance and record keeping time. *Br J Anaesth* 1995;**74**:619–26.

8. Wax DB, Lin HM, Reich DL. Intraoperative non-record-keeping usage of anesthesia information

management system workstations and associated hemodynamic variability and aberrancies. *Anesthesiology* 2012;**117**:1184–9.

9. Thrush DN. Are automated anesthesia records better? *J Clin Anesth* 1992;**4**:386–9.

10. Lerou JG, Dirksen R, van Daele M, Nijhuis GM, Crul JF. Automated charting of physiological variables in anesthesia: a quantitative comparison of automated versus handwritten anesthesia records. *J Clin Monit* 1988;**4**:37–47.

11. Devitt JH, Rapanos T, Kurrek M, Cohen MM, Shaw M. The anesthetic record: accuracy and completeness. *Can J Anaesth* 1999;**46**:122–8.

12. Reich DL, Wood RK Jr, Mattar R, et al. Arterial blood pressure and heart rate discrepancies between handwritten and computerized anesthesia records. *Anesth Analg* 2000;**91**:612–16.

13. Feldman JM. Do anesthesia information systems increase malpractice exposure? Results of a survey. *Anesth Analg* 2004;**99**:840–3.

14. Vigoda MM, Lubarsky DA. The medicolegal importance of enhancing timeliness of documentation when using an anesthesia information system and the response to automated feedback in an academic practice. *Anesth Analg* 2006;**103**:131–6.

15. Wanderer JP, Gruss CL, Ehrenfeld JM. Using visual analytics to determine the utilization of preoperative anesthesia assessments. *Appl Clin Inform* 2015;**6**:629–37.

16. Bowman S. Impact of electronic health record systems on information integrity: quality and safety implications. *Perspect Health Inf Manag* 2013;**10**:1c.

17. Meeks DW, Smith MW, Taylor L, Sittig DF, Scott JM, Singh H. An analysis of electronic health record-related patient safety concerns. *J Am Med Inform Assoc* 2014;**21**:1053–9.

18. Shaarani I, Taleb R, Antoun J. Effect of computer use on physician-patient communication using a validated instrument: patient perspective. *Int J Med Inform* 2017;**108**:152–7.

19. Blijleven V, Koelemeijer K, Jaspers M. Identifying and eliminating inefficiencies in information system usage: a lean perspective. *Int J Med Inform* 2017;**107**:40–7.

20. Denham CR, Classen DC, Swenson SJ, Henderson MJ, Zeltner T, Bates DW. Safe use of electronic health records and health information technology systems: trust but verify. *J Patient Saf* 2013;**9**:177–89.

21. Tsou AY, Lehmann CU, Michel J, Solomon R, Possanza L, Gandhi T. Safe practices for copy and paste in the EHR. Systematic review, recommendations, and novel model for health IT collaboration. *Appl Clin Inform* 2017;**8**:12–34.

22. Gálvez JA, Rothman BS, Doyle CA, Morgan S, Simpao AF, Rehman MA. A narrative review of meaningful use and anesthesia information management systems. *Anesth Analg* 2015;**121**:693–706.

23. McWilliams JM. MACRA: big fix or big Problem? *Ann Intern Med* 2017;**167**:122–4.

24. Epstein RH, Dexter F, Patel N. Influencing anesthesia provider behavior using anesthesia information management system data for near real-time alerts and post hoc reports. *Anesth Analg* 2015;**121**:678–92.

25. Simpao AF, Tan JM, Lingappan AM, Gálvez JA, Morgan SE, Krall MA. A systematic review of near real-time and point-of-care clinical decision support in anesthesia information management systems. *J Clin Monit Comput* 2017;**31**:885–94.

26. Nair BG, Gabel E, Hofer I, Schwid HA, Cannesson M. Intraoperative clinical decision support for anesthesia: a narrative review of available systems. *Anesth Analg* 2017;**124**:603–17.

27. Belard A, Buchman T, Forsberg J, et al. Precision diagnosis: a view of the clinical decision support systems (CDSS) landscape through the lens of critical care. *J Clin Monit Comput* 2017;**31**:261–71.

28. Sadeghi-Bazargani H, Tabrizi JS, Azami-Aghdash S. Barriers to evidence-based medicine: a systematic review. *J Eval Clin Pract* 2014;**20**:793–802.

29. Kumanan W. Evidence-based medicine. The good the bad and the ugly. A clinician's perspective. *J Eval Clin Pract* 2010;**16**:398–400.

30. Prasad V, Cifu A. Medical reversal: why we must raise the bar before adopting new technologies. *Yale J Biol Med* 2011;**84**:471–8.

31. Varghese J, Kleine M, Gessner SI, Sandmann S, Dugas M. Effects of computerized decision support system implementations on patient outcomes in inpatient care: a systematic review. *J Am Med Inform Assoc* 2018;**25**(5):593–602.

32. O'Reilly M, Talsma A, VanRiper S, Kheterpal S, Burney R. An anesthesia information system designed to provide physician-specific feedback improves timely administration of prophylactic antibiotics. *Anesth Analg* 2006;**103**:908–12.

33. Wax DB, Beilin Y, Levin M, Chadha N, Krol M, Reich DL. The effect of an interactive visual reminder in an anesthesia information management system on timeliness of prophylactic antibiotic administration. *Anesth Analg* 2007;**104**:1462–6.

34. Nair BG, Newman SF, Peterson GN, Wu WY, Schwid HA. Feedback mechanisms including real-time electronic alerts to achieve near 100% timely prophylactic antibiotic administration in surgical cases. *Anesth Analg* 2010;**111**:1293–300.

35. Nair BG, Newman SF, Peterson GN, Schwid HA. Automated electronic reminders to improve redosing of antibiotics during surgical cases: comparison of two approaches. *Surg Infect* 2011;**12**:57–63.

36. Schwann NM, Bretz KA, Eid S, et al. Point-of-care electronic prompts: an effective means of increasing compliance, demonstrating quality, and improving outcome. *Anesth Analg* 2011;**113**:869–7.

37. Kooij FO, Klok T, Hollmann MW, Kal JE. Decision support increases guideline adherence for prescribing postoperative nausea and vomiting prophylaxis. *Anesth Analg* 2008;**106**:893–8.

38. Kappen TH, Vergouwe Y, van Wolfswinkel L, Kalkman CJ, Moons KG, van Klei WA. Impact of adding therapeutic recommendations to risk assessments from a prediction model for postoperative nausea and vomiting. *Br J Anaesth* 2015;**114**:252–60.

39. Nair BG, Horibe M, Newman SF, Wu WY, Peterson GN, Schwid HA. Anesthesia information management system-based near real-time decision support to manage intraoperative hypotension and hypertension. *Anesth Analg* 2014;**118**:206–14.

40. McCormick PJ, Levin MA, Lin HM, Sessler DI, Reich DL. Effectiveness of an electronic alert for hypotension and low bispectral index on 90-day postoperative mortality: a prospective, randomized trial. *Anesthesiology* 2016;**125**:1113–20.

41. Vigoda MM, Lubarsky DA. Failure to recognize loss of incoming data in an anesthesia record-keeping system may have increased medical liability. *Anesth Analg* 2006;**102**:1798–802.

42. Ehrenfeld JM, Epstein RH, Bader S, Kheterpal S, Sandberg WS. Automatic notifications mediated by anesthesia information management systems reduce the frequency of prolonged gaps in blood pressure documentation. *Anesth Analg* 2011;**113**:356–63.

43. Nair BG, Horibe M, Newman SF, Wu WY, Schwid H. Near real-time notification of gaps in cuff blood pressure recordings for improved patient monitoring. *J Clin Monit Comput* 2013;**27**:265–71.

44. Freundlich RE, Grondin L, Tremper KK, Saran KA, Kheterpal S. Automated electronic reminders to prevent miscommunication among primary medical, surgical and anaesthesia providers: a root cause analysis. *BMJ Qual Saf* 2012;**21**:850–4.

45. Sanborn KV, Castro J, Kuroda M, Thys DM. Detection of intraoperative incidents by electronic scanning of computerized anesthesia records. Comparison with voluntary reporting. *Anesthesiology* 1996;**85**:977–87.

46. Benson M, Junger A, Fuchs C, et al. Using an anesthesia information management system to prove a deficit in voluntary reporting of adverse events in a quality assurance program. *J Clin Monit Comput* 2000;**16**:211–17.

47. Grant C, Ludbrook G, Hampson EA, Semenov R, Willis R. Adverse physiological events under anaesthesia and sedation: a pilot audit of electronic patient records. *Anaesth Intensive Care* 2008;**36**:222–9.

48. Wax DB, McCormick PJ, Joseph TT, Levin MA. An automated critical event screening and notification system to facilitate preanesthesia record review. *Anesth Analg* 2018;**126**:606–10.

49. Pedersen NE, Rasmussen LS, Petersen JA, Gerds TA, Østergaard D, Lippert A. A critical assessment of early warning score records in 168,000 patients. *J Clin Monit Comput* 2018;**32**:109–16.

50. Blankush JM, Freeman R, McIlvaine J, Tran T, Nassani S, Leitman IM. Implementation of a novel postoperative monitoring system using automated Modified Early Warning Scores (MEWS) incorporating end-tidal capnography. *J Clin Monit Comput* 2017;**31**:1081–92.

51. Breighner CM, Kashani KB. Impact of e-alert systems on the care of patients with acute kidney injury. *Best Pract Res Clin Anaesthesiol* 2017;**31**:353–9.

52. Schmidt PE, Meredith P, Prytherch DR, Watson D, Watson V. Impact of introducing an electronic physiological surveillance system on hospital mortality. *BMJ Qual Saf* 2015;**24**:10–20.

53. Ljungqvist O, Scott M, Fearon KC. Enhanced recovery after surgery: a review. *JAMA Surg* 2017;**152**:292–8.

54. Kruger GH, Tremper KK. Advanced integrated real-time clinical displays. *Anesthesiol Clin* 2011;**29**:487–504.

55. Nair BG, Newman SF, Peterson GN, Schwid HA. Smart Anesthesia Manager™ (SAM) – a real-time decision support system for anesthesia care during surgery. *IEEE Trans Biomed Eng* 2013;**60**:207–10.

56. Kheterpal S, Shanks A, Tremper KK. Impact of a novel multiparameter decision support system on intraoperative processes of care and postoperative outcomes. *Anesthesiology* 2018;**128**:272–82.

57. Wetmore D, Goldberg A, Gandhi N, Spivack J, McCormick P, DeMaria S Jr. An embedded checklist in the anesthesia information management system improves pre-anaesthetic induction setup: a randomised controlled trial in a simulation setting. *BMJ Qual Saf* 2016;**25**:739–46.

58. Shear T, Deshur M, Avram MJ, et al. Procedural timeout compliance is improved with real-time clinical decision support. *J Patient Saf* 2018;**14**(3):148–52.

59. Patel S, Carmichael JM, Taylor JM, Bounthavong M, Higgins DT. Evaluating the impact of a clinical decision support tool to reduce chronic opioid dose

and decrease risk classification in a veteran population. *Ann Pharmacother* 2018;**52**:325–31.

60. Quan KA, Cousins SM, Porter DD, et al. Electronic health record solutions to reduce central line-associated bloodstream infections by enhancing documentation of central line insertion practices, line days, and daily line necessity. *Am J Infect Control* 2016;**44**:438–43.

61. Kahn SR, Morrison DR, Cohen JM, et al. Interventions for implementation of thromboprophylaxis in hospitalized medical and surgical patients at risk for venous thromboembolism. *Cochrane Database Syst Rev* 2013;7:CD008201.

62. Jenkins I, Doucet JJ, Clay B, et al. Transfusing wisely: clinical decision support improves blood transfusion practices. *Jt Comm J Qual Patient Saf* 2017;**43**:389–95.

63. Nair BG, Grunzweig K, Peterson G, et al. Intraoperative blood glucose management: impact of a real-time decision support system on adherence to institutional protocol. *J Clin Monit Comput* 2016;**30**:301–12.

64. Schulz L, Osterby K, Fox B. The use of best practice alerts with the development of an antimicrobial stewardship navigator to promote antibiotic de-escalation in the electronic medical record. *Infect Control Hosp Epidemiol* 2013;**34**:1259–65.

65. Chen YY, Chi MM, Chen YC, Chan YJ, Chou SS, Wang FD. Using a criteria-based reminder to reduce use of indwelling urinary catheters and decrease urinary tract infections. *Am J Crit Care* 2013;**22**:105–14.

66. Karbing DS, Allerød C, Thomsen LP, et al. Retrospective evaluation of a decision support system for controlled mechanical ventilation. *Med Biol Eng Comput* 2012;**50**:43–51.

67. Nair BG, Peterson GN, Newman SF, Wu WY, Kolios-Morris V, Schwid HA. Improving documentation of a beta-blocker quality measure through an anesthesia information management system and real-time notification of documentation errors. *Jt Comm J Qual Patient Saf* 2012;**38**:283–8.

68. Krasowski MD, Chudzik D, Dolezal A, et al. Promoting improved utilization of laboratory testing through changes in an electronic medical record: experience at an academic medical center. *BMC Med Inform Decis Mak* 2015 February 22;**15**:11.

69. Schneider E, Zelenka S, Grooff P, Alexa D, Bullen J, Obuchowski NA. Radiology order decision support: examination-indication appropriateness assessed using 2 electronic systems. *J Am Coll Radiol* 2015;**12**:349–57.

70. Epstein RH, Gratch DM, Grunwald Z. Development of a scheduled drug diversion surveillance system based on an analysis of atypical drug transactions. *Anesth Analg* 2007;**105**:1053–60.

71. Epstein RH, Gratch DM, McNulty S, Grunwald Z. Validation of a system to detect scheduled drug diversion by anesthesia care providers. *Anesth Analg* 2011;**113**:160–4.

72. Wax DB, McCormick PJ. A real-time decision support system for anesthesiologist end-of-shift relief. *Anesth Analg* 2017;**124**:599–602.

73. Bhutiani M, Jablonski PM, Ehrenfeld JM, McEvoy MD, Fowler LC, Wanderer JP. Decision support tool improves real and perceived anesthesiology resident relief. *Anesth Analg* 2018;**127**(2):513–19.

74. Wanderer JP, Charnin J, Driscoll WD, Bailin MT, Baker K. Decision support using anesthesia information management system records and accreditation council for graduate medical education case logs for resident operating room assignments. *Anesth Analg* 2013;**117**:494–9.

75. Was A, Wanderer J. Matching clinicians to operative cases: a novel application of a patient acuity score. *Appl Clin Inform* 2013;**4**:445–53.

76. Blum JM, Kheterpal S, Tremper KK. A comparison of anesthesiology resident and faculty electronic evaluations before and after implementation of automated electronic reminders. *J Clin Anesth* 2006;**18**:264–7.

77. Rusa R, Klatil F, Fu R, Swide CE. Impact of faculty-specific electronic reminders on faculty compliance with daily resident evaluations: a retrospective study. *J Clin Anesth* 2009;**21**:159–64.

78. Sessler DI, Makarova N, Riveros-Perez R, Brown DL, Kimatian S. Lack of association between blood pressure management by anesthesia residents and competence committee evaluations or in-training exam performance: a cohort analysis. *Anesthesiology* 2016;**124**:473–82.

79. Lubarsky DA, Sanderson IC, Gilbert WC, et al. Using an anesthesia information management system as a cost containment tool. Description and validation. *Anesthesiology* 1997;**86**:1161–9.

80. Nair BG, Peterson GN, Neradilek MB, Newman SF, Huang EY, Schwid HA. Reducing wastage of inhalation anesthetics using real-time decision support to notify of excessive fresh gas flow. *Anesthesiology* 2013;**118**:874–84.

81. Wax DB, Hill B, Levin MA. Ventilator data extraction with a video display image capture and processing system. *J Med Syst* 2017;**41**:101.

82. Reich DL, Kahn RA, Wax D, Palvia T, Galati M, Krol M. Development of a module for point-of-care charge capture and submission using an anesthesia

information management system. *Anesthesiology* 2006;**105**:179–86.

83. Spring SF, Sandberg WS, Anupama S, Walsh JL, Driscoll WD, Raines DE. Automated documentation error detection and notification improves anesthesia billing performance. *Anesthesiology* 2007;**106**:157–63.

84. Kheterpal S, Gupta R, Blum JM, Tremper KK, O'Reilly M, Kazanjian PE. Electronic reminders improve procedure documentation compliance and professional fee reimbursement. *Anesth Analg* 2007;**104**:592–7.

85. Foglia RP, Alder AC, Ruiz G. Improving perioperative performance: the use of operations management and the electronic health record. *J Pediatr Surg* 2013;**48**:95–8.

86. Van Winkle RA, Champagne MT, Gilman-Mays M, Aucoin J. Operating room delays: meaningful use in electronic health record. *Comput Inform Nurs* 2016;**34**:247–53.

87. Reich DL, Galati M, Krol M, Bodian CA, Kahn RA. A mission-based productivity compensation model for an academic anesthesiology department. *Anesth Analg* 2008;**107**:1981–8.

Future Monitoring Technologies: Wireless, Wearable, and Nano

Ira S. Hofer and Myro Figura

Introduction

Advances in technology permit monitoring of an increasing array of physiological parameters in near real-time in diverse environments, by healthcare providers, their patients, and even consumers interested in self-monitoring. Miniaturization and nanotechnology engender monitors that are more portable and allow for the measurement of previously unobtainable physiological parameters. These advances allow us to glean much more physiological data, and when combined with improved data analytic capabilities, are on the verge of creating a system that gives providers the ability to monitor patients accurately and continuously, without geographic limitations.

Sophisticated monitoring is no longer restricted to hospitalized patients. Advances in sensors, battery technology, and connectivity of previously hospital-based "professional" monitors may now be packaged into consumer products. The fitness and wellness industry has already showcased devices that can be purchased anywhere and quantify heart rate, caloric expenditure, cardiac rhythm, pulse oximetry, and other measures with an accuracy that approaches that of medical grade devices. Further, startups and large companies alike are delving into the current gap between consumer and healthcare products, developing noninvasive and minimally invasive technologies and applications for home telemetry, glucose monitoring, control of infusion pumps, medication adherence, and symptom tracking for various medical diseases (e.g., shortness of breath in lung disease). As these technologies emerge, the volume of data generated is growing exponentially, and we are beginning to see the early integration of these technologies into existing health systems' care delivery.

Implementation of these technologies faces a number of new challenges. They not only have to be dependable, reliable, and accurate, but they must also be deployed on a secure and robust infrastructure with reporting and monitoring features. Some challenges that face wired technologies are amplified, and new ones are introduced once connectivity and device interoperability is incorporated. As solutions to these challenges are being developed, what remains to be answered is how clinicians will access and utilize the wide breadth of this information. Outstanding questions include: How will monitoring data from wearables and remote sensors interface with current systems? How secure can and will this communication be? Will the data from wireless sensors be accurate and reliable enough to be the basis for remotely ordered medical interventions? And ultimately, will this newly acquired information reduce morbidity and mortality, or at least improve the quality of life? One thing is for certain, clinicians will begin to acquire insight into patients' daily lives, communicate and connect with them in new ways, and for the first time obtain data that are not limited to a hospital stay or brief office visit.

Wireless Technologies in the Healthcare Sector

The most basic advantage of wireless monitors is the untethering of patients from the walls and electrical outlets of clinical settings. Wires, cables, and tubing form a web around patients that clinicians often need to untangle, taking time and attention away from more critical patient care activities.[1] In high-stake locations like the operating room or intensive care unit (ICU), this diverts precious resources away from heuristic critical tasks. This web, sometimes also referred to as "spaghetti", may pose potential physical hazards. Tripping on tangled wires may remove intravenous (IV) catheters and result in lost access, blood loss and air embolus, damage the monitors themselves, or harm patients and providers due to heavy falling objects. Wireless technology should reduce these hazards.

Wireless technology may also reduce the risk of complications that come with immobility (e.g., thromboembolism, delirium). The ability to ambulate and not be subject to sedentary care due to monitoring is associated with improved patient outcomes.[2] In the ambulatory setting, wireless technology allows patients to get out of bed and ambulate, and perform activities of daily living while being monitored continually without interruption.

Further development of wireless technology may eventually enable remote monitoring of patients from their homes via monitors that communicate with a telemedicine center through an app on patients' smartphones. This, however, will depend on a number of advances in the monitors themselves and the supportive infrastructure.

Cardiac Telemetry

Noninvasive electrocardiography (ECG) monitoring devices use electrodes attached to the skin with electro-conductive gel. The electrodes record signals that are sent to a main console, which processes and optimizes the data and displays them on a screen in real-time, sometimes with a suggested interpretation. Several wireless iterations of the ECG already exist, and most involve communications between a fixed base station and multiple mobile stations located within a coverage area. Battery-powered portable wireless consoles perform most of the signal processing locally and transmit results remotely. This processing and transmission normally consume a lot of power, relative to what can be supplied by current battery sources. Current research is geared toward addressing tradeoffs between range limitations, power consumption, and immobility of the local fixed home station.

Recent years have introduced several wearable ECG monitoring devices into mainstream use. There are Adhesive ECG patches (AECG) with integrated microelectronics, such as the ZIO® XT Patch and those incorporated into the NUVANT™ and SEEQ™ mobile cardiac telemetry (MCT) systems. These systems are indicated for short- to medium-term (days to weeks) monitoring. They solve the problem of power consumption by storing the data internally and only transmitting it at set intervals. There also are handheld smartphone-enabled systems with electrode-embedded attachment modules (such

as AliveCor and ECG Check) for very short-term (seconds to minutes) monitoring. These address the power consumption issue by using a second device, the smartphone, for data storage and transmission.

Systems like AliveCor and ECG Check are able to record single lead ECG by sensing electrical activity from a separate small recording device that connects wirelessly to the smartphone. The user places the fingers of both hands on the recording device, which then displays the single lead ECG on the smartphone screen. The device then interfaces with the smartphone and is able to provide a snapshot of the patient's cardiac rhythm viewable on screen. The AliveCor and ECG Check applications are currently able to detect atrial fibrillation without human need for interpretation in real-time.

Adhesive ECG patch devices are more complex and are composed of a sensor system, a microelectronic circuit with a recorder and memory storage, and an internal battery embedded in a relatively flexible synthetic matrix, resin, or other material. They are usually intended for medium-term use ranging from days to several weeks. AECG system patches are leadless, minimally intrusive to daily activities, water-resistant, and are designed for single use only. These systems have the capability to detect clinically relevant arrhythmias and conduction system abnormalities and may soon support analysis of the QT intervals and ST segment changes. A limitation of these devices, however, is that they do not process data in real-time. Clinicians and patients ultimately depend on the device company to process the data collected from these devices, and this may take weeks after data collection is complete. Some systems, such as the ZIO® XT system, actually require that the user return the device in a postage-paid envelope upon study completion, further adding to the lag time between data collection, analysis, and physician interpretation. Such barriers make these devices unsuitable for real-time monitoring.

Further research is geared toward wearable monitoring systems (WMS) such as textile-based smart systems that collect ECG data from a wearable garment. Thus far, ECG data have been collected using smart shirts, harnesses, and other body wear. These systems are being optimized to record ECG signals without the use of a gel, and reduce baseline noise and motion artifacts thorough hardware-implemented high-pass, low-pass, and notch filters.[3] Improvements in the sensors utilized in these systems are often coupled with software that harnesses the processing power and communications capabilities of existing mobile devices. One advantage of these systems is that by spreading the "leads" across a garment the overall size of the device is increased, allowing more space to place the necessary batteries, transmitters, and processors.

These systems are changing the landscape of cardiac diagnosis. Truly wireless mobile ECG monitoring systems with real-time transmission may eventually address convenience and comfort, reduce cost and travel time, and enable immediate medical assistance in case of emergency. To meet a medical standard as a clinically accepted monitoring system, these systems will have to incorporate high-quality real-time data acquisition, early detection of abnormal conditions, and accurate decision support. In order to be accepted by consumers, they must also be user-friendly and easy to wear. They must also have fast processing, low power consumption, and small size, and therefore likely will be smartphone based.

Blood Pressure Monitoring

Wireless blood pressure monitoring is already in mainstream use and automatic portable blood pressure cuffs are readily available to consumers. These battery powered devices often provide results comparable to those of hospital-grade devices and classic auscultation. Data transmission to smartphones and computer-based applications is relatively easy and monitoring of large groups of patients in this intermittent manner is viable. Although chronic monitoring of blood pressure in ambulatory patients provides useful telehealth and alarm functionality, blood pressure may vary widely and continuous blood pressure measurements, possibly using minimally invasive implants, might present a new opportunity to improve management and outcomes.

Wearable cuffless blood pressure monitoring devices are currently under development. The underlying principle of this technology is based on the time it takes for a volume of blood to travel from the heart to the measurement location, such as wrist.[4-8] Algorithmic models predict blood pressure from the time delay, usually obtained from the cardiac electrical signal acquired by ECG and the recording device at the peripheral site such as a pulse oximeter.[9-12] There are several practical limitations, however, that must be overcome before wearable cuffless blood pressure monitoring devices are adopted for clinical practice. Many existing systems do not provide continuous

data, as most approaches to ECG acquisition require the user to touch an electrode on the wearable device. Additionally, in order to maintain accuracy, all existing models require intermittent calibration with standard blood pressure measurement.[13,14] The variance of blood pressure due to other factors, such as changes in vasomotor tone and heart rate, require additional parameters to be incorporated into the algorithm to achieve accuracy.[15,16] Currently, the accuracy of these technologies measured via the regression coefficient (R^2) is low, with significant variations even at the same activity level within the same subject.[17] Future advances will likely overcome these limitations and produce the higher accuracy and precision necessary for a medical-grade device.

There is also promise for invasive and minimally invasive blood pressure monitoring devices. Microelectromechanical system (MEMS)-based pressure sensors have been implanted into the live canine aorta and coupled with magnetic telemetry. Rozenman et al. (2007) implanted a miniature device into both animals and a patient cohort.[18] The sensor was based on an acoustically powered piezoelectric transducer with a custom-built, low-power control chip able to transmit pressure measurements continuously for 5–10s. Readings were simultaneously taken with a catheter tip transducer advanced to the same location. Good agreement was found between the two methods, with a maximum deviation of less than 5 mmHg.

A similar protocol was used by Verdejo et al. (2007) to evaluate the accuracy of the CardioMEMSTM[TM] heart failure sensor that is also based on a MEMS pressure-sensitive capacitor.[19] The sensor was electromagnetically coupled to an external antenna that both powers the device and captures a resonant frequency that reflects the arterial pressure. The method was validated against standard care, and in a randomized controlled trial proved to result in a significant and large reduction in the rate of heart-failure-related hospitalizations at 6 months.[20] Although these implantable devices show promise, they are quite invasive and therefore carry risk. A proposed alternative to intra-arterial pressure measurement is extra-arterial blood pressure monitoring using similar technology.[21] This technology, however, is quite nascent today.

Pulse Oximetry

Pulse oximetry is a robust tool that allows for the simultaneous measurement of perfusion, oxygenation,

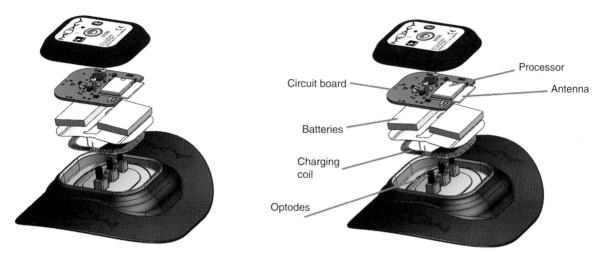

Figure 17.1 The Moxy Monitor System muscle oxygenation monitor consists of a spectrometer (light emitting diodes and photo detectors), a battery for power, a microprocessor for operating the spectrometer, a memory chip for storing data, and a radio transmitter for sending live data to other devices. From www.moxymonitor.com/device/.

heart rate, and heart rhythm. Wireless pulse oximeters have long been available to consumers and can be purchased for less than $20.00. Some of these devices can be connected to smartphones and thereby allow transmission of data.

The trend in pulse oximetry has been the conversion of a stand-alone monitor into a wearable continuous fitness tracker. Beginning in 2012, watches with optical heart rate monitors (OHRMs) have been directly available to consumers. Since then the industry's leading companies (i.e., Apple, Fitbit, and Garmin) have steadily moved toward the addition of pulse oximetry to their devices. Many of these monitors currently use the principle of photoplethysmography (PPG). The PPG signal may contain valuable information about the cardiovascular system, such as oxygen saturation (SpO_2), heart rate, blood pressure, and respiratory rate. Devices utilizing PPG currently are able to measure heart rate; however, the green light wavelength (typically 540 nanometers) used in PPG is readily absorbed by human tissue and is affected by hydration, hemoglobin concentration, the ambient environment, and other factors. These limitations have reduced the ability to provide healthcare-grade continuous home oxygen saturation monitoring by OHRMs.

Traditional wavelengths used in pulse oximetry, red light and infra-red light (600 and 900nm, respectively), penetrate tissue with much more ease than green light wavelengths. However, continous device use at these wavelength requires a large supply of power, which today has prohibied it's use in a small device such as a watch. Two companies, BSX Athletics (Austin, TX) and Moxy Monitor (Hutchinson, MN), are producing slightly larger wearable monitors using near-infrared wavelengths to measure muscle oxygenation for athletes (Figure 17.1). Further, Apple and Garmin are believed to be designing smaller sensors to integrate into their wearables. As this technology develops it likely will become reliable enough for healthcare use.

Consumer Wearables

Until recently, cardiac telemetry and blood pressure and pulse oximeter monitors were only available to the medical community; however, these modalities are increasingly available to consumers. Rapid advances in semiconductor technology are shrinking the gap between consumer and medical grade devices in terms of diversity and quality. In fact, one of the biggest changes in the healthcare market has been the proliferation of direct-to-consumer marketing of wearable devices that currently range from simple fitness trackers to more advanced devices such as continuous ECG and pulse oximeter devices. Micro-sensors may be seamlessly integrated into textiles, and consumer electronics are being embedded in clothes, watches, belts, eye-glasses, and contact lenses. This direct-to-consumer monitoring device industry may soon surpass that geared toward hospitals.

Smartwatches

Smartwatches are currently the dominant wearable in consumer health. To accurately monitor motion, 3-axis accelerometers, magnetometers and gyroscope sensors obtain data, and in combination have the capability to sense in 9 degrees of freedom. Although very small in size, each monitor contains several parts that typically use piezoelectric and capacitance sensors that utilize microscopic crystal structures to generate a voltage current in response to accelerative forces. Algorithms based on combined motion-sensing are able to measure step count and sometimes approximate distance traveled.

There are a number of such products currently on the market, and research has demonstrated these trackers to be accurate with a step count error rate of less than 1.3%.[22] Many consumer wearables additionally measure heart rate utilizing the PPG signal with acceptable results for consumer use. As previously stated, PPG is based on reflection or transmission of light that changes with blood volume in the microvascular tissue. For example, Fitbit demonstrates a moderately strong correlation with ECG for heart rate ($r = 0.83$, $p < 0.001$), with an average mean bias of -8.8 beats per minute (95% LoA 24.2, -41.8). These technologies, however, tend to be less accurate and reliable at heart rates greater than 110 beats per minute.[23] Further research is geared toward inclusion of additional sensors to monitor SpO_2, estimate VO_2 (typically via a variation of Cooper run test or Rockport walk test), and heart rate variability. The accuracy and reliability of these monitoring technologies, however, must improve in order to gain acceptance for healthcare use.

E-textiles

E-textiles are a futuristic wearable modality. Special weaving can be used to incorporate electrically conductive yarn into a fabric that becomes a "wearable motherboard" and can connect multiple sensors on the body (e.g., ECG electrodes and pulse oximetry) to signal acquisition bases. Many uses for e-textiles have been proposed and some have entered into clinical trials. Products have been developed that integrate pressure sensors into a bedsheet or mattress in order to manage and prevent bed sores, bioimpedance sensors into a vest measuring extravascular lung water to track congestive heart failure, and smart-lights into therapy blankets for infants with neonatal jaundice. Washable stockings that measure lower extremity edema utilizing ankle circumference and tissue elasticity sensors. The circumference sensor is composed of two magnets and an electromagnet that respond to the difference in position of these sensors as a result of change in circumference. The tissue elasticity sensor requires the user to push on a small lever in the sock that compresses the skin, and then measures elasticity based on the applied force and produced tissue displacement.[24]

The basic requirements of e-textile technologies are that they must be washable and durable, connect to information repositories such as smartphones, and be highly reliable in order to be fit for medical grade use. Ultra-low power advanced reduced instruction set computing machine microcontrollers (ARM MCUs) seem to be ideal for this emerging technology. Their architecture combines ultralow power, high-signal processing functionality, and ease of use. Fiberoptics are ideal, as they can connect multiple sensors and carry no risk of electroshock. Sensors, including light, heat, oximetry, pressure, and bioimpedance, are sufficiently developed in terms of functionality, but must be adapted to reduce size and power consumption to make them practical. These challenges are not insurmountable and smart clothing could completely replace bedside monitoring in hospitals, with shirts that track heart rate, temperature, position, blood pressure, and oxygen saturation.

Ocular Devices

Other wearables in development have focused on incorporation of sensors into eyeglasses and contact lenses. Contact lens sensors have already been developed for analysis of glucose composition of tears as a surrogate for blood glucose, and for the diagnosis of glaucoma by measuring intraocular pressure. With further advances in electronics, connectivity, polymer synthesis, and micro-nanofabrication, contact lenses with sensors to monitor concentrations of other ocular fluid contents such as electrolytes, lactate, urea, and albumin are in development.[25]

There are a number of challenges to overcome before contact lens monitoring technologies become mainstream. The relationship between the concentration of several analytes in tear fluid and blood has been difficult to establish and may not be consistent. Rates of tear production and type of tear production can vary. The low sample volumes and low solute concentrations require high sensitivity for analysis.[26] Wearing contact lenses itself alters the fluid profile in a complex but consistent manner.[27,28] Although these challenges seem insurmountable, the prospect of a contact lens sensor that is powered externally and permits wireless reporting using an auxiliary device has generated significant interest from Google, Novartis, Microsoft, and other companies, and it is an active area of research.

Sensors incorporated into eyeglasses and contact lenses to track eye and head movements with accelerometers and cameras are also under development. These wearables may not only have monitoring potential (e.g., hemi-neglect, seizures) but may also project images to the wearer that can be used for patient education, therapy, or health notifications.

Overall, consumer wearables have the potential to incorporate vital information about our patients into the current decision-making processes. These technologies provide the opportunity to monitor patients after discharge, perhaps reducing length of stay and alerting providers of complications before they are clinically apparent. This increase in data collection may guide differential diagnosis, aid in risk stratification, and assist in algorithm-based management in the hospital. Lastly, this new database of information may be mined, and analytics developed that allow for development of better predictive models. For example, a simple Fitbit may be used to count steps per postoperative day, and those data may be used to develop an independent marker of readiness for discharge or to set target activity levels for patients.

Insight from Analytics and Technology Convergence

A powerful and rapidly evolving trend in monitoring technology is the application of analytic techniques to data that are already being obtained via smartphones, wearables, and other devices. One example is Leaf (Leaf Healthcare, Pleasonton, CA), a small, lightweight, waterproof patch equipped with accelerometers that are very similar to those used in smartphones. The patch has the capability of determining the position and movement of the patient. The data are transferred to a dashboard that provides patient positioning analytics and presents continuous results to providers and caretakers in acute and chronic care facilities, alerting them to patients who have been immobile for an excessive period of time. The device aims to increase mobility and avoid complications related to immobility such as pressure ulcers.

In addition to the creation of new types of monitors, previously unconnected monitors are leveraging smartphones and other devices to become connected to the "internet of things." Many glucometers, weight scales, fitness trackers, and symptom trackers now connect to iOS and Android systems, allowing these disparate data to be pooled and thus generating new insights from their analysis. For example, Propeller (Propeller Health, Madison, WI) is an attachment to an inhaler that serves as a symptom tracker for asthma and chronic obstructive pulmonary disease. The Propeller device attaches to an already existing inhaler, tracks its use, and then sends that information to the application installed on a smartphone. Cloud analytics track inhaler use (i.e., frequency, time of day, and context), set medication reminders, and provide analytics to patients and providers. This allows real-time tracking of disease exacerbation, and simplifies previously complicated associations such as frequency of inhaler use and the amount and type of pollen predominant in a particular geographical location. This kind of tracking and analytics allows Propeller's system to reduce short-acting bronchodilator use,[29] healthcare system utilization,[30] and asthma symptoms.[31]

Another example is a platform called Livongo (Mountainview, CA), a combination of a cellular-connected blood-sugar monitor and artificial intelligence–driven data analytics and coaching. Depending on the blood glucose reading, the patient receives smartphone-enabled suggestions tailored to the patient and the situation, such as drinking a glass of fruit juice if hypoglycemic or adjusting insulin dosing if a particular time of the day always yields a high value. If the values stray too much from the norm, Livongo connects the user to a live coach or refers them to specialist. This integrated approach is improving patient care. After one year, Livongo members show an average 18.4% decrease in the likelihood of having a day with hypoglycemia (BG < 70 mg/dL) and an average 16.4% decrease in hyperglycemia (BG > 180 mg/dL).[32] It is also estimated to save as much as $100 per month per patient to payers in healthcare utilization.[33] Similar platforms are in various stages of development for a wide variety of other chronic diseases.

Other approaches have focused on continuous collection of data that were previously only available as intermittent measurements, and then applying a layer of data analytics. One disease that has been particularly amenable to this approach is diabetes mellitus. Implantable sensors coupled with insulin pumps have been developed and combined with advanced analytics to predict times of hypo- and hyperglycemia. The combined monitoring-delivery devices can then dose the insulin, as well as generate nutrition and exercise recommendations that can help prevent such episodes. Many systems are currently in development, with MiniMed™ by Medtronic (Minneapolis, MN) approved by the FDA in 2017, and devices by BigFoot Medical (Milpitas, CA), Tandem (San Diego, CA), Insulet (San Diego, CA), and Beta Bionics (Boston, MA) currently undergoing clinical trials with planned approval and commercial availability in the next few years. In the meantime, a number of motivated patients have adapted delivery systems utilizing OpenAPS and Loop frameworks that enable patient-programmed closed-loop systems or automatic adjustment of output (insulin administration) based on inputted glucose readings.

Altogether, consistently recorded measurements drive analytic platforms to determine associations and insights that providers and patients previously did not consider. The power of these technologies will be amplified when used in concert (e.g., weight scale, glucometer, calorie counter).

Improved monitoring and advanced analytics will drive telehealth and the shift from patient hospitalization toward ambulatory care, and will ward off readmission. Close follow up with simple remote video monitoring session programs are already reducing hospital readmission for heart failure patients.[34] In select patient populations, total joint replacements are being performed as same-day surgeries. Tele-rehabilitation programs[34] have been implemented for total knee replacement patients who have difficulty attending in-person therapy sessions. This trend will continue and expand to many procedures and medical diagnosis that previously required hospitalization.

Challenges

In recent years there have been great strides in the development of new sensors and wireless technologies. How these technologies will be used and integrated, however, remains to be seen. There are many potential barriers to adoption, including concerns about privacy and security. Wireless technologies create a potential door for intruders which, in addition to posing privacy concerns, can actually result in

physical danger to a patient. An increasingly common concern is that pacemakers and insulin pumps connected to a wireless network can potentially be hacked and reprogrammed to change treatment or reported results and cause harm. Thus, integration of future devices into the "internet of things" requires advanced security protocols to ensure that the devices cannot be modified without appropriate approval.

Another potential challenge in implementing these systems is their reliability. Dead zones and interference zones will cause monitoring or at least data reporting failures. Even the most widely used electronic medical record in the United States has a frequent downtime requirement, during which storage of data is interrupted and paper orders and record keeping need to be implemented. A blackout or an internet outage could impact tens of thousands of patients all at once. Thus, successful development of these technologies requires appropriate fail-safes and backup systems that may include household batteries and generators.

Additional challenges relate to integration of various monitoring technologies and protocol standardization. Most medical devices are simply not interoperable because they provide output that is proprietary. Even publicly available healthcare taxonomies used by these devices such as Systematized Nomenclature of Medicine Clinical Terms (SNOMED), Logical Observation Identifiers Names and Codes (LOINC), International Organization for Standardization (ISO), and others are not designed to be interoperable with one another. A single parameter, such as a heart rate or temperature, may be represented differently in each system, and thus each proprietary system must be translated into a common format such as HL7. Although widely accepted as a standard, HL7 is also inherently inflexible, and each data system even in a single hospital may still use a slightly different standard. Thus, all HL7 messages may need to pass through an interface engine that facilitates exchange, translation, and sharing of data, in order to integrate into the electronic health record. All of these processes prevent sharing of high-resolution data and hinder real-time applications and advances.

Initiatives such as Integrating the Healthcare Enterprise's (IHE) Patient Care Device (PCD) and the Fast Healthcare Interoperability Resources (FHIR) are advocating for new standards in interoperability and device communication. FHIR specifications are evolving, with significant changes proposed to accompany each new version's release. Vendors and hospitals are therefore postponing elective adoption of FHIR standards until the industry firmly commits to a more permanent standard.

Conclusions

New healthcare monitoring technologies are developing at an increasingly rapid pace, mirroring the larger overall technology revolution. New problems including integration, stability, and hacking have accompanied these developments. A new set of associated ethical issues is arising too. For example, if a patient is monitored at home several questions quickly arise: Who should have access to the data – physician, healthcare system, employer, and/or the health insurance company? What is the patient–physician contract for acting on abnormal data? Does the patient have the right to share data that are generated by (and at some expense to) one provider and health system with other providers and health systems?

New technologies have been developed to include sensors in medication tablets that monitor medication compliance that is known to be inadequate in many medical diseases and in specific subsets of patients. With the viability of this technology, what will be the repercussions for non-compliant patients? Can a health system participating in value-based care dismiss the patient from their practice? Can the insurer raise their rates or perhaps change their co-pay requirements for complications related to non-compliance?

What is certain is that these devices will be commonplace in the very near future, their sophistication will likely exceed most of our imaginations, the quantity of data generated will be enormous, and a new medical paradigm will be required.

References

1. Kalisch BJ, Lee S, Dabney BW. Outcomes of inpatient mobilization: a literature review. *J Clin Nurs* 2014;**23** (11–12):1486–501.

2. Hofer I, Cannesson M. Is wireless the future of monitoring? *Anesth Analg* 2016;**122**(2):305–6.

3. Baig MM, Gholamhosseini H, Connolly MJ. A comprehensive survey of wearable and wireless ECG monitoring systems for older adults. *Med Biol Eng Comput* 2013;**51**(5):485–95.

4. Thomas SS, Nathan V, Chengzhi, et al. BioWatch – a wrist watch based signal acquisition system for physiological signals including blood pressure. *Conf Proc IEEE Eng Med Biol Soc* 2014;**2014**: 2286–9.

5. Kim J, Park J, Kim K, et al. Development of a nonintrusive blood pressure estimation system for computer users. *Telemed J E Heal [Internet]* 2007;**13** (1):57–64.

6. Kim JS, Chee YJ, Park JW, Choi JW, Park KS. A new approach for non-intrusive monitoring of blood pressure on a toilet seat. *Physiol Meas* 2006;**27**(2):203–11.

7. Baek HJ, Lee HB, Kim JS, et al. Nonintrusive biological signal monitoring in a car to evaluate a driver's stress and health state. *Telemed e-HEALTH 183* 2009;**15** (2):182–9.

8. Gu WB, Poon CCY, Leung HK, et al. A novel method for the contactless and continuous measurement of arterial blood pressure on a sleeping bed. *Conf Proc IEEE Eng Med Biol Soc* 2009;**2009**(c):6084–6.

9. Nye ER. The effect of blood pressure alteration on the pulse wave velocity. *Br Heart J* 1964;**26**(2):261–5.

10. Gribbin B, Steptoe A, Sleight P. Pulse wave velocity as a measure of blood pressure change. *Psychophysiology* 1976;**13**(1):86–90.

11. Ahmad S, Chen S, Soueidan K, et al. Electrocardiogram-assisted blood pressure estimation. *IEEE Trans Biomed Eng* 2012;**59**(3):608–18.

12. Lass J, Meigas K, Karai D, et al. Continuous blood pressure monitoring during exercise using pulse wave transit time measurement. *Conf Proc IEEE Eng Med Biol Soc* 2004;**3**:2239–42.

13. McCarthy BM, O'Flynn B, Mathewson A. An investigation of pulse transit time as a non-invasive blood pressure measurement method. *J Phys Conf Ser* 2011;**307**(1): 012060.

14. Singh RB, Cornélissen G, Weydahl A, et al. Circadian heart rate and blood pressure variability considered for research and patient care. *Int J Cardiol* 2003;**87**(1):9–28.

15. Liu Q, Yan BP, Yu CM, Zhang YT, Poon CC. Attenuation of systolic blood pressure and pulse transit time hysteresis during exercise and recovery in cardiovascular patients. *IEEE Trans Biomed Eng [Internet]*. 2014;**61**(2):346–52. Available from: http://ieeexplore.ieee.org/document/6645391/

16. Wong YM, Zhang YT. The effects of exercises on the relationship between pulse transit time and arterial blood pressure. *2005 IEEE Eng Med Biol 27th Annu Conf [Internet]*. 2005;**5**:5576–8. Available from: http://ieeexplore.ieee.org/lpdocs/epic03/wrapper.htm?arnumber=1615748

17. Wong MY, Pickwell-MacPherson E, Zhang YT. The acute effects of running on blood pressure estimation using pulse transit time in normotensive subjects. *Eur J Appl Physiol [Internet]*. 2009;**107**(2):169–75. Available from: http://link.springer.com/10.1007/s00421-009-1112-8

18. Rozenman Y, Schwartz RS, Shah H, Parikh KH. Wireless acoustic communication with a miniature pressure sensor in the pulmonary artery for disease surveillance and therapy of patients with congestive heart failure. *J Am Coll Cardiol* 2007;**49**(7):784–9.

19. Verdejo HE, Castro PF, Concepción R, et al. Comparison of a radiofrequency-based wireless pressure sensor to Swan-Ganz catheter and echocardiography for ambulatory assessment of pulmonary artery pressure in heart failure. *J Am Coll Cardiol* 2007;**50**(25):2375–82.

20. Abraham WT, Adamson PB, Bourge RC, et al. Wireless pulmonary artery haemodynamic monitoring in chronic heart failure: a randomised controlled trial. *Lancet* 2011;**377**(9766):658–66.

21. Potkay JA. Long term, implantable blood pressure monitoring systems. *Biomed Microdevices* 2008;**10**(3):379–92.

22. Alharbi M, Bauman A, Neubeck L, Gallagher R. Validation of Fitbit-Flex as a measure of free-living physical activity in a community-based phase III cardiac rehabilitation population. *Eur J Prev Cardiol* 2016;**23**(14):1476–85.

23. Jo E, Lewis K, Directo D, Kim MJ, Dolezal BA. Validation of biofeedback wearables for photoplethysmographic heart rate tracking. *J Sport Sci Med* 2016;**15**(3):540–7.

24. De Rossi DE, Paradiso R. Future direction: E-textiles. In: Bonfiglio A, De Rossi D (eds) *Wearable Monitoring Systems*. Boston, MA: Springer, 2011.

25. Farandos NM, Yetisen AK, Monteiro MJ, Lowe CR, Yun SH. Contact lens sensors in ocular diagnostics. *Adv Healthc Mater* 2015;**4**(6):792–810.

26. Fullard RJ, Snyder C. Protein levels in nonstimulated and stimulated tears of normal human subjects. *Investig Ophthalmol Vis Sci* 1990;**31**(6):1119–26.

27. Grus FH, Sabuncuo P, Augustin AJ. Quantitative Analyse der Tränenproteinmuster bei weichen Kontaktlinsen – Klinische Studie 1. 2001;239–42.

28. Mann A, Tighe B. Contact lens interactions with the tear film. *Exp Eye Res [Internet]*. 2013;**117**:88–98.

29. Merchant RK, Inamdar R, Quade RC. Effectiveness of population health management using the Propeller health asthma platform: a randomized clinical trial. *J Allergy Clin Immunol Pract [Internet]*. 2016;**4**(3):455–63.

30. Merchant R, Tuffli M, Barrett M, Hogg C, Van Sickle D. Interim results of the impact of a digital health intervention on asthma healthcare utilization. *J Allergy Clin Immunol [Internet]*. 2017;**139**(2):AB250. Available from: http://linkinghub.elsevier.com/retrieve/pii/S0091674916323235

31. Barrett MA, Humblet O, Marcus JE, et al. Effect of a mobile health, sensor-driven asthma management platform on asthma control. *Ann Allergy, Asthma Immunol [Internet]*. 2017;**119**(5):415–421.e1. Available from: http://linkinghub.elsevier.com/retrieve/pii/S1081120617306415

32. Downing J, Bollyky J, Schneider J. Use of a connected glucose meter and certified diabetes educator coaching to decrease the likelihood of abnormal blood glucose excursions: the Livongo for Diabetes Program. *J Med Internet Res* 2017;**19**(7):1–6.

33. June P, Health L. Livongo Clinical and Financial Outcomes Report Diabetes to Live a Better Life. 2016;(June).

34. Jiang S, Xiang J, Gao X, Guo K, Liu B. The comparison of telerehabilitation and face-to-face rehabilitation after total knee arthroplasty: a systematic review and meta-analysis. *J Telemed Telecare [Internet]*. 2016 December 27;1357633X16686748.

Downside and Risks of Digital Distractions

Peter J. Papadakos and Albert Yu

Introduction

This chapter will focus on two issues that have arisen in our newly electronicized workplace: (1) digital distraction and (2) alarm fatigue. Digital distraction due to personal electronic devices (PEDS) and, paradoxically, electronic medical records can undermine our ability to pay attention to one task for more than a few minutes. Alarm fatigue refers to a desensitization to alarm stimuli that clinicians experience in the context of frequent alarms and alerts, causing a delayed or missed response to an alarm. The combination of digital distraction and alarm fatigue is particularly disruptive and potentially injurious to patients.

There has been a marked evolution in the modern operating room (OR) over the last 20 years. Not so long ago there was genuine one-on-one engagement with patients. Anesthesiologists were literally tethered to their patient with a custom molded earpiece, which itself was almost a rite of passage into the specialty. Now, the term "earpiece" in the context of monitoring respiration and breath sounds is likely unknown to any graduate from this millennium, and would be more likely mistaken for an earbud. Patients were routinely touched without gloves to assess temperature and the presence or absence of diaphoresis, and describing the patient as "cold and clammy" immediately conveyed serious concern. With the typical latex-free gloves worn to suppress transmission of infection, this assessment is now near impossible. Written paper records in triplicate form required entry of vital signs, medications, notation of processes and procedures, and other critical information. Now nearly 80% of larger anesthesiology practices utilize Anesthesia Information Management Systems (AIMS) that automatically download and chart vital signs, allow quickly charted groups of phrases, and use dozens to hundreds of click boxes, resulting in charts that are exponentially larger (especially in intensive care units) but may actually convey less information.

The practice of medicine in general has similarly evolved to the point where the physician–patient relationship may never even occur in-person or require physical presence in the same city, state, or country. Telemedicine allows for the care of our sickest patients in intensive care units by doctors sitting in their own homes, or in monitoring centers, sometimes thousands of miles away. When there is intent to provide in-person care and have an "old-fashioned" physician–patient relationship, over the course of a workday, an individual provider will interact and respond to hundreds of alarms, emails, texts, and alerts from their AIMS and Electronic Medical Records (EMRs), as well as PEDs such as phones, tablets, watches, and fitness trackers. From these devices a plethora of information related to patient care and personal life is constantly intermingled. These changes have occurred very rapidly over the past ten years and have had a dramatic effect on workplace behavior, yet there has been little effort to quantify and understand their impact on patient care or establish an appropriate "code of conduct."

Anesthesiologists traditionally consider vigilance as their primary responsibility. The word "Vigilance" appears over the picture of a lighthouse in the emblem of the American Society of Anesthesiologists, signifying the central element of the specialty. Anesthesiologists, therefore, must take the lead in understanding digital distraction and alarm fatigue, minimize their impact on patient care, and establish an appropriate culture of electronic etiquette. This requires that a new educational experience be incorporated into the curriculum of all health personnel that would likely need to evolve over time as new digital distractions emerge.

Computers and smartphones (which are really just computers more powerful than those that were used to land man on the moon shrunken into a handheld device) give us a wide array of information that was simply not available as recently as 2008, when the first iPhone was released and the US government pushed for EMRs, resulting in the widespread appearance of computer workstations everywhere that patients are cared for. This has resulted in information pushed to us and pulled by us, arriving in our virtual in-boxes faster than was ever imaginable a decade ago. Pushed amber alerts, weather warnings, breaking news, sales advertisements, journal article e-releases, hospital announcements, and departmental updates are coming in all day, every day. Our reliance on pulled information, including drug dosages, guidelines, protocols, scoring systems, and remote viewing of the EMR, is so total that without PEDs providing access to this information, current medical care might come to a standstill. In addition to pure information, text messaging, Skype, Instagram, Snapchat, Facebook, and other social media designed to connect us instantly to our family, friends, colleagues, and sometimes patients have also weaved their way into the work environment.

Use of these applications is addictive, may result in the creation and need to maintain a personal avatar (a virtual digital identity), can interfere with job performance, and may even promote dangerous levels of inattentiveness and a complete lapse in the vigilance that anesthesiologists uphold as their main virtue. PED "dependency" is a genuine problem. In 2017, the average time spent on social media worldwide was reported to be 135 minutes per day, and young adults have been reported to use their phones an average of 5 hours a day, or almost one-third of all their awake time! The current zeitgeist of device speed and dependence is termed "hyperculture,"[1] to reflect the rapid change in technology's impact on society; this of course also applies to the microcosm of healthcare.

Physical ailments secondary to PED use like "blackberry thumb" seem antediluvian. This dependency on PEDs has spawned a whole new set of psychological phenomena, including "nomophobia" (the fear of having no mobile phone handy),[2,3] "phantom vibration and ringing syndrome" (the sensation that a phone has vibrated in our pocket or rung when in fact it has not),[4] and "FOMO" (the fear of missing out).[5] While these new words and acronyms may be amusing, it is possible that healthcare workers, including anesthesiologists, are "addicted"[6] to their PEDs and that the addiction interferes with vigilance and increases medical errors, morbidity, and mortality. This behavior and the possible risk that it poses have given rise to the term *distracted doctoring*.

Distracted Doctoring

There is a growing literature that addiction to technology is endemic and as a result the physician–patient relationship has decayed. In his 2011 *New York Times* front-page medical exposé, Matt Richtel wrote:[7]

> Hospitals and doctors' offices, hoping to curb medical error, have invested heavily to put computers, smartphones and other devices into the hands of medical staff for instant access to patient data, drug information and case studies. But like many cures, this solution has come with an unintended side effect: doctors and nurses can be focused on the screen and not the patient, even during moments of critical care.

Distracted doctoring has greatly affected the care of patients. Until recently, the focus was on the impact of EMRs and entry of data infringing on the patient–doctor relationship. Failure to make eye contact, sitting with one's back to the patient, and copying and pasting of prior notes all seemed to dramatically change the typical office and bedside encounter. Doctors distracted by their electronic record keeping abandon traditional verbal and body language cues and often physical examination as well. PEDs, FOMO, and the need to participate in social media in order to market one's practice and maintain a brand have become part and parcel of daily practice.

In 2012, 37% of residents and 12% of faculty admitted that during hospital rounds they read and responded to personal texts and e-mails.[8] Even more concerning, 19% of residents and 12% of attendings believed they had missed important information because of distraction from their smartphones. In 2020, it is highly likely these percentages have at least doubled.[9] If critical care physicians and residents are inappropriately focused on their PEDs while in the group setting of patient rounds, then lone anesthesia providers without peer pressure or group surveillance are likely more affected. Anesthesia training would seem to require some education in the risk of distracted doctoring and applicable mitigation strategies.[9] Another study published in 2012 reported that use of the anesthesia workstation for non-patient care activity (e.g., internet surfing) occurred for 29% of the total case time in cases with a duration of more than

4 hours.[10] Again, in 2020, the combination of PEDs and workstation use for nonmedical activity has likely driven the proportion of time spent in this behavior much higher.

An environment that is laden with distractions is conducive to medical error.[11] A good analogy is auto safety – imagine driving at night on a rainy night while at the same time your beeper is going off, someone is calling on your cell phone, the navigation system is informing you to turn, and your tire pressure alarm alerts you to the possibility of a flat tire. Are you more prone to have an accident then, compared to driving on a sunny day with no electronic signals at all? That is not too dissimilar from the state of affairs in our operating rooms today. A 2011 study described distractions that were present during critical phases of anesthesia[12] and included auditory alarms, conversations, music, and other equipment sounds. Notably, conversation unrelated to the procedure occurred during 28 of 30 emergences, and loud noise (> 70 dB) during emergence in almost every case! These distractions' potential negative impact on communication, concentration, and situational awareness was noted by the authors who cited the aviation literature and suggested a "sterile cockpit" strategy to eliminate them. In the current environment there is an even wider array of distractions because of the ubiquitous presence of PEDs and the stream of e-mail, texts, news alerts, tweets, and social media that compete for attention.

This focus on PEDs decreases reaction time and degrades performance of tasks requiring attention, concentration, and decision-making.[12] Furthermore, distractions from PEDs can degrade the entire team's performance. According to Attri et al., smartphones impair short-term memory, vigilance, and other aspects of cognitive performance.[13]

The problem of the distracted anesthesiologist is not new, but it has escalated over the years. Early concerns revolved around reading and use of anesthesia OR computer stations for non-patient care activities. The ubiquitous presence of PEDs in the OR raises greater concerns, as their portability presents an ever-present source of distraction as users are typically in a state of readiness to respond quickly to every incoming signal. The nearly constant stream of sounds and/or vibrations signaling incoming messages demands the individual to attend to the PED screen[14–16] and distracts them from attending to the patient and monitors.

Changing the Culture

Since PED technology is here to stay, an organization-wide and profession engagement model can help promote a culture of patient safety through improved focus on patient care. Widespread education on how technology can be addictive and detract from patient care must be introduced in school and in training programs.[9] Such training should incorporate simulation scenarios that illustrate to trainees the power of PEDs to distract and affect their ability to focus on the task at hand. Electronic distractions need to be included in all clinical scenarios so that trainees can see how they affect the vigilance and response time. For example, a simulation scenario in which a caregiver is receiving a barrage of text and social media alerts as they are caring for a patient who is slowly declining. Post-simulation analysis of how rapidly the caregiver reacted to the changing clinical climate would be a very clear educational tool to point out how PEDs affect focus and attention to the environment around them. Through such education we can train healthcare workers to use PED technology in a way that enhances their professional performance, rather than diminishing their performance by distraction. Healthcare institutions, facilities, departments, professional groups, and insurers also need to address this growing issue of patient safety, professionalism, legal implications, and costs – the caregiver is not the only stakeholder. Similar to the development of the "time out" in a past era, there is a need for increased awareness, education, and guidelines that cross professional boundaries, with the overriding goal of patient safety.

Alarm Fatigue

Electronic distractions not only come from devices that we bring on our person into the clinical setting, but also alarms that have always had a place in the care of patients. The increased digitalization of medicine has led to an increase in monitors, LED screens, robots, and other devices in the operating room, all of which compete for our attention. These electronic devices are an integral part of patient care, especially in operating rooms and ICUs, but every advance is accompanied by a new risk. This increase in the variety and quantity of alarms, however, results in "alarm fatigue," desensitization to alarm stimuli that results in delayed and missed responses. Alarms have been identified as a factor that increases the risk of adverse patient events, due to auditory overload and its distracting from other "important" alarms and duties. Clinicians may be exposed to hundreds of alarms per patient per day, with 74–99% being "nonactionable,"[17] meaning that there is no mechanical or clinical response required of the clinician to resolve the alarming. As the awareness of alarm fatigue and distraction is increasing, however, so is the number of devices and alarms in our environment that we must attend to, and the task to minimize their potential for harm seems Sisyphean. While there is no gold standard for measuring alarm fatigue, most studies have used surrogate measures such as total alarm count or response time to alarm (i.e., alarm duration). There are no studies, however, that have quantified the combined burden of digital distraction by PEDs and EMRs coupled with alarm fatigue on clinical performance.

The Association for the Advancement of Medical Instrumentation (AAMI) Alarm Standards Committee defines alarm fatigue as a condition that occurs when a user is desensitized by the presence of excessive alarm signals, many of which are nonactionable or in some cases false, and no or delayed response to the alarm signal occurs and harm to the patient could result. Factors contributing to alarm fatigue can include false alarms, nonactionable alarms, confusing alarms or inability to discriminate alarm sounds from background noise, distressing sounds, and more.[18]

In 2013, the Joint Commission identified the recognition of alarm fatigue and the need for clinical alarm management as a National Patient Safety Goal by 2016.[19] This call for action was in response to 98 alarm-related sentinel events reported from 2009 to 2012, including 8 deaths and 13 patients with permanent loss of function. The US Food and Drug Administration has reported over 566 deaths where alarm fatigue was a contributing factor in just a five-year time span.[19] The Emergency Care Research Institute has identified missed alarms as one of the top health technology hazards since 2012 and continues to track it as it remains in the top ten.

Clinical alarms usually indicate a derangement in the patient's physiologic state that requires attention by a provider.[20] Most physiologic alarms have their threshold set to be sensitive in order to not miss a clinically significant physiologic derangement. Technical alarms indicate that something related to our biomedical equipment requires attention. Both

physiologic and technical alarms can issue true and false positive alarms.[21] False alarms can also occur when the monitor receives signals that it interprets as pathological when the clinical condition of the patient is normal (e.g., a tachycardia alarm when electrocautery is used during surgery). Nuisance alarms are nonactionable alarms that occur when a physiologic parameter exceeds set levels but does not require any action on the part of the clinician because it self-resolves in a clinically insignificant amount of time (e.g., when a healthy patient's heart rate transiently dips below a preset of 60 BPM).[22]

It is normal human behavior to deprioritize or even disregard signals that in the past proved to be false. A clinician's response to an alarm is related to the perceived likelihood that the alarm represents a genuine urgency to be addressed.[23,24] The positive predictive value (PPV) of an alarm is the probability that there is a true clinical event associated with the alarm: PPV = true positive alarms/(true positive alarms + false positive alarms).[25] If the alarm has a low PPV due to a large percentage of false alarms, clinicians will be desensitized over time and respond less frequently and with decreased speed to these alarms. An observational study performed in a postoperative care unit of nurse response times to pulse oximetry desaturation alarms found that response times increased (i.e., worsened) incrementally as the number of nonactionable alarms increased in the previous 120 minutes.[26]

In the operating room multiple mental and physical tasks need to be performed simultaneously. Primary tasks include continuous physical assessment, operating room table optimization, draping, administration of medications and fluids, and performance of procedures. Secondary tasks include documentation, responding to alarms, and team communication. It has been shown that as primary workload increases secondary task performance decreases, and multitasking simply results in less attention paid to each individual task, especially when the PPV of an alarm is low. This is appropriate as time and effort spent on responding to alarms would detract from the primary tasks.[27,28] Alarms, however, are designed to be disturbing and get the attention of the provider. Simply recognizing (e.g., hearing or seeing), evaluating (e.g., what exactly is alarming – blood pressure monitor, respirator, pulse oximeter), and responding to an alarm can interfere with the primary tasks of the clinician and add to workload, even if there is nothing required to be done other than attending to the alarm and resetting it. Interrupted tasks also increase the chance for error. If a clinician is interrupted during a medication-related task, the chance of making an error after resuming the task approaches 25%.[25] Newer alarms with easily differentiable signals utilizing volume and pitch variation help stratify the alarm's importance and alert the clinician when immediate attention is absolutely necessary.

Optimizing appropriate use of alarms can of course potentially mitigate alarm fatigue. Many newer monitors and devices have preprogrammed settings for specific clinical situations (e.g., pediatric profiles); however, many times the profiles are outdated, not selected, or not adjusted appropriately to the patient's baseline status. Alarm technology can leverage its sophistication to generate signals based on physiological trends and/or multiple variables, reducing the false alarm rate, and increasing the clinician's response rate to alarms. For example, a pulse oximetry waveform displayed in addition to the digital readout can easily clue the observer into the data's validity.

Setting alarm parameters individualized for the patient's condition is one of the most frequently described methods for decreasing alarm fatigue; it decreases the total number of alarms.[26] Allowing clinicians to individualize alarm settings to their patient is another possible means of decreasing the risk of alarm fatigue. In a systemic review published in 2016, the proportion of alarms requiring intervention ranged from < 1% to 36%, with rates of < 1%–26% in adult ICU settings and 20–36% in adult ward settings.[27] A study from the 1990s showed the PPV of a pulse oximetry alarm and a ventilator alarm to be 1% and 3%, respectively, and demonstrated that less than 10% of all alarms in a pediatric ICU setting influenced clinical care.[27] Intelligently and consciously adjusting alarm parameters for individual patients may lead to less total alarms and fewer false or nuisance alarms. Examples of over-monitoring that can lead to diluting the PPV of alarms include arrhythmia monitoring on every floor patient and high oxygen saturation alarms in adults on room air. The oxygen saturation alarms for premature cyanotic patients with congenital heart disease need to be significantly different than that of a healthy adult. Another potential means to decrease alarm fatigue is to move the alarm parameter further away from the normal zone and more clearly into the abnormal and potentially dangerous zone. This will increase the PPV but potentially decrease the sensitivity of the alarm, as sensitivity = true positive alarms/(true positive alarms + false negative alarms); thus, a true actionable event becomes more likely to not alarm. One should consider that risk really equals probability multiplied by consequence in order to determine the setting of alarm thresholds, because all "actionable" events are not equal. If the consequence of an event not triggering an alarm is minimal (e.g., an alarm designed to trigger if the urine output is less than .5 ml/kg over one hour) this strategy is acceptable, but if the consequence is potentially lethal, even if the probability is low (e.g., abnormal electrocardiogram may be interference or ventricular fibrillation), then this strategy is not acceptable. A randomized trial showed that reducing a pulse oximeter alarm parameter from 90% to 85% resulted in 61% fewer alarms, but tripled the number of patients who indeed desaturated to less than 85%.[29]

Other potential solutions to reduce the number of nonactionable alarms is to apply a delay, so that self-resolving conditions are not audibly alarmed at all, while non-latching alarms are programmed to stop signaling when the alarmed parameter returns to normal without requiring manual resetting. These potential solutions may be used when the alarmed parameter is expected to have a large proportion of time-limited, clinically insignificant derangements. In a prospective investigation of pulse oximetry, the impact of lowering the SpO_2 alarm trigger from $\leq 90\%$ to $\leq 85\%$ and adding a time delay was investigated. Simply lowering the trigger of course reduced alarms, but patients experience triple the incidence of $SpO_2 \leq 85\%$ and a six-fold increase at $SpO_2 \leq 80\%$; review of the data revealed that a 15-second alarm delay for $SpO_2 \leq 90\%$ might be an effective means of reducing false alarms without increasing the risk of significant hypoxemia.[29]

The next generation of monitors and alarms are being integrated into multi-parameter formats that allow for programmed cross-checking of physiologic parameters and decrease the number of false, nonactionable alarms. Intelligent alarms that are triggered by trends rather than a single value and can potentially decrease the number of nonactionable alarms (see Chapter 4 describing the Oxygen Reserve Index), especially when combined with programmed patient history, are being introduced into new anesthesia systems. Other systems may use novel means of notification such as voice alerts, as well as differential routing of alarm notifications whereby if an alarm is not acted upon by the first-tier responder it can be sent to a backup responder. Another option is to prioritize alarm signals by assigning soft alerts to low-priority self-limiting conditions and loud noxious alarms for significant conditions only.

Optimizing the technology for the desired result is another way to decrease total alarms and false alarms. For example, there are several ways to monitor for respiratory insufficiency (see Chapter 16), including visual examination, end tidal CO_2 detection, bioimpedance of the chest wall, respiratory-induced movement of the bed surface, pulse oximetry, and continuous acoustic respiratory rate monitoring. In one study, acoustic monitoring produced fewer false alarms and detected more apnea events than did capnography,[29] but good data comparing all of these potential monitoring modalities are lacking.

One basic intervention to decrease nonactionable alarms is to optimize physiologic monitors and check sensor placement. Changing the EKG electrodes prior to the start of a procedure will potentially decrease artifacts from motion, electromagnetic interference, and poor electrode contact. Use of disposable pulse oximeter probes that stick on the finger significantly reduces probe displacement and time spent trouble-shooting simple sensor disconnects. Disposable ECG wires for single-patient use have been shown to lead to a significant decrease in the total number of alarms, without negative implications for patient safety or cost-effectiveness.[31]

Conclusion

The information and communications technology revolution has brought many advances that have led to improved patient care, but like many advances in the past, they have come with unforeseen consequences. Digital distractions are here to stay; EMRs and PEDs are not going away, and the array of digital physiological monitors and their associated alarms is only growing. The impact of digital distractions on physician behavior and the physician–patient relationship and the risks posed by digital distraction and alarm fatigue require further investigation, innovation, and education.

Reference

1. Bertman S. *Hyperculture: The Human Cost of Speed*, Westport: Greenwood, 1998, p. 267.

2. Farooqui IA, Pore P, Gothankar J. Nomophobia: an emerging issue in medical institutions? *J Ment Health* 2017;**22**:1–4.

3. Bragazzi NL, Del Puente G. A proposal for including nomophobia in the new DSM-V. *Psychol Res Behav Manag* 2014;**7**:155–60.

4. Deb A. Phantom vibration and phantom ringing among mobile phone users: a systematic review of literature. *Asia Pac Psychiatry* 2015;**7**(3):231–9.

5. Dossey L. FOMO, digital dementia and our dangerous experiment. *Explore* 2015;**10**(2):69–73.

6. Roberts J, Pullig C, Manolis C. I need my smartphone: a hierarchical model of personality and cell-phone addiction. *Personal Individ Differ* 2015;**79**:13–19.

7. Richtel M. As doctors use more devices, potential for distraction grows. New York Times 2011 December 15:A1,4. Available from www.NYtimes.com

8. Katz-Sidlow RJ, Ludwig A, Miller S, Sidlow R. Smartphone use during inpatient attending rounds: prevalence, patterns and potential for distraction. *J Hosp Med* 2012;**7**(8):595–9.

9. Papadakos PJ. Electronic etiquette: a curriculum for health professionals. In: Papadakos PJ, Bertman S., eds. *Distracted Doctoring: Returning to Patient-Centered Care in the Digital Age*. Cham, Switzerland: Springer International Publishing AG, 2017;219–27.

10. Wax DB, Lin HM, Reich DL. Intraoperative non-record-keeping usage of anesthesia information management system workstations and associated hemodynamic variability and aberrancies. *Anesthesiology* 2012;**117**:1184–9.

11. Kalisch BJ, Aebersold M. Interruptions and multitasking in nursing care. *Jt Comm J Qual Patient Saf* 2010;**36**(3):126–32.

12. Broom MA, Capek AL, Carachi P, Akeroyd MA, Hilditch G. Critical phase distractions in anesthesia and the sterile cockpit concept. *Anaesthesia* 2011;**66**:175–9.

13. Attri J, Kheptarpal R, Chatrath V, Kaur J. Concerns about usage of smartphones in the operating room and critical care scenario. *Saudi J Anesth* 2016;**10** (1):87–94.

14. Piscotty R, Voepel-Lewis T, Lee SH, et al. To tweet or not to tweet? Nurses, social media, and patient care. *Nurs Manag* 2013;**44**(5):52–3.

15. Cohn TA, Shappell SA, Reeves ST, Boquet AJ. Distracted doctoring: the role of personal electronic devices in the operating room.

Perioperative Care and Operating Room Management 2018;**10**:10–13.

16. Papadakos PJ. Electronic distractions of the respiratory therapist and their impact on patient safety. *Respir Care* 2014;**59**(8):1306–9.

17. Paine CW, Goel VV, Ely E, et al. Systematic review of physiologic monitor alarm characteristics and pragmatic interventions to reduce alarm frequency. *J Hosp Med* 2016;**11**(2):136–44.

18. Winters BD, Cvach MM, Bonafide CP. Technologic distractions (part 2): a summary of approaches to manage clinical alarms with intent to reduce alarm fatigue. *Crit Care Med* 2018;**46**(1):130–7.

19. The Joint Commission Sentinel Event Alert. Medical device alarm safety in hospitals. www.jointcommission.org/sea_issue_50/

20. Ruskin KJ, Hueske-Kraus D. Alarm fatigue: impacts on patient safety. *Curr Opin Anaesthesiol* 2015;**28**(6):685–90.

21. Manzey D, Gerals N, Wiczorek R. Decision-making and response strategies interaction with alarms: the impact of alarm reliability, availability of alarm validity information and workload. *Ergonomics* 2014;**57**(12):1833–55.

22. Bonafide CP, Lin R, Zander M, et al. Association between exposure to nonactionable physiologic monitor alarms and response times in a children's hospital. *J Hosp Med* 2015;**10**(6):981–5.

23. Bliss JP, Dunn MC. Behavioral implications of alarm mistrust as a function of task workload. *Ergonomics* 2002;**43**(9):1283–300.

24. Edworthy J, Hellier E. Alarms and human behavior: implications for medical alarms. *Br J Anaesth* 2006;**97**(1):12–17.

25. Westbrook JI, Coiera E, Dundmuir WE. The impact of interruptions on clinical task completion. *Qual Saf Healthcare* 2010;**19**:284–9.

26. Graham KC, Cvach M. Monitor alarm fatigue: standardizing use of physiologic monitors and decreasing nuisance alarms. *Am J Crit Care* 2010;**19**:28–34.

27. Paine CW, Goel VV, Ely E, et al. Systematic review of physiologic monitor alarm characteristics and pragmatic interventions to reduce alarm frequency. *J Hosp Med* 2016;**11**(2):136–44.

28. Lawless ST. Crying wolf: false alarms in a pediatric intensive care unit. *Crit Care Med* 1994;**22**(6):981–5.

29. Rheineck-Leyssius AT, Kalkman CJ. Influence of pulse oximeter lower limit on the incidence of hypoxemia in the recovery room. *Br J Anaesth* 1997;**79**(4):460–4.

30. Tanaka PP, Tanaka M, Drover DR. Detection of respiratory compromise by acoustic monitoring, capnography and brain function monitoring during monitored anesthesia care. *J Clin Monit Comput* 2014;**28**:561–6.

31. Albert NM, Murry T, Bena JF, et al. Differences in alarm events between disposable and reusable electrocardiography lead wires. *Am J Crit Care* 2015;**24**(1):67–74.

Index